Handbook of Settings-Based Health Promotion

Sami Kokko • Michelle Baybutt

Editors

Handbook of Settings-Based Health Promotion

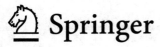 Springer

Editors
Sami Kokko
Research Center for Health Promotion,
Faculty of Sport and Health Sciences
University of Jyväskylä
Jyväskylä, Länsi-Suomi, Finland

Michelle Baybutt
Healthy and Sustainable Settings Unit
School of Community Health and
Midwifery
University of Central Lancashire
Preston, Lancashire, UK

ISBN 978-3-030-95858-9   ISBN 978-3-030-95856-5   (eBook)
https://doi.org/10.1007/978-3-030-95856-5

This Springer imprint is published by the registered company Springer Nature Switzerland AG
The registered company address is: Gewerbestrasse 11, 6330 Cham, Switzerland

Foreword

I welcome the publication of the *Handbook of Settings-Based Health Promotion* and applaud the editors and contributing authors in producing such a comprehensive and scholarly overview of the field. This handbook tracks the evolution of the settings-based approach to health promotion over the last 30-plus years, providing readers with in-depth and novel insights into the core concepts, principles, and theoretical underpinnings for settings-based health promotion and its application in practice and policy.

This impressive collection of work provides up-to-date specialist knowledge and guidance on the development and application of a settings-based approach to health promotion. The handbook articulates from a theoretical and practical perspective how the settings and places where people live their lives can foster the creation of health and well-being, address the interrelated determinants of health, and enable individuals and populations to flourish. While enhancing a common understanding of a settings-based approach, this handbook also seeks to generate new thinking on its application in both traditional and new and emerging contexts. Challenges and opportunities for future developments from a global perspective are also presented.

The settings approach builds on the socio-ecological model of health promotion, as articulated in the Ottawa Charter for Health Promotion and subsequent WHO declarations, and emphasizes the fundamental and inextricable link between people and their environments. As such, it provides a powerful conceptual framework for health promotion practice and has given rise to some of the most innovative and sustainable health promotion initiatives globally. Health promotion emphasizes that health is created where people live their lives and that these everyday contexts or settings such as the home, school, workplace, and community are where health can be promoted. Adopting a settings-based approach means appreciating that the setting itself is crucially important in determining health and calls for systems-based, multi-level strategies that will create healthy, supportive, and sustainable environments. The development of healthy settings movements, such as health-promoting schools, healthy cities and communities, and health-promoting hospitals, has successfully translated into practice the aim of creating supportive environments for health, and these initiatives have been successfully implemented in many countries globally.

Implementing a settings-based approach is, however, complex and not without its challenges. As there are different interpretations and ideological understandings of what applying a settings-based approach means, the handbook is intended to provide clarity on the distinction between actions focused on modifying individual behaviors within a setting and actions aimed at modifying the setting itself and the conditions underlying the setting. A settings-based approach, therefore, implies that the setting itself must be the entry point for health promotion. A clear conceptual and practical framework is needed to plan and deliver multilevel, integrated interventions that are aimed at the whole setting and its underlying conditions. The complexity of implementing such a multilevel systems-based approach is addressed in this handbook, including the importance of connecting between different settings to maximize impact and effectiveness. Critical perspectives are also presented on the challenge of evaluating settings-based interventions and generating robust evidence on the effectiveness of this approach.

The handbook is structured in three parts. Part I outlines the conceptual basis and key principles for a settings-based approach and explores the theoretical links with systems thinking, complexity, and ecological and salutogenic orientations. Issues of governance and supportive policy structures are also addressed, together with an exploration of the challenges of evaluating and building evidence of the effectiveness of a settings-based approach.

Part II of the handbook brings a focus on the practical application of the settings-based approach, illustrated through practice examples and case studies from across diverse settings, including cities, schools, hospitals, universities, workplaces, prisons, sports clubs and stadia, and new and emerging settings. In Part III, the challenges facing practitioners, policymakers, and academics engaged in implementing and evaluating a healthy setting approach are considered. These challenges include addressing sustainability and planetary health and taking effective health promotion action in the Anthropocene.

Developing the settings-based approach for health promotion practice, research, and policy has been, and continues to be, an important focus for the IUHPE. Many of the authors of this handbook are members of the IUHPE Global Working Group on Healthy Settings, which brings together health promoters from different world regions to advance and further develop the study and practice of a settings-based approach to health promotion. The collective efforts of the group, through publications such as this handbook, contribute to the scientific base of health promotion and to the core mission of the IUHPE, which is to promote global health and well-being and to contribute to the achievement of equity in health between and within countries of the world. The IUHPE's mission is translated into practice through scientific and professional activities developed through a global network of members and organizations who are specialized in and committed to health promotion (further details of which can be found at https://www.iuhpe.org/).

I congratulate the editors and authors on this important publication, which makes a significant contribution to the field of health promotion and to deepening our understanding and appreciation of the settings-based approach. This handbook will be a valuable resource for all academic scholars, practitioners, and policymakers interested in understanding the theoretical base and practical applications of healthy settings and advancing the field of health promotion.

International Union for Health Promotion   Margaret M. Barry
and Education (IUHPE)
National University of Ireland Galway,
Galway, Ireland

Preface

Origins and Purpose of the Book

This handbook on settings-based health promotion originated during a meeting of the Global Interest Group[1] on Healthy Settings during the 22nd IUHPE World Conference, on May 24th, 2016, in Curitiba, Brazil. The Global Interest Group acknowledged the opportunity to work together and share their expertise in producing a book that would build on the previous influential book written by Green et al. (2000). Other health promotion texts that followed do not have the settings approach as the primary focus or they are limited in scope, especially in relation to theoretical basis and mutual understanding across settings. The editors believe that this new publication is timely and novel. It comprehensively sets out reflections on the history and development of the approach with contemporary perspectives for academics, students, policymakers, and practitioners alike.

The healthy settings approach, as it is defined in this handbook, has been evolving more than 30 years now. The main aim of the handbook is to provide clarity amidst different interpretations and ideological understandings of what the settings-based approach is and what it means in practice today. During this time, the research and practice around the approach have continued to be active; however, the emphasis has tended to be on traditional institutional settings, such as schools, cities, and hospitals, with newcomers, often non-traditional ones, being less recognized. Also, settings-based health promotion has tended to vary significantly with some working with comprehensive and dynamic aims and means while others have been limited and static—the latter representing more "health promotion *in* settings," rather than being more comprehensive and holistic settings-based health promotion. Therefore, this book explores how the settings approach to health promotion strives for change in the structure and ethos of the setting—detailing how changes and developments in people's health and health behavior are easier to achieve if health promoters focus

---

[1] Interest Group at that time. It is the "Global Working Group on Healthy Settings" currently.

on the environments (settings) where people live their lives rather than on the individuals themselves.

Overview of the Book

This book comprises 15 chapters divided between three parts. Part I is made up of four chapters, which explore the history and origins of the healthy settings approach and the theoretical concepts that underpin it and set out the key principles for practice. This part also presents governance, policy, and evaluation perspectives to the approach. Part II of the book consists of nine chapters, which explore the history, development, and application of the approach in different well-established settings. Also, some emerging settings are introduced. Part III of the book has two chapters, which explore Gaia and health promotion in the Anthropocene discussing Earth as the ultimate setting and determinant of health and therefore argues for a transition from social determinants to planetary health.

Each chapter explores implications for practice and considerations for practitioners working in a range of settings. The book intends to be a supportive handbook with guidance for both studying and delivering settings-based health promotion around the world.

Part I: Evolution, Foundations and Key Principles of the Settings-Based Approach

Part I of the book investigates determinants and provides the rationale for the settings-based health promotion approach. In this part, the key characteristics of the settings approach are discussed with a specific focus on the evolution, approaches and key concepts, theoretical grounds, practical principles, governance, and evaluation. This part of the book also explores the relationship of the settings approach to wider public health and health promotion theory.

1. **Evolution of the Settings-Based Approach**
   This chapter provides a background to the settings-based approach to health promotion, examining the evolution of the approach and highlighting issues for further consideration. Adopting a largely chronological approach, it looks at (a) international policy development as a context for healthy settings, (b) emergence and consolidation of the approach and its application in different contexts, and (c) key emerging themes for critical reflection, debate, and research.
2. **Theoretical Grounds and Practical Principles of the Settings-Based Approach**
   This chapter introduces the theoretical basis and fundamentals of the settings-based approach, complementing Chap. 1 by tracing the evolution of thinking

over time. While there have been multiple attempts to establish models, typolo-gies, and frameworks for the settings-based approach, a recurring theme has been the absence of a shared understanding of the theoretical foundations of the approach. This chapter summarizes key advances, presents an expanded concep-tual framework that can be used to guide future policy and practice, considers how theory can be usefully translated into practice, and identifies key themes for critical reflection.

3. **Governance and Policies for Settings-Based Work**
   Using insights from practice, research, and theory, this chapter argues that policy (and more precisely, the policy *process*) is a unique setting for health develop-ment, social discourse, and setting the conditions for societies and ecosystems to thrive in support of (planetary) health. A policy setting is, by its very nature, a form of governance with implications for health, well-being, and equity. Using insights from practice, research, and theory, this chapter works through what policy or political institutions are made up of. Positioning of health as an idea for public policy and the governance that goes behind this need to be better articu-lated, and governance strategies should be developed to progress "healthy public policy" objectives. The chapter then goes on to define "policy for health" before unpacking the historical journey and differences between "healthy public pol-icy" and "health in all policies" objectives, to suggest that "public policy" remains core despite these health-named diversions. The chapter then details governance as the interrelated dimensions and trajectories of systems, organiza-tions, and individual-driven actions and what this means for settings-based health promotion. The chapter concludes by presenting a graphic heuristic, the policy cube, that articulates the varied dimensions of "healthy" public policy as a dynamic system.

4. **Assessment for and Evaluation of Healthy Settings**
   Given the multidimensional nature of issues addressed in healthy settings initia-tives, a multilevel set of interconnected and often innovative assessment, moni-toring, and evaluation methods are needed to address the complex nature of evaluating healthy settings. The chapter argues that to look comprehensively at how a setting might be influential in promoting or maintaining health, it is neces-sary to look at the complexity of relationships, structures, and processes and to examine the connections among systems, environments, people, and behaviors. Since settings-based health promotion seeks to address issues of equity and power relations within, outside, and across settings, assessment and evaluation efforts must address these issues as well. This chapter reviews two approaches to conducting an assessment of a healthy setting, basic elements to include in a healthy settings evaluation, some of the most common and effective evaluation types and tools, a few examples of monitoring and evaluation, and some of the challenges faced in monitoring and evaluating healthy settings and provides overall conclusions.

Part II: Applying the Settings-Based Approach to Key Settings

Part II of the book provides the reader with a comprehensive overview to the key settings initiatives—traditional and nontraditional, and emerging—with their developments and specific features. This section discusses how these various setting initiatives have developed over time and how the settings approach recognizes that many health determinants and influences are interrelated and can be best tackled through comprehensive, integrated programs and/or actions in the contexts and places where people live their lives.

5. **Healthy Cities**
   This chapter reviews the historical and current foundations of one of the original "settings for health": healthy cities. It demonstrates that urban development has always gone hand in hand with health considerations. This is true for the planning and design (i.e., the morphology) of cities, as well as the human, social, and cultural dimensions. These were adopted in a development from the early 1960s that culminated into a formalization of healthy city qualities in the 1980s. This development is characterized by a strong emphasis on values in urban health. The chapter outlines these and then moves on to describe emergent global networks of cities, "theme cities." They all qualify as settings for health to a greater or lesser extent. The chapter concludes with an analysis of the future of local perspectives in global context.

6. **Health-Promoting Schools**
   The school as a setting for health-promoting initiatives has been demonstrating for over three decades that school communities can improve both health and education of students in an integrated way. This only works if initiatives are continually well resourced, local school communities are involved, common values such as student empowerment and active participation are practiced, and external acknowledgement of schools through award systems is sustained. Reports from three global regions, Europe, the Middle East, and Asia, are described and analyzed in this chapter. The authors draw on the considerable emerging evidence from international studies that shows that the future of the HPS needs to always recognize the close connection of health and education priorities. Fundamental to success is working with students as pivotal change agents, recognizing the nature of schools as complex systems, and enabling them to shape their own ongoing HPS that is based on easily understood research evidence and adequate financial resources for continued implementation.

7. **Health-Promoting Hospitals**
   Health-promoting hospitals (HPH) as a concept, a project, a network, and a movement have its roots in the Ottawa Charter (WHO 1986). With its call for "reorienting health services," the Ottawa Charter implicitly diagnosed that health services had a too narrow mandate and mission on treatment of diseases and therefore were in need of reform. Health promotion philosophy offered a widening of the understanding of health care towards disease prevention, health

protection, and health promotion that goes beyond the hospital's focus on cure and care. And that not just for patients' health gain, but also for staff's health and the health of the residents in the community a hospital serves. Yet, a concrete and comprehensive concept for hospitals as a health-promoting setting and for strategies to implement this concept into already existing hospital structures, cultures, and processes had to be developed and piloted before a network of health-promoting hospitals could be established. This chapter first reconstructs and describes the historical development of HPH, second reflects on how successful HPH has been so far in terms of its reproduction and production, and third concludes with some thoughts on the future of HPH and next steps.

8. **Health-Promoting Higher Education**
   Health-promoting universities are a growing global movement and one important application of settings-based health promotion. This chapter contextualizes and provides a brief overview of the development of health-promoting universities and then goes on to review and discuss key conceptual and theoretical considerations, emphasizing the importance of comprehensive whole institution and systemic approaches. It then moves on to look at the translation of theory into practice, presenting three contrasting examples from different regions of the world. It concludes by looking to the future in the context of the International Okanagan Charter for Health Promoting Universities and Colleges—outlining key opportunities and challenges and spotlighting the following: the importance of whole system working, the need to maximize leverage for transformative change through future-oriented and outward-focused engagement with civic and global challenges, the willingness to advocate and live countercultural values such as compassion and respect, and the commitment to positive-focused approaches that integrate salutogenesis and regenerative sustainability.

9. **Health-Promoting Workplaces**
   This chapter sets out how the concept of workplace health promotion (WHP) has evolved, influenced by the ILO's international standards and the WHO's health promotion principles and in response to the rapid transformation of the world of work, the globalized world economy, and the development of management principles. It highlights how the concept of WHP has shifted away from a narrow focus on health education and individual responsibility to a broader, more comprehensive, integrative approach to health and health determinants. The world of work is undergoing profound changes, not least the transformative effect of new technology, changing demographics, and climate change and the shift towards the green economy. These mega-trends are affecting ideas of what a job is, what work is, and how the workplace is designed. These changes will bring about new challenges and opportunities for the safety and health of the world's workers. Workplace health promotion has been shown to have a number of beneficial outcomes for workers and companies including improving productivity, decreasing sickness absence, improving working relationships and employee morale, and creating a better public image for organizations that implement WHP programs.

10. **Prisons as a Setting for Health**

Prison is a home to some people and a workplace for others. It is a setting with significant interaction with the wider community through family and legal visits and service provision. Prisoners tend to come from marginalized and socially disadvantaged sections of society, exhibiting a disproportionately high incidence of ill health. Prison is therefore a key setting to intervene for both individual and wider public health benefit. This chapter seeks to explore prisons as settings for health. It outlines the historical developments of the health-promoting prison concept and discusses how the idea has developed over the past number of years. The chapter also highlights some of the challenges and tensions that have faced policy and practice in this environment, including the challenges of translating the strategy into practical action. The chapter provides a case study illustrating the health and wellbeing benefits of whole system working, before concluding with a discussion of the future role of prisons as settings for health.

11. **Health Promotion in Sports Settings**

This chapter focuses on sports-related settings and represents both sports clubs and stadia. Sports clubs reach a large population across life stages and socioeconomic levels. They play an important role in their members' health through their informal education nature. While sports clubs' core business is offering physical activity, a well-acknowledged health determinant, their potential to go further is enormous, by being health-promoting sports clubs (HPSC) and promoting the physical, social, and mental health of their members. In the last decade, the state of the art has evolved including renewing the theoretical model, providing an intervention framework and guidelines, developing new measurement instruments and some interventions, and conducting several cross-sectional studies. Sports stadiums/stadia have also been identified as potential settings for health promotion. Stadiums reach large numbers of people with wide variation in their background. Healthy Stadia was established in 2005, and in 2006 European-level network started. This chapter introduces the evolvement of the Healthy Stadia, its current activities, and future aims.

12. **Digital Environment and Social Media as Settings for Health Promotion**

The digital world has reshaped the traditional definition of health-promoting settings, as increasing online resources are offering opportunities, across the life span, for people to work, learn, play, establish relationships ("love"), and essentially live a great proportion of their lives. As in other settings, it is critical that the digital environment be viewed as a health-promoting setting. Digital health literacy is a key skill enabling individuals, families, communities, and societies to maximize the health-promoting benefits the digital world offers while seeking to mitigate the potential physical, mental, and social risks. The Internet, social media, and Avatars are the case examples described and analyzed for their potential health-promoting contribution, including cultural responsiveness. In addition, health-promoting media, whether online or offline, may easily be joined with another appropriate health-promoting setting, thereby enhancing a systems approach to healthy settings. Finally, future research on innovation and health-promoting settings is proposed.

13. **Emerging Settings**
    This chapter offers some reflections on the development of different types of
    settings and focuses on the potential of new and emerging settings presented as
    three case studies. These case studies offer fresh perspectives and renewed
    efforts to develop the settings-based approach in new and emerging settings
    while responding to contemporary issues that relate to health and well-being.
    Examples of these are set out and include the development of healthy airports
    with action that respond to the global climate change agenda, places of worship
    as "nested" settings and central in communities, and the paradox of health and
    the coast for developing healthy coastal communities in the UK, post the
    COVID-19 pandemic. The chapter proposes that any setting has the potential to
    be health promoting while recognizing the challenges this may entail.

Part III: Gaia—The Ultimate Setting for Health Promotion

Part III of the book discusses the Earth as the ultimate determinant of and setting for
health. This section of the book sets out the need for a transition from social determinants to integrate both social and ecological sustainability and justice in the context of the emerging field of planetary health.

14. **Gaia and the Anthropocene: The Ultimate Determinant of Health**
    This chapter focuses on Gaia—the Earth, our home—to be understood as a living
    entity in its own right. As the ultimate determinant of our health, it is the ultimate
    setting for health promotion. The Earth provides us, and the myriad of species
    with whom we share the Earth, a set of vitally important ecosystem goods and
    services: air, water, food, fuel, materials, waste detoxification and disposal, pro-
    tection from UV radiation, and a generally stable climate—at least for the past
    11,000 years of the Holocene. These are the ecological determinants of our
    health, and they are even more fundamental to our health, and indeed to our very
    survival, than the social determinants of health with which they interact.

    But on Earth, humans have become a force of nature equal to or greater than
    natural forces, creating massive and rapid global ecological changes. This is
    resulting in a new geologic epoch—the Anthropocene—that is replacing the
    Holocene. These changes in turn are driven by the sociocultural phenomenon of
    a globalized twenty-first-century industrial and postindustrial/digital age, with
    a focus on progress understood largely as growth in material and financial
    wealth. But human-driven global ecological changes, which are crossing plan-
    etary boundaries, threaten our health and stability and perhaps even survival of
    our societies.

15. **Health Promotion in the Anthropocene**
    The Ottawa Charter called for a socio-ecological approach in health promotion,
    but in practice we have until recently paid little attention to the ecological deter-
    minants of health. Yet, if we understand public health as a branch of human and
    social ecology, what we might call "Health Promotion 2.0" needs to integrate

both social and ecological sustainability and justice in the context of the emerging field of planetary health. This chapter sets out the need to create a future where governance is focused not on unsustainable—and thus unattainable— growth in material prosperity, but on sustainable, equitable human development. Among other things, this calls for a new set of core values that will lead us to an economics for well-being.

Jyväskylä, Länsi-Suomi, Finland   Sami Kokko
Preston, Lancashire, UK   Michelle Baybutt

Reference

Green, L. W., Poland, B. D., & Rootman, I. (2000). The settings approach to health promotion. In B. D. Poland, L. W. Green, & I. Rootman (Eds.), Settings for health promotion: Linking theory and practice (pp. 1–43). London: Sage.

Acknowledgments

The editors would like to thank the following bodies and people:

We would like to thank all of the authors for their important contribution. Particularly, we would like to acknowledge the contributions from members of the IUHPE Global Working Group for Healthy Settings in providing direction and constructive feedback and for patience, support, and commitment to this project. In addition, we would like to express our gratitude to Professor Mark Dooris and Professor Evelyne de Leeuw for their significant contribution to the book and its various chapters.

We would also like to thank Springer for commissioning this book and supporting us to develop the material and navigate the production process.

The work on Chap. 11, Sect. 11.2, was partially funded by the Erasmus + Collaborative Partnerships grant (ref: 613434-EPP-1-2019-1-HR-SPO-SCP) as part of the Sports Club for Health (SCforH) 2020–2022 project.

Contents

Part I   Evolution, Foundations and Key Principles of the Settings-Based Approach

1   **Evolution of the Settings-Based Approach**   3
    Mark Dooris, Sami Kokko, and Evelyne de Leeuw

2   **Theoretical Grounds and Practical Principles
    of the Settings-Based Approach**   23
    Mark Dooris, Sami Kokko, and Michelle Baybutt

3   **Governance and Policies for Settings-Based Work**   45
    Evelyne de Leeuw and Patrick Harris

4   **Assessment for and Evaluation of Healthy Settings**   67
    Marilyn E. Rice

Part II   Applying the Settings-Based Approach to Key Settings

5   **Healthy Cities**   91
    Evelyne de Leeuw

6   **Health-Promoting Schools**   105
    Lawrence St. Leger, Goof Buijs, Nastaran Keshavarz Mohammadi,
    and Albert Lee

7   **Health-Promoting Hospitals**   119
    Jürgen M. Pelikan, Birgit Metzler, and Peter Nowak

8   **Health-Promoting Higher Education**   151
    Mark Dooris

9   **Health-Promoting Workplaces**   167
    Karl Kuhn and Cordia Chu

10   **Prisons as a Setting for Health**   177
    James Woodall and Michelle Baybutt

11 Health Promotion in Sports Settings 189
Aurélie Van Hoye, Susanna Geidne, Jan Seghers,
Aoife Lane, Alex Donaldson, Matthew Philpott, and Sami Kokko

**12 Digital Environment and Social Media as Settings
for Health Promotion** 205
Diane Levin-Zamir, Isabella C. Bertschi, Evelyn McElhinney,
and Gill Rowlands

13 Emerging Settings 225
Michelle Baybutt, Sami Kokko, Alana Crimeen, Evelyne de Leeuw,
Emma Tomalin, Jo Sadgrove, and Ursula Pool

Part III   Gaia—The Ultimate Setting for Health Promotion

**14 Gaia and the Anthropocene: The Ultimate Determinant
of Health** 241
Trevor Hancock

15 Health Promotion in the Anthropocene 259
Trevor Hancock

Index 283

Contributors

Margaret M. Barry, PhD International Union for Health Promotion and Education (IUHPE), National University of Ireland Galway, Galway, Ireland

Michelle Baybutt, BA (Hons), MA and PrD Healthy and Sustainable Settings Unit, School of Community Health and Midwifery, University of Central Lancashire, Preston, Lancashire, UK

Isabella C. Bertschi, MSc Department of Psychology, Clinical Psychology for Children/Adolescents & Couples/Families, University of Zurich, Zurich, Switzerland

Goof Buijs, MSc UNESCO Chair Global Health and Education, Paris, France

Cordia Chu, PhD Centre for Environment and Population Health, Griffith University, Nathan, QLD, Australia

Alana Crimeen, MPH School of Built Environment, Faculty of Arts, Design and Architecture, University of New South Wales (UNSW), and the Centre for Health Equity Training, Research and Evaluation (CHETRE), part of the Centre for Primary Health Care and Equity, University of New South Wales, Sydney, Australia

Alex Donaldson, PhD Centre for Sport and Social Impact, La Trobe University, Melbourne, Australia

Mark Dooris, BA(Hons), PhD Institute of Citizenship, Society and Change/ Healthy and Sustainable Settings Unit, University of Central Lancashire, Preston, Lancashire, UK

Susanna Geidne, PhD School of Health Sciences, Örebro University, Örebro, Sweden

Trevor Hancock, PhD School of Public Health and Social Policy, University of Victoria, Victoria, BC, Canada

Patrick Harris, PhD, MPH Centre for Health Equity Training, Research & Evaluation (CHETRE), Part of the UNSW Australia Research Centre for Primary Health Care & Equity, A Unit of Population Health, South Western Sydney Local Health District, NSW Health, A member of the Ingham Institute, Liverpool Hospital, University of New South Wales, Sydney, Australia

Aurélie Van Hoye, PhD EA4360 APEMAC, Université de Lorraine, Nancy, France

Nastaran Keshavarz Mohammadi, PhD Shahid Beheshti University of Medical Sciences, Tehran, Iran

Sami Kokko, PhD Research Center for Health Promotion, Faculty of Sport and Health Sciences, University of Jyväskylä, Länsi-Suomi, Finland

Karl Kuhn, MA European Network for Workplace Health Promotion (ENWHP), Fröndenberg, North Rhine-Westphalia, Germany

Aoife Lane, PhD Department of Sport and Health Sciences, SHE Research Group, Technological University of the Shannon, Athlone, Ireland

Albert Lee, PhD Centre for Health Education and Health Promotion, Lek Yuen Health Centre, Shatin, NT, Hong Kong

Evelyne de Leeuw, MSc, MPH, PhD Centre for Health Equity Training, Research and Evaluation, University of New South Wales, Sydney, NSW, Australia

Diane Levin-Zamir, PhD, MPH, MCHES School of Public Health, University of Haifa, Haifa, Israel

Department of Health Education and Promotion, Clalit Health Services, Tel Aviv, Israel

Evelyn McElhinney, PhD Department of Nursing and Community Health, School of Health and Life Sciences, Glasgow Caledonian University, Glasgow, Scotland

Birgit Metzler, MA Competence Centre Health Promotion and Health System (Austrian National Public Health Institute), Gesundheit Österreich GmbH, Vienna, Austria

Peter Nowak, PhD WHO Collaborating Centre for Health Promotion in Hospitals and Health Care, Department of Health Literacy and Health Promotion (Austrian National Public Health Institute), Gesundheit Österreich GmbH, Vienna, Austria

Jürgen M. Pelikan, PhD WHO Collaborating Centre for Health Promotion in Hospitals and Health Care, Department of Health Literacy and Health Promotion (Austrian National Public Health Institute), Gesundheit Österreich GmbH, Vienna, Austria

Matthew Philpott, PhD European Healthy Stadia Network, Liverpool, UK

Ursula Pool, PhD Healthy and Sustainable Settings Unit, School of Community Health and Midwifery, Faculty of Health and Care, University of Central Lancashire, Preston, Lancashire, UK

Marilyn E. Rice, MPH, MA, CEO Consulting International, LLC (merci), Fairfax, VA, USA

Gill Rowlands, MBBS, MD, FRCP, FRCGP Population Health Sciences Institute, Newcastle University, Newcastle upon Tyne, UK

Jo Sadgrove, BA, MA, PhD Centre For Religion and Public Life, University of Leeds, Leeds, West Yorkshire, UK

Jan Seghers, PhD Physical Activity, Sport & Health Research Group, Department of Movement Sciences, University of Leuven (KU Leuven), Leuven, Belgium

Lawrence St. Leger, BA, MEd St, PhD, TSTC Faculty of Health, Deakin University, Melbourne, VIC, Australia

Emma Tomalin, PhD Centre for Religion and Public Life, School of Philosophy, Religion and History of Science, University of Leeds, Leeds, West Yorkshire, UK

James Woodall, PhD School of Health, Leeds Beckett University, Leeds, UK

About the Editors

Sami Kokko is an Associate Professor in Health Promotion and the Director of Research Center for Health Promotion at the Faculty of Sport and Health Sciences at the University of Jyväskylä, Finland. He is a member of the Nordic Health Promotion Research Network and the Global Working Group on Healthy Settings at the International Union for Health Promotion and Education (IUHPE).

Sami's main research interests are settings-based health promotion, especially in sports club settings, and physical activity/sports-related topics. He has worked at the University of Jyväskylä 20 years, and his publications have contributed not only to science but also to health and physical activity promotion policy and practice.

Michelle Baybutt is a Reader (Associate Professor) in Sustainable Health and Justice, Co-director of the Healthy and Sustainable Settings Unit (HSSU), and Prisons Strand Lead for the Centre for Criminal Justice Research Partnerships at the University of Central Lancashire in the UK. She is a member of the Global Working Group on Healthy Settings at the International Union for Health Promotion and Education (IUHPE) and is Editor of the *International Journal of Health Promotion and Education.*

Michelle's academic expertise linking health promotion practice with research and knowledge exchange forms an academic narrative around *prisons as a setting for fostering health and well-being*, notably the duality of governance/prison health systems and implementation of sustainable public health interventions. Michelle has extensive health promotion and public health expertise working with people in prisons and those with experience of prison in the wider community. She is committed to improving the health and opportunities of people who are socially excluded or marginalized and to addressing health inequalities and social injustice.

Part I
Evolution, Foundations and Key Principles of the Settings-Based Approach

Chapter 1
Evolution of the Settings-Based Approach

Mark Dooris, Sami Kokko, and Evelyne de Leeuw

1.1 Introduction

In considering the historical development of the settings-based approach to health promotion, it is useful to focus on the three domains of policy, practice and theory, which are inherently interconnected. Thus, policy both guides and reflects practice; practice both informs and is informed by theory; and theory can emerge from and contribute to the development of policy (de Leeuw, 2016). Focusing on the emergence and evolution of Healthy Settings over time, this chapter highlights policy perspectives, and Chap. 2 focuses on theory and on principles for practice.

Educational, workplace, healthcare and other settings have long been used as a means of targeting health promotion interventions (Mullen et al., 1995; Tones & Tilford, 1994). However, what has become known as the settings-based approach to health promotion goes beyond this – understanding that context can have direct and indirect influences on well-being and seeking to embed health within the culture, ethos and core business of settings. Understood in this way, St Leger (1997) and Green et al. (2000) have traced how insights from sociology, organizational and

M. Dooris (✉)
Institute of Citizenship, Society and Change/Healthy and Sustainable Settings Unit, University of Central Lancashire, Preston, Lancashire, UK
e-mail: mtdooris@uclan.ac.uk

S. Kokko
Research Center for Health Promotion, Faculty of Sport and Health Sciences, University of Jyväskylä, Länsi-Suomi, Finland
e-mail: sami.p.kokko@jyu.fi

E. de Leeuw
Centre for Health Equity Training, Research and Evaluation, University of New South Wales, Sydney, NSW, Australia
e-mail: e.deleeuw@unsw.edu.au

© Springer Nature Switzerland AG 2022
S. Kokko, M. Baybutt (eds.), *Handbook of Settings-Based Health Promotion*, https://doi.org/10.1007/978-3-030-95856-5_1

environmental psychology, geography and other disciplines laid the ecological foundations for the healthy settings approach.

1.2   The 1980s: The Emergence of the Healthy Settings Approach

1.2.1   Setting the Scene: The Liberation After the Second World War

Social developments in the wake of the Second World War formed fertile ground for the emergence of a new and different approach to health promotion. This has been called by some the 'fourth wave' in public health (De Leeuw, 2016). After the first (infrastructural sewage systems and piped water), second (clinical—vaccination programmes) and third (social—lifestyle change through health education), we reached a 'health cultural' stage that exists in parallel with the others. What the fourth stage adds is a recognition of social movements (e.g. women's health movement, sustainability engagement), a systems view (first expressed in the reports by the Club of Rome) and an emancipatory gaze (e.g. anti-colonialism, feminism, equal rights for lesbian, gay, bisexual, transgender, intersex, and questioning—LGBTIQ—people). In the health field, these shifts were championed by people like Halfdan Mahler (De Leeuw, 2017a). Under their leadership, they set the stage for the Declaration of Alma Ata on Primary Health Care (WHO, 1978), the associated Health for All by the Year 2000 WHO programme developed globally (WHO, 1981) as well as regionally and nationally, and a recognition of wider social, economic, physical and political determinants of health.

1.2.2   Ottawa Charter for Health Promotion

Within this context, the first International Health Promotion Conference was held, culminating in the Ottawa Charter for Health Promotion (WHO, 1986). Building on a new perspective established in Canada and elsewhere (LaFramboise, 1973; Lalonde, 1974; McKeown, 1976), the conference was tagged as 'the move toward a new public health'. It set out a new manifesto for health promotion with an explicit focus on settings. Describing health promotion as the process of enabling people to increase control over, and to improve, their health, the Charter highlighted the need for advocacy, mediation and enablement strategies and presented five action areas—building healthy public policy, creating supportive environments, strengthening community action, developing personal skills and reorienting health services. In considering implications of moving into the future, the Charter stated:

Health is created and lived by people within the settings of their everyday life; where they learn, work, play and love. Health is created by caring for oneself and others, by being able to take decisions and have control over one's life circumstances, and by ensuring that the society one lives in creates conditions that allow the attainment of health by all its members. Caring, holism and ecology are essential issues in developing strategies for health promotion. (WHO, 1986, pp. 3–4)

Whilst not articulating an explicit theory for the healthy settings approach, the Ottawa Charter encapsulated broader conceptual thinking and policy development that had developed during the late 1970s and early 1980s. In a well-crafted process (de Leeuw & Harris-Roxas, 2016), it built on an earlier discussion document (WHO, 1984) to present a holistic socioecological model of health and reflect a focus on salutogenesis (Antonovsky, 1985, 1996). As Kickbusch (1996, p. 5) has commented, this led to the settings approach becoming the starting point for the WHO's lead health promotion programmes, with a commitment to 'shifting the focus from the deficit model of disease to the health potentials inherent in the social and institutional settings of everyday life' and pioneering strategies that 'strengthened both sense of place and sense of self'.

1.2.3   Healthy Cities

Building on a working conference held in Toronto in 1984 (Beyond Health Care, 1985) and influenced by the ideas of Duhl (1963), Healthy Cities (see also Chap. 5) was the first of these programmes to take shape, 'shifting from a linear disease model to an open, learning, inquiring system which is complex and holistic' (Duhl, 1988, p. 10) and setting out a process-based vision of a healthy city as one

that is continually creating and improving those physical and social environments and expanding those community resources which enable people to mutually support each other in performing all the functions of life and in developing to their maximum potential... (Hancock & Duhl, 1988, cited in Tsouros, 1991, p. 20)

The European Office of the WHO intended 'Healthy Cities' to be a small-scale experimental project with a handful of cities (de Leeuw, 2017b). It aimed 'to put health on the agenda of decision-makers in the cities of Europe' (Tsouros, 1995, p. 133). The project sought to translate the rhetoric of Health for All and the Ottawa Charter into tangible action—serving as a 'testing ground for developing and implementing these new public health approaches at the local level' (Tsouros, 1991, p. 18). Informed by modern management theory and practice, the project recognized that success requires experimentation, learning, adaptation and change. It thus aimed to realize the vision of the healthy city through a process of political commitment, visibility for health, institutional change and innovative action for health—supported by partnership working, networking, evaluation and dissemination. The approach quickly fired the imagination of professionals, politicians and citizens in Europe and beyond worldwide. By the end of the decade, Healthy Cities was set to become a major global movement for the new public health, having not only expanded within Europe but having taken root in a variety of forms (e.g. as Healthy Communities) within other parts of the 'developed' world such as Australia, Canada, Japan, New Zealand and the United States of America (Baum, 2002; Tsouros, 1991; WHO, 2003).

1.3   The 1990s: The Consolidation, Expansion and Wider Application of the Healthy Settings Approach

The 1990s was characterized by the expansion of Healthy Cities beyond High-Income Countries and its further development and adaptation to other area-based settings, the wider application of the healthy settings approach to 'organizational' settings, the emergence of praxis-based theory, and the further strengthening of international and national policy.

1.3.1   The Expansion of Healthy Cities and Its Further Development and Adaptation

The expansion of Healthy Cities to the Global South quickly followed its launch within Europe and its development in other parts of the Global North. In some regions, developments were led by the WHO. For instance, the local government emphasis aligned very well with the Pan-American Health Organization's programme on Sistemas Integrales Locales para la Salud, the SILOS. In the Eastern Mediterranean, the WHO used Healthy Cities to further sustain it local hygiene and sanitation projects. in other regions, developments were led by external countries working with the WHO—an example being the Francophone network of Healthy Cities established in the African region with support from Québec in Canada; and in yet others, the WHO involvement followed a burgeoning of grassroots activity—an example being South-East Asia Healthy Cities Programme (Goldstein, 1996). Recognizing the success of the European experience and its rapid expansion, the WHO Global Management Development Committee in 1995 encouraged the WHO to endorse an interregional programme on Healthy Cities (WHO, 2002a).

Looking back, three interrelated factors are particularly pertinent in understanding the popularity of the approach: First, the rapid urbanization that affected (and still affects) developing countries; second, the focus on combining top-down political commitment, bottom-up community participation and inter-sectoral collaboration to bring about change for health and equity; and third, the convergence of health and sustainable development agendas. This convergence was highlighted by the Sundsvall Statement on Supportive Environments (WHO, 1991b), which was presented at the Rio Conference on Environment and Development (the 'Earth Summit') in 1992 and contributed to the resulting Agenda 21 (United Nations, 1993).

Agenda 21 included a major focus on the need to integrate health and sustainability into community-based urban planning and development, a focus taken forward at the Second United Nations Conference on Human Settlements in 1996. The growing concern to coordinate action for health and sustainable development had an immediate resonance with many developing countries, but also influenced the development and implementation of Healthy Cities more generally. Working with the European Sustainable Cities and Towns Campaign, the WHO published a series of reports on sustainable development and health (Price & Dubé, 1997; WHO, 1997a, 2002b) and incorporated in its Healthy Cities Phase III designation criteria a commitment to sustainable development and a requirement to link city health plans to local Agenda 21 strategies (WHO, 1998a). The challenge of enhancing coordination between the two agendas was explored in depth by Dooris (1999).

Although there was no doubting the appeal and rapid spread of Healthy Cities, the assertion that it had become a social movement was questioned by some. Baum (1993), in particular, explored the possible contradiction between Healthy Cities as a movement for radical social change and Healthy Cities as a WHO-led programme—echoing earlier critiques of Health for All (Navarro, 1984; Strong, 1986) and Healthy Cities (Dooris, 1988). The interesting issue that such critiques fail to fully appreciate, though, is that local governance for health, and relations between how 'health' is constructed by people and institutions in settings on the one hand, and higher governance levels (regions, provinces, oblasts, states, nation-states, or federations such as Australia or Canada) on the other, is uniquely determined at street level. This resonates with the idea of street level bureaucracies that create unique policy and programme approaches for each context—or setting (e.g. Delaney, 1994). In some cases this creates activities that are wholly community owned and driven, in others they turn into state-sponsored delivery projects.

1.3.2 The Wider Application of the Healthy Settings Approach

Drawing on the experience of Healthy Cities and on related activity in a range of sectors, in the 1990s, developments in settings-based health promotion took root within a wide range of area-based and organizational settings (Catford & St Leger, 1996; Kickbusch, 1997; St Leger, 1997).

At a geographical level, the decade was characterized by the adaptation of Healthy Cities to other area-based settings—examples being **Healthy Villages** initiatives in Africa and the Eastern Mediterranean (de Leeuw & Simos, 2017; Khosh-Chashm, 1995; Kickbusch, 1997), **Healthy Islands** projects in the Western Pacific and other regions (de Leeuw, Martin, & Waqanivalu, 2018; Galea et al., 2000) and, less explicitly, the **Regions for Health** Network in Europe. A vision for Healthy Islands was first proposed in the Yanuca Declaration (WHO, 1995a), in response to the WHO Western Pacific Region's health policy framework—New Horizons in Health (WHO, 1995b). Focused on national-level developments and reflecting a holistic and ecological model of health promotion and a respect for cultural and environmental diversity, Healthy Islands were conceptualized as places where children are nurtured in body and mind, environments invite learning and leisure, people work and age in dignity, and ecological balance is a source of pride. This initial concept of Healthy Islands—based on a commitment to community empowerment, capacity building and cultural sensitivity—proved to be a powerful catalyst for change. Ministers reaffirmed their commitment to the pursuit of Healthy Islands in the Rarotonga Agreement (WHO, 1997b), which presented a framework for coordinating health promotion strategies, health protection strategies and issue-based programmes across the island setting and within smaller settings, such as villages, schools, workplaces and markets (Galea et al., 2000).

In parallel with the growth of area-based activity, the approach quickly came to be adapted to and applied within organizational settings. As Squires and Strobl (1996, p. 16) explain:

> A natural stage in the development of the Healthy Cities movement was to move towards focusing on more discrete "settings" in both urban and rural environments where effective health promotion principles might be applied…The rationale for this approach was that all settings in which people live, interact, work and play are overlapping and therefore action is necessary in all 'settings' in order to achieve effective and lasting change.

As highlighted by Young (2005), the conceptual origins of **Health Promoting Schools** (see also Chap. 6) can be traced back to a European symposium titled 'The Health Promoting School', held in Scotland in 1986. This led to the publication of a report on 'The Healthy School' (Young & Williams, 1989), so-called because the WHO Regional Office for Europe was keen to make links to its Healthy Cities Project. Following this, the European Health Promoting Schools Network was established formally in 1992 as a tripartite venture of the WHO, the European Commission and the Council of Europe (Barnekow Rasmussen, 2005)—initially involving pilot schools in four countries. Around the same time (in 1983), a new school-based cross-national health behaviour survey, namely Health Behaviour among School-aged Children (HBSC) was established by the WHO (see more http://www.hbsc.org/), which enabled evidence moving beyond education for health in schools to creating more systems-based environments of health in schools. The concept of the Health Promoting School went beyond a focus on the formal curriculum to highlight the role of the staff/pupil/community relationships, the school environment and health-related services—pointing the way to what later became known as the 'whole school approach'. These developments were paralleled in North America, with the term 'comprehensive school health programme' being coined there to reflect a similar broadening of vision beyond mere health instruction. As with Healthy Cities, the idea quickly spread—with the Australian Health Promoting Schools Association being launched in 1994, the WHO Global School Health Initiative being established in 1995, and further Health Promoting Schools and Healthy Schools programmes taking shape across the Western Pacific, and in Southeast Asia, Africa, the Americas and the Eastern Mediterranean Region.

Building on conceptual developments and modelling carried out in Vienna in 1989, the WHO **Health Promoting Hospitals** Network was initially launched in

1990 (see also Chap. 7), as a multi-city action plan of the WHO European Healthy Cities Project (Tsouros, 1995). The Budapest Declaration (WHO, 1991c) proposed 17 criteria, focusing not only on clinical tasks but also on the physical environment, living and working conditions, educational programmes and collaboration with the community. These criteria provided strategic direction to the European Pilot Health Promoting Hospitals Project, within which 20 hospitals from eleven countries participated from 1993 to 1997. The resulting Vienna Recommendations (WHO, 1997c) set out six fundamental principles and four strategies for implementation, which have guided the future development of Health Promoting Hospitals as the International Network has steadily expanded. In parallel with European developments, the idea of Health-Promoting Hospitals also gained ground in Australia during the 1990s (Johnson & Paton, 2007), with a concern to build on the European experience but to develop an approach relevant to the Australian context. Of these, the most significant in terms of research and conceptual development proved to be a project in Adelaide, which emphasized the need to combine infrastructure development to support health promotion and organizational change with health promotion activity related to patients/families, staff, organization, physical environment and community. Through research conducted as part of this Health-Promoting Hospital initiative, a typology of health-promoting hospitals later emerged, as discussed in Chap. 2 (Johnson & Baum, 2001).

Discussing the concept of the **Health-Promoting Workplace** (see also Chap. 9), Chu et al. (2000) have suggested that the 1990s saw a shift towards an interdisciplinary approach reflecting an increased understanding of the multi-determinants of workers' health. Looking beyond the workplace as a location for individually focused behaviour-change interventions, this involved workers and management collectively endeavouring to change the workplace into a health-promoting setting. These shifts in understanding were influenced by and reflected in developments across the globe. For example, the European Foundation for the Improvement of Living and Working Conditions (EFILWC) conducted research and development projects focused on workplace health promotion (e.g. EFILWC, 1997a, 1997b), the WHO Regional Office for Europe published a guidance manual (Demmer, 1995), and the European Network for Workplace Health Promotion was formed in 1996— subsequently adopting the Luxembourg Declaration (*European Network for Workplace Health Promotion*, 1997). This defined workplace health promotion as 'the combined efforts of employers, employees and society to improve the health and well-being of people at work'—to be achieved through improving the work organization and the working environment, promoting active participation and encouraging personal development. Building on work within countries such as China and Australia, a Western Pacific Regional Network for the Health Promoting Workplace was established in 1997, supported by the publication of Guidelines for Healthy Workplaces (WHO, 1999a). This diverse regional activity was complemented by the WHO's Global Healthy Work Approach (WHO, 1997d), which called for a comprehensive perspective to promoting health of all working populations.

In 1995, the WHO Regional Office for Europe built on its experience in relation to cities, schools and hospitals by establishing its Health in Prisons Project (HIPP), launching an international movement concerned to promote health and tackle health inequalities in the prison setting (Gatherer et al., 2005; Woodall, 2016) (see also Chap. 10). The first international conference on **Healthy Prisons**, held in Liverpool in March 1996 (Squires & Strobl, 1996), proposed a framework comprising five spheres of influence:

• The physical, social and political environment of the prison
• The organizational culture of the prison
• Specific health issues associated with prisons and the demographic characteristics of the prison population
• Improving prisoners' practical and life skills
• Establishing and developing links with the outside community

At its inception, the HIPP identified three priority issues—communicable diseases, mental health and drug misuse. These formed the focus for subsequent conferences, producing a number of landmark documents to guide national policy and practice, including the Consensus Statement on Mental Health Promotion in Prisons (WHO, 1999b).

Health-Promoting Universities (see also Chap. 8) grew out of the local application of the healthy settings approach within English universities. Inspired by a WHO-sponsored international symposium on settings-based health promotion held at the University of Central Lancashire in 1993 (Theaker & Thompson, 1995), Lancaster University and the University of Central Lancashire established Health-Promoting University initiatives. Around the same time, the UK's Faculty of Public Health Medicine (1995) published an issue of its newsletter that took Health-Promoting Universities as its focus topic. In the editorial, Beattie (1995) noted that

> initiatives in universities have emerged more or less in parallel with projects on the health-promoting workplace, school and hospital, but – without the benefit of any national or international infrastructure – they are only just beginning to generate a momentum of research and development… (p. 2)

The WHO Regional Office for Europe, through its Healthy Cities office, subsequently sponsored the First International Conference on Health-Promoting Universities in 1996, holding a round table meeting in 1997 and publishing a book, *Health Promoting Universities: Concept, Experience and Framework for Action* the following year (Tsouros et al., 1998). Explicitly rooted in the principles of Health for All, sustainable development and the Ottawa Charter, this drew on the experience of other settings-based programmes and on insights from universities themselves to provide conceptual and practical guidance. The strategic framework proposed to guide local practice sought to enable integration of health into the culture, structures and processes of the university—with a focus on creating healthy working, learning and living environments; increasing the health promotion aspects of teaching and research; and developing links with and supporting health development in the community. Alongside this, the book presented a framework for action by a European Network of Health Promoting Universities. Although Health-Promoting Universities was incorporated within the Healthy Cities Phase III strategic plan (WHO, 1998a), plans to establish a European Network and WHO-led programme did not materialize—and instead, theory and practice development continued to be led by a small number of universities committed to applying the settings approach and developing a 'whole university' model.

As the decade progressed, the healthy settings approach continued to be adapted and applied within different regions of the world, responsive to particular economic, political and cultural contexts and sowing the seeds for new developments in the next decade.

1.3.3 The Further Strengthening of International Policy

Whilst global and regional strategies for Health for All published in the early 1980s did not mention healthy settings as an approach, there was a more explicit policy focus by the early 1990s. For example, the revised European Health for All Policy (WHO, 1991a, p. 77) included as Target 14, 'By the year 2000, all settings of social life and activity, such as the city, school, workplace, neighbourhood and home, should provide greater opportunities for promoting health'. Furthermore, the Sundsvall Statement coming out of the Third Global Conference on Health Promotion, reinforced the Ottawa Charter, argued that 'a call for the creation of supportive environments is a practical proposal for public health action at the local level, with a focus on settings for health that allow for broad community involvement and control' (WHO, 1991b, p. 4). Although perhaps best remembered for controversy regarding the legitimacy of the private sector's involvement in health-promotion collaborations, the fourth Global Conference on Health Promotion—through the resulting Jakarta Declaration on Leading Health Promotion into the twenty-first Century (WHO, 1997e)—served a pivotal role in reaffirming the importance of the healthy settings approach within the arena of international policy. Viewing health promotion as an investment not only for human health but also for social and economic development, this suggested that settings 'represent the organisational base of the infrastructure required for health promotion' (p. 4)—going on to highlight the need for intersectoral collaboration through new and diverse networks facilitating exchange of information and experience on which strategies are effective in which settings. While the Declaration did not attempt to articulate a theory for healthy settings, it explicitly endorsed the approach as offering practical opportunities for the implementation of effective and comprehensive strategies (combining a focus on building healthy public policy, creating supportive environments, strengthening community action, developing personal skills and reorienting health services). Furthermore, it specifically highlighted the experience gained through geographical settings (mega-cities, islands, cities, municipalities and local communities) and their component organizational or 'micro' settings (markets, schools, workplaces, healthcare facilities).

1.4 Healthy Settings Into the New Millennium

The importance of healthy settings was also confirmed in regional policy documents published by the WHO in the lead-up to the new millennium. For instance, the settings approach was included under Target 13 of the WHO's new European Health for All Policy Framework, Health 21 (WHO, 1998b); in its 'Healthy Urbanization' policy programme, the Western Pacific Region looked at a range of settings including workplaces, marketplaces and schools (WHO, 2011, 2016a); and in the Americas, the Healthy Settings movement was inspired by the emerging development of the 'Health in All Policies' approach which came to full fruition in the 2000s (Buss et al., 2016; Jackson et al., 2013; Rudolph et al., 2013).

Thus, by the end of the twentieth century, the healthy settings approach was well established worldwide with international, regional and national programmes and networks covering a wide range of contexts. The new millennium has been characterized by a number of developments, including the application of the approach to a wider range of settings; documentation, guidance and cross-setting collaboration; and the identification of emerging themes for critical reflection, debate and research.

1.4.1 Application to New Settings

Building on the rapid expansion that characterized the 1990s, the new millennium saw the settings-based approach being applied to further new settings (see also Chaps. 11, 12 and 13)—some through formalized initiatives led by the WHO and other bodies, others emerging through pilot studies and projects. These included villages (Howard, 2002), marketplaces (WHO, 2004), sports clubs (Geidne et al., 2013; Kokko et al., 2006; Kokko et al., 2014) and sports stadia (Drygas et al., 2013); early years (Mooney et al., 2008; Welsh Government, 2011), further education (Warwick et al., 2008), general practice and primary care (Watson, 2008); aged home and residential care (Harris et al., 2008; Krajic et al., 2015; Mahler et al., 2014); libraries (Whitelaw et al., 2016); airports (de Leeuw, Crimeen, et al., 2018); nature-based settings such as wetlands and watersheds (Bunch et al., 2011; Horwitz & Finlayson, 2011); and social media and digital settings (Loss et al., 2014).

1.4.2 Documentation, Evidence, Guidance and Cross-Setting Collaboration

At the level of global policy, settings continued to feature in the WHO's health-promotion conferences, with the Bangkok Charter (WHO, 2005), calling for all sectors and settings to advocate for, invest in and build capacity for health; and the Shanghai Declaration (WHO, 2016b) reaffirming but slightly revising the Ottawa

Charter's original statement to argue that 'health is created in the settings of everyday life – in the neighbourhoods and communities where people live, love, work, shop and play' (p. 3).

For those programmes that had already taken root, the 2000s were important in documenting their stories and building and communicating evidence of effectiveness, often linked to the production of further guidance. For example:

- The International Union of Health Promotion and Education (IUHPE) (2000) issued the second edition of *The Evidence of Health Promotion Effectiveness*, which included a focus on healthy settings, specifically schools, health services and workplaces.
- The WHO published *Evaluation in Health Promotion* (Rootman et al., 2001), which likewise included a section on healthy settings, focusing on cities, communities, schools, workplaces and health services.
- The Department of Health for England published a guidance document, *Health Promoting Prisons: A Shared Approach* (Department of Health, 2002), which explored the meaning of a whole prison approach and drew on the experience of the WHO European Health in Prisons Project; and concurrently, the Scottish Prison Service developed their strategic position for the health promoting prison (Scottish Prison Service, 2002).
- The WHO Regional Office for Europe prepared a compilation of papers on progress and achievements within Europe together with an overview of the Healthy Cities movement in the six WHO regions (Tsouros & Farrington, 2003; WHO, 2003) and systematically evaluated each Phase of its Healthy City evolution (Tsouros et al., 2015; Tsouros & Green, 2009; Tsouros & Green, 2013).
- IUHPE issued a special edition of its journal on Global School Health Promotion and the following year published Protocols and Guidelines for Health Promoting Schools (International Union of Health Promotion, 2005, 2006).
- The WHO Regional Office for Europe reviewed the progress of Health-Promoting Hospitals, publishing *Health Promotion in Hospitals: Evidence and Quality Management* (Groene & Garcia-Barbero, 2005)
- IUHPE followed up its earlier work by coordinating a publication on *Global Evidence of Health Promotion Effectiveness* (McQueen & Jones, 2007), which included a focus on schools together with an exploration of the challenges involved in building evidence for the effectiveness of the settings approach (Dooris et al., 2007).
- IUHPE issued a special supplement of its journal on health-promoting settings around the world (Global Health Promotion, 2016).

Poland et al. (2009) were influential in taking a broader approach to programme design and delivery. They presented an analytic framework that put context to the fore, arguing that while different settings have commonalities, they are each distinct. They proposed a nested series of guiding questions concerned with understanding settings, changing settings, and developing and translating knowledge, set within a set of principles for practice. Reflecting on this framework, Kokko et al. (2014) use the sports club as a focus to consider the shared and specific characteristics of different settings. Additionally, they present a model exploring the reciprocal relationship between individuals and settings, while examining the social, economic, environmental and cultural determinants of health promotion that operate at micro, meso and macro levels.

The last two decades have also seen the incorporation of healthy settings within academic books—both through dedicated texts (e.g. Johnson & Paton, 2007; Poland et al., 2000; Scriven & Hodgins, 2011) and through chapters and sections within generic publications (e.g. Baum, 2002; Naidoo & Wills, 2000; Scriven & Orme, 2001; Green et al., 2019; Baybutt et al., 2006; Dooris & Hunter, 2007; Dooris, 2012a; Mittelmark et al., 2016).

1.5   Identifying Emerging Themes for Critical Reflection, Debate and Research

As already indicated, the twenty-first century has been characterized by the identification of emerging themes for critical reflection, debate and research. These include the following:

Developing coherent frameworks for healthy settings that recognize interrelationships, strengthen linkages and enhance synergy: As discussed above, developments in the conceptualization of healthy settings have highlighted the practical importance of acknowledging and understanding the interrelationships between different types and scales of settings. Poland et al. (2000) and Dooris (2004, 2006b) have presented a rationale for greater coordination and connectedness based on the fact that people live their lives across a range of settings, that there can be synergistic effects between settings, and that a problem manifest in one setting may have its roots in another. Going one step further, Galea et al. (2000) have proposed the hierarchical categorization of contextual and elemental settings, a consideration that has been further developed by Dooris (2009, 2013); Kokko et al. (2014); and Bloch et al. (2014), and facilitated by the work of IUHPE.

Ensuring that the healthy settings approach tackles inequalities in health and promotes social inclusion: Concern that the healthy settings approach could serve to exacerbate health inequalities and social exclusion was highlighted in the 1990s by Kickbusch (1995, 1997) and Galbally (1997). The challenge has been further discussed during the past two decades, with calls for the approach to be extended to informal and less well-defined settings, to acknowledge and take account of power relations within and between settings, and to work upwards and outwards, influencing organizational policies that really matter and advocating for macro-level political, economic and social change (Dooris, 2004, 2009; Dooris & Hunter, 2007; Green et al., 2000). More recently, Shareck et al. (2013) have argued for an equity-oriented settings approach and, reflecting concerns raised in the WHO's Commission on Social Determinants of Health (2008), Newman et al. (2015) have called for health promotion to shift the focus of settings-based work further upstream and to evaluate programmes for differential equity impacts.

Locating healthy settings in a globalized world: The relationship between healthy settings practice and macro policy has become increasingly important in the context of twenty-first century globalization. Ziglio et al. (2000, p. 149) have convincingly argued the case for the Investment for Health and Development approach, with its shift of focus to strategies 'which maintain and create health equitably and are integral to sustainable social, economic and human development policies'. Highlighting the opportunities and challenges of globalization and the need to make the promotion of health central to the global development agenda, the Bangkok Charter (WHO, 2005) called for all sectors and settings to advocate for health; invest in sustainable policies, action and infrastructure to address the determinants of health; build capacity for health promotion; regulate and legislate for health and well-being; and build partnerships to create sustainable actions. Significantly, Kickbusch has also explored the 'deterritorialization' of health and the implications of globalization for healthy settings (Kickbusch, 2007a, 2007b).

Connecting health, sustainability and social justice agendas: As discussed earlier, the publication of Agenda 21 strongly influenced the future direction of Healthy Cities. More generally, a number of WHO regions (e.g. Southeast Asia, Americas) have led their healthy settings programmes within the context of their sustainable development work. Growing concern about the health consequences of climate change have further highlighted the imperative of connecting public health and sustainable development within the context of particular settings such as cities, schools and universities (Bentley, 2007; Davis & Cooke, 2007; Orme & Dooris, 2010; Rice & Hancock, 2016). More broadly, there have been strong calls for the settings-based approach to connect agendas by coordinating and integrating action for health, sustainability and social justice, thereby achieving co-benefits across policy domains (Dooris, 2012b, 2013; Poland et al., 2011; Poland & Dooris, 2010). At a global level, the Shanghai Declaration on Promoting Health in the 2030 Agenda for Sustainable Development (WHO, 2016b) was highly significant in affirming the centrality of health within the Sustainable Development Goals (United Nations, 2015) and in positioning health promotion as a crucial mechanism going forward.

Evaluating healthy settings initiatives and building evidence of effectiveness: Kickbusch (2003, p. 386) reflected that the success of the healthy settings approach does 'not fit easily into an epidemiological framework of "evidence" but needs to be analyzed in terms of social and political processes'. In addition to the general difficulties faced by public health and health promotion in responding to the demand for evidence, it has been argued that a number of specific challenges make it difficult to undertake robust evaluation and to build a convincing evidence base for the settings approach. These concern the funding and construction of the evidence base for public health and health promotion; the diversity characterizing both conceptualization and practice; and the complexity of evaluating ecological whole system approaches (Dooris, 2006a; Dooris & Hunter, 2007). Dooris et al. (2007) have explored these challenges and discussed the potential value of critical realism and complexity theory for overcoming the limitations of traditional evaluation models and helping generate evidence of effectiveness (see Chap. 4).

1.6 Summary

Taking a historical perspective, this chapter has sought to distil and provide an overview of how Healthy Settings has emerged and evolved over time. While touching on theoretical and practice developments—considered in detail in the following chaps. 2 and 3—the focus has been on the establishment and development of the approach across the globe, highlighting the role of both policy and critical commentary in guiding, legitimizing and honing settings-based health promotion from its inception in the mid-1980s to the current day.

References

Antonovsky, A. (1985). *Health, stress and coping.* Jossey Bass.

Antonovsky, A. (1996). The salutogenic model as a theory to guide health promotion. *Health Promotion International, 11*(1), 11–18.

Barnekow Rasmussen, V. (2005). The European Network of Health Promoting Schools – from Iceland to Kyrgyzstan. *Promotion & Education, XII*(3–4), 169–172.

Baum, F. (1993). Healthy Cities and change: Social movement or bureaucratic tool? *Health Promotion International, 8*(1), 31–40.

Baum, F. (2002). *The new public health* (2nd ed.). Oxford University Press.

Baybutt, M., Hayton, P., & Dooris, M. (2006). A reader in promoting public health: Challenge and controversy. In J. Douglas, S. Earle, S. Handsley, C. Lloyd, & S. Spurr (Eds.), *Prisons in England and Wales: An important public health opportunity?* (pp. 237–245). Sage/Milton Keynes: Open University Press.

Beattie, A. (1995). Editorial: New agendas for student health. *Health for All 2000 News, 31*, 2–3.

Bentley, M. (2007). Healthy Cities, local environmental action and climate change. *Health Promotion International, 22*(3), 246–253.

Beyond Health Care. (1985). Proceedings of a working conference on healthy public policy. *Canadian Journal of Public Health, 76*(S1), 1–104.

Bloch, P., Toft, U., Reinbach, H. C., Clausen, L. T., Mikkelsen, B. E., Poulsen, K., et al. (2014). Revitalizing the setting approach – supersettings for sustainable impact in community health promotion. *International Journal of Behavioral Nutrition and Physical Activity, 11*, 118.

Bunch, M. J., Morrison, K. E., Parkes, M. W., & Venema, H. D. (2011). Promoting health and wellbeing by managing for social–ecological resilience: The potential of integrating ecohealth and water resources management approaches. *Ecology and Society, 16*(1), 6.

Buss, P. M., Fonseca, L. E., Galvão, L. A. C., Fortune, K., & Cook, C. (2016). Health in all policies in the partnership for sustainable development. *Revista Panamericana de Salud Publica, 40*, 186–191.

Catford, J., & St Leger, L. (1996). Moving into the next decade—and a new dimension? *Health Promotion International, 11*(1), 1–3.

Chu, C., Breucker, G., Harris, N., Stitzel, A., Gan, X., Gu, X., et al. (2000). Health promoting workplaces – international settings development. *Health Promotion International, 15*(2), 155–167.

Commission on Social Determinants of Health (CSDH). (2008). *Closing the gap in a generation: Health equity through action on the social determinants of health.* Final Report of the Commission on Social Determinants of Health. World Health Organization.

Davis, J., & Cooke, S. (2007). Educating for a healthy, sustainable world: an argument for integrating Health Promoting Schools and Sustainable Schools. *Health Promotion International, 22*(4), 346–353.

de Leeuw, E. (2016). From research to policy and practice in public health. In P. Liamputtong (Ed.), *Public health. Local and global perspectives* (pp. 213–234). Cambridge University Press.

de Leeuw, E. (2017a). A tribute to Dr Halfdan Mahler, 1923–2016. *Health Promotion International, 32*(1), 1.

de Leeuw, E. (2017b). Cities and health from the Neolithic to the Anthropocene. In E. de Leeuw & J. Simos (Eds.), *Healthy Cities – The theory, policy, and practice of value-based urban planning* (pp. 3–30). Springer.

de Leeuw, E., Crimeen, A., Freestone, R., Jalaludin, B., Sainsbury, P., Hirono, K., et al. (2018). *Healthy airports*. Centre for Health Equity Training, Research and Evaluation (CHETRE), University of New South Wales.

de Leeuw, E., & Harris-Roxas, B. (2016). Crafting health promotion: From Ottawa to beyond Shanghai. *Environ Risque Sante, 15*, 1–4.

de Leeuw, E., Martin, E., & Waqanivalu, T. (2018). Healthy Islands. In M. Van den Bosch & W. Bird (Eds.), *Oxford textbook of nature and public health: The role of nature in improving the health of a population* (pp. 285–290). Oxford University Press.

de Leeuw, E., & Simos, J. (Eds.). (2017). *Healthy Cities - The theory, policy, and practice of value-based urban planning*. Springer.

Delaney, F. G. (1994). Muddling through the middle ground: Theoretical concerns in intersectoral collaboration and health promotion. *Health Promotion International, 9*(3), 217–225.

Demmer, H. (1995). *Worksite health promotion: How to go about it*. European Health Promotion Series Number 4. WHO Regional Office for Europe/Essen: WHO Collaborating Centre – European Information Centre, Company Health Promotion.

Department of Health. (2002). *Health promoting prisons: A shared approach*. Department of Health.

Dooris, M. (1988). The pursuit of Healthy Cities: A case of David and Goliath? *Radical Health Promotion, 9*, 4–9.

Dooris, M. (1999). Healthy cities and local agenda 21: The UK experience – Challenges for the new millennium. *Health Promotion International, 14*(4), 365–375.

Dooris, M. (2004). Joining up settings for health: A valuable investment for strategic partnerships? *Critical Public Health, 14*(1), 49–61.

Dooris, M. (2006a). Healthy settings: Challenges to generating evidence of effectiveness. *Health Promotion International, 21*(1), 55–65.

Dooris, M. (2006b). Editorial – Healthy settings: Future directions. *Promotion & Education, XIII*(1), 1–5.

Dooris, M. (2009). Holistic and sustainable health improvement: The contribution of the settings-based approach to health promotion. *Perspectives in Public Health, 129*(1), 29–36.

Dooris, M. (2012a). Settings for promoting health. In L. Jones & J. Douglas (Eds.), *Public health: Building innovative practice*. Sage.

Dooris, M. (2012b). The settings approach: An overview – looking back, looking forward. Chapter. In A. Scriven & M. Hodgins (Eds.), *Health promotion settings: Principles and practice*. Sage.

Dooris, M. (2013). Expert voices for change: Bridging the silos – Towards healthy and sustainable settings for the 21st century. *Health & Place, 20*, 39–50.

Dooris, M., & Hunter, D. (2007). Organisations and settings for promoting public health. In C. Lloyd, S. Handsley, J. Douglas, S. Earle, & S. Spurr (Eds.), *Policy and practice in promoting public health* (pp. 95–125). Sage/Milton Keynes: Open University.

Dooris, M., Poland, B., Kolbe, L., de Leeuw, E., McCall, D., & Wharf-Higgins, J. (2007). Healthy settings: Building evidence for the effectiveness of whole system health promotion – Challenges and future directions. In D. McQueen & C. Jones (Eds.), *Global perspectives on health promotion effectiveness* (pp. 327–352). Springer Science and Business Media.

Drygas, W., Ruszkowska, J., Philpott, M., Björkström, O., Parker, M., Ireland, R., et al. (2013). Good practices and health policy analysis in European sports stadia: Results from the 'Healthy Stadia' project. *Health Promotion International, 28*(2), 157–165.

Duhl, L. (Ed.). (1963). *The urban condition: People and policy in the metropolis*. Basic Books, Inc.

Duhl, L. (1988). The mind of the city: the context for urban life. *Environments, 19*(3), 1–13.

European Foundation for the Improvement of Living and Working Conditions (EFILWC) (Ed.). (1997a). *Workplace health promotion in Europe. Program summary.* Office for Official Publications of the European Communities.

European Foundation for the Improvement of Living and Working Conditions (EFILWC) (Ed.). (1997b). *Manual for training in workplace health promotion.* Office for Official Publications of the European Communities.

European Network for Workplace Health Promotion. (1997). *Luxembourg declaration on workplace health promotion in the European Union.* ENWHP.

Faculty of Public Health Medicine (1995). *Health for All 2000 News, 31.*

Galbally, R. (1997). Health-promoting environments: Who will miss out? *Australian and New Zealand Journal of Public Health, 21*(4), 429–430.

Galea, G., Powis, B., & Tamplin, S. (2000). Healthy islands in the Western Pacific – international settings development. *Health Promotion International, 15*(2), 169–178.

Gatherer, A., Moller, L., & Hayton, P. (2005). WHO European Health in prisons project after ten years: Persistent barriers and achievements. *American Journal of Public Health, 95*(10), 1696–1700.

Geidne, S., Quennerstedt, M., & Eriksson, C. (2013). The youth sports club as a health-promoting setting: An integrative review of research. *Scandinavian Journal of Public Health, 41*(3), 269–283.

Global Health Promotion (2016). *23i Special supplement on approaches to health-promoting settings around the world.*

Goldstein, G. (1996). WHO healthy cities: Towards an interregional programme framework. In C. Price & A. Tsouros (Eds.), *Our cities, our future: Policies and action plans for health and sustainable development* (pp. 193–202). WHO Regional Office for Europe. Retrieved April 8, 2021, from https://www.euro.who.int/__data/assets/pdf_file/0010/100999/wa38096OU.pdf

Green, J., Cross, R., Woodall, J., & Tones, K. (2019). *Health promotion: Planning and strategies* (4th ed.). Sage.

Green, L. W., Poland, B. D., & Rootman, I. (2000). The settings approach to health promotion. In B. D. Poland, L. W. Green, & I. Rootman (Eds.), *Settings for health promotion: Linking theory and practice* (pp. 1–43). Sage.

Groene, O., & Garcia-Barbero, M. (Eds.). (2005). *Health promotion in hospitals: Evidence and quality management.* WHO Regional Office for Europe.

Hancock, T., & Duhl, L. (1988). *Promoting health in the urban context.* WHO Healthy Cities Papers, 1. WHO Regional Office for Europe.

Harris, N., Grootjans, J., & Wenham, K. (2008). Ecological aging: The settings approach in aged living and care accommodation. *Ecohealth, 5*, 196–204.

Horwitz, P., & Finlayson, M. (2011). Wetlands as settings for human health: Incorporating ecosystem services and health impact assessment into water resource management. *Bioscience, 61*(9), 678–688.

Howard, G. (2002). *Healthy villages: A guide for communities and community health workers.* WHO.

International Union for Health Promotion and Education (IUHPE). (2000). *The evidence of health promotion effectiveness. Shaping public health in a new Europe. Part Two: Evidence book* (2nd ed.). ECSC-EC-EAEC.

International Union for Health Promotion and Education (IUHPE). (2005). *Promotion & Education, XII*(3–4).

International Union for Health Promotion and Education (IUHPE). (2006). *Protocols and guidelines for Health Promoting Schools.* IUHPE.

Jackson, S. F., Birn, A. E., Fawcett, S. B., Poland, B., & Schultz, J. A. (2013). Synergy for health equity: Integrating health promotion and social determinants of health approaches in and beyond the Americas. *Revista Panamericana de Salud Publica, 34*, 473–480.

Johnson, A., & Baum, F. (2001). Health promoting hospitals: A typology of different organizational approaches to health promotion. *Health Promotion International, 16*(3), 281–287.

Johnson, A., & Paton, K. (2007). *Health promotion and health services: Management for change.* Oxford University Press.

Khosh-Chashm, K. (1995). Healthy Cities and Healthy Villages. *Eastern Mediterranean Health Journal, 1*(2), 103–111.

Kickbusch, I. (1995). An overview to the settings-based approach to health promotion. In T. Theaker & J. Thompson (Eds.), *The settings-based approach to health promotion.* Report of an international working conference, 17-20 November 1993 (pp. 3–9). Hertfordshire Health Promotion.

Kickbusch, I. (1996). Tribute to Aaron Antonovsky – 'what creates health'? *Health Promotion International, 11*(1), 5–6.

Kickbusch, I. (1997). Health-promoting environments: The next steps. *Australian and New Zealand Journal of Public Health, 21*(4), 431–434.

Kickbusch, I. (2003). The contribution of the World Health Organization to a new public health and health promotion. *American Journal of Public Health, 93*(3), 383–388.

Kickbusch, I. (2007a). Responding to the health society. *Health Promotion International, 22*(2), 89–91.

Kickbusch, I. (2007b). Health governance: The health society. In D. McQueen, I. Kickbusch, L. Potvin, J. Pelikan, L. Balbo, & T. Abel (Eds.), *Health and modernity: The role of theory in health promotion* (pp. 144–161). Springer Science and Business Media.

Kokko, S., Green, L., & Kannas, L. (2014). A review of settings-based health promotion with applications to sports clubs. *Health Promotion International, 29*, 494–509.

Kokko, S., Kannas, L., & Villberg, J. (2006). The health promoting sports club in Finland – a challenge for the settings-based approach. *Health Promotion International, 21*(3), 219–229.

Krajic, K., Cichocki, C., & Quehenberger, V. (2015). Health-promoting residential aged care: A pilot project in Austria. *Health Promotion International, 30*(3), 769–781.

Laframboise, H. L. (1973). Health policy: Breaking the problem down into manageable segments. *Canadian Medical Association Journal, 108*, 388–393.

Lalonde, M. (1974). *A new perspective on the health of Canadians.* Information Canada.

Loss, J., Lindacher, V., & Curbach, J. (2014). Online social networking sites—A novel setting for health promotion? *Health & Place, 26*, 161–170.

Mahler, M., Sarvimäki, A., Clancy, A., Stenbock-Hult, B., Simonsen, N., Liveng, A., et al. (2014). Home as a health promotion setting for older adults. *Scandinavian Journal of Public Health, 42*(S15), 36–40.

McKeown, T. (1976). *The role of medicine: Dream, mirage, or nemesis?* Nuffield Provincial Hospitals Trust.

McQueen, D., & Jones, C. (Eds.). (2007). *Global perspectives on health promotion effectiveness.* Springer Science and Business Media.

Mittelmark, M. B., Sagy, S., Eriksson, M., Bauer, G., Pelikan, J. M., Lindström, B., et al. (Eds.). (2016). *The handbook of Salutogenesis.* Springer. Retrieved April 8, 2021, from https://www.springer.com/gp/book/9783319045993

Mooney, A., Boddy, J., Statham, J., & Warwick, I. (2008). Approaches to developing health in early years settings. *Health Education, 108*(2), 163–177.

Mullen, P., Evans, D., Forster, J., Gottlieb, N., Kreuter, M., Moon, R., et al. (1995). Settings as an important dimension in health education/promotion policy, programs, and research. *Health Education Quarterly, 22*(3), 329–345.

Naidoo, J., & Wills, J. (2000). *Health promotion: Foundations for practice* (2nd ed.). Baillière Tindall.

Navarro, V. (1984). A critique of the ideological and political positions of the Willy Brandt Report and the WHO Alma Ata Declaration. *Social Science and Medicine, 18*(6), 467–474.

Newman, L., Baum, F., Javanparast, S., O'Rourke, K., & Carlon, L. (2015). Addressing social determinants of health inequities through settings: A rapid review. *Health Promotion International, 30*(S2), ii126–ii143.

Orme, J., & Dooris, M. (2010). Integrating health and sustainability: The higher education sector as a timely catalyst. *Health Education Research, 25*(3), 425–437.

Poland, B., & Dooris, M. (2010). A green and healthy future: a settings approach to building health, equity and sustainability. *Critical Public Health, 20*(3), 281–298.

Poland, B., Dooris, M., & Haluza-Delay, R. (2011). Securing 'supportive environments' for health in the face of ecosystem collapse: Meeting the triple threat with a sociology of creative transformation. *Health Promotion International, 26*(S2), ii202–ii215.

Poland, B., Green, L., & Rootman, I. (2000). *Settings for health promotion: Linking theory and practice*. Sage.

Poland, B., Krupa, G., & McCall, D. (2009). Settings for health promotion: An analytic framework to guide intervention design and implementation. *Health Promotion Practice, 10*(4), 505–516.

Price, C., & Dubé, P. (1997). *Sustainable development and health: Concepts, principles and framework for action for European cities and towns*. WHO Regional Office for Europe. Retrieved April 9, 2021, from https://www.euro.who.int/__data/assets/pdf_file/0016/43315/E53218.pdf

Rice, M., & Hancock, T. (2016). Equity, sustainability and governance in urban settings. *Global Health Promotion, 23*(S1), 94–97.

Rootman, I., Goodstadt, M., Hyndman, B., McQueen, D., Potvin, L., Springett, J., et al. (Eds.). (2001). *Evaluation in health promotion: Principles and perspectives*. WHO Regional Office for Europe.

Rudolph, L., Caplan, J., Ben-Moshe, K., & Dillon, L. (2013). *Health in all policies: A guide for state and local governments*. American Public Health Association and Public Health Institute.

Scottish Prison Service. (2002). *The health promoting prison. A framework for promoting health in the Scottish prison service*. Health Education Board for Scotland.

Scriven, A., & Hodgins, M. (2011). *Health promotion settings: Principles and practice*. Sage.

Scriven, A., & Orme, J. (Eds.). (2001). *Health promotion: Professional perspectives* (2nd ed.). Macmillan.

Shareck, M., Frohlick, K., & Poland, B. (2013). Reducing social inequities in health through settings-related interventions — A conceptual framework. *Global Health Promotion, 20*(2), 39–52.

Squires, N., & Strobl, J. (Eds.). (1996). *Healthy prisons – A vision for the future*. Report of the 1st International Conference on Healthy Prisons, Liverpool, 24-27 March 1996. University of Liverpool.

St Leger, L. (1997). Health promoting settings: From Ottawa to Jakarta. *Health Promotion International, 12*(2), 99–101.

Strong, M. (1986). A new modelled medicine? Comments on the WHO's Regional Strategy for Europe. *Social Science and Medicine, 22*(2), 193–199.

Theaker, T., & Thompson, J. (Eds.). (1995). *The settings-based approach to health promotion*. Report of an International Working Conference, 17-20 November 1993. Hertfordshire Health Promotion.

Tones, K., & Tilford, S. (1994). *Health education: Effectiveness, efficiency and equity* (2nd ed.). Chapman Hall.

Tsouros, A. (Ed.). (1991). *World Health Organization Healthy Cities Project: A project becomes a movement. Review of progress 1987-1990*. FADL Publishers/SOGESS.

Tsouros, A. (1995). The WHO Healthy Cities Project: State of the art and future plans. *Health Promotion International, 10*(2), 133–141.

Tsouros, A., de Leeuw, E., & Green, G. (2015). Evaluation of the fifth phase (2009–2013) of the WHO European Healthy Cities network: Further sophistication and challenges. *Health Promotion International, 30*(S1), i1–i2.

Tsouros, A., Dowding, G., Thomson, J., & Dooris, M. (Eds.). (1998). *Health promoting universities: Concept, experience and framework for action*. WHO Regional Office for Europe. Retrieved April 9, 2021, from http://www.euro.who.int/document/e60163.pdf

Tsouros, A., & Farrington, J. (Eds.). (2003). *WHO Healthy Cities in Europe: A compilation of papers on progress and achievements*. WHO Regional Office for Europe.

Tsouros, A., & Green, G. (2009). *Health Promotion International, 24*(suppl_1). Special supplement on European Healthy Cities.

Tsouros, A., & Green, G. (2013). Healthy cities in Europe. *Journal of Urban Health, 90*(1), 1–3.

United Nations (UN). (1993). *Earth Summit – Agenda 21*. United Nations.

United Nations (UN). (2015). *Transforming our World: The 2030 Agenda for Sustainable Development*. UN.

Warwick, I., Statham, J., & Aggleton, P. (2008). *Healthy and health promoting colleges – An evidence base*. Project Report. Thomas Coram Research Unit, University of London. Retrieved April 9, 2021, from https://discovery.ucl.ac.uk/id/eprint/10000064/1/Healthy_colleges.pdf

Watson, M. (2008). Going for gold: The health promoting general practice. *Quality in Primary Care, 16*, 177–185.

Welsh Government. (2011). *Healthy and sustainable pre-school scheme National Award criteria*. Welsh Government.

Whitelaw, S., Coburn, J., Lacey, M., McKee, M., & King, C. (2016). Libraries as 'everyday' settings: The Glasgow MCISS project. *Health Promotion International, 32*(5), 891–900.

Woodall, J. (2016). A critical examination of the health promoting prison two decades on. *Critical Public Health, 26*(5), 615–662.

World Health Organization (WHO). (1978). *Declaration of Alma-Ata*. International Conference on Primary Health Care, Alma-Ata, USSR, 06-12 September. WHO.

World Health Organization (WHO). (1981). *Global strategy for health for all by the year 2000*. WHO.

World Health Organization (WHO). (1984). *Health promotion: A discussion document on concepts and principles*. WHO Regional Office for Europe.

World Health Organization (WHO). (1986). *Ottawa Charter for Health Promotion*. Adopted at an International Conference on Health Promotion – The Move Towards a New Public Health (co-sponsored by the Canadian Public Health Association, Health and Welfare Canada and the World Health Organization), 17-21 November, Ottawa, Canada. WHO.

World Health Organization (WHO). (1991a). *Health for all targets: The health policy for Europe – Updated Edition*. (European Health For All Series, No 4). WHO Regional Office for Europe.

World Health Organization (WHO). (1991b). Sundsvall statement on supportive environments for health. In *Adopted at the 3ʳᵈ International Conference on Health Promotion, 09-15 June 1991*. WHO.

World Health Organization (WHO). (1991c). *Budapest declaration for health promoting hospitals*. WHO Regional Office for Europe.

World Health Organization (WHO). (1995a). *Yanuca Island Declaration*. WHO Regional Office for the Western Pacific.

World Health Organization (WHO). (1995b). *New Horizons in Health*. WHO Regional Office for the Western Pacific.

World Health Organization (WHO). (1997a). *City planning for health and sustainable development*. (European Sustainable Development and Health Series: 2). WHO Regional Office for Europe.

World Health Organization (WHO). (1997b). *The Rarotonga Agreement: Towards Healthy Islands*. WHO Regional Office for the Western Pacific.

World Health Organization (WHO). (1997c). *Vienna recommendations for health promoting hospitals*. WHO Regional Office for Europe.

World Health Organization (WHO). (1997d). *WHO's global healthy work approach*. WHO.

World Health Organization (WHO). (1997e). *Jakarta Declaration on Leading Health Promotion into the 21ˢᵗ Century*. Adopted at the 4th International Conference on Health Promotion, 21-25 July. WHO.

World Health Organization (WHO). (1998a). *Strategic Plan: Urban Health/Healthy Cities Programme (1998-2002): Phase III of the WHO Healthy Cities Project*. WHO Regional Office for Europe.

World Health Organization (WHO). (1998b). *Health 21. The health for all policy for the WHO European Region – 21 targets for the 21st century*. WHO Regional Office for Europe.

World Health Organization (WHO). (1999a). *Regional guidelines for the development of healthy workplaces*. WHO Regional Office for the Western Pacific.

World Health Organization (WHO). (1999b). *Consensus statement on mental health promotion in prisons*. WHO Regional Office for Europe.

World Health Organization (WHO). (2002a). *Healthy Cities initiative: Approaches and experience in the African Region*. WHO Regional Office for Africa.

World Health Organization (WHO). (2002b). *Community participation in local health and sustainable development – Approaches and techniques*. WHO Regional Office for Europe.

World Health Organization (WHO). (2003). *Healthy Cities around the world: An overview of the Healthy Cities movement in the Six WHO Regions*. WHO Regional Office for Europe.

World Health Organization (WHO). (2004). *Healthy marketplaces in the Western Pacific: Guiding future action. Applying a settings approach to the promotion of health in marketplaces*. WHO Regional Office for the Western Pacific.

World Health Organization (WHO). (2005). *Bangkok Charter for Health Promotion in a Globalized World*. World Health Organization.

World Health Organization (WHO). (2011). *Healthy Urbanization: Regional Framework for Scaling Up and Expanding Healthy Cities in the Western Pacific 2011-2015*. WHO Regional Office for the Western Pacific.

World Health Organization (WHO). (2016a). *Regional framework for urban health in the Western Pacific 2016-2020: Healthy and Resilient cities*. WHO Regional Office for the Western Pacific.

World Health Organization (WHO). (2016b). *Shanghai Declaration on Promoting Health in the 2030 Agenda for Sustainable Development*. World Health Organization.

Young, I. (2005). Health promotion in schools – A historical perspective. *Promotion & Education, XII*(3–4), 112–117.

Young, I., & Williams, T. (Eds.). (1989). *The Healthy School*. Scottish Health Education Group.

Ziglio, E., Hagard, S., & Griffiths, J. (2000). Health promotion development in Europe: Achievements and challenges. *Health Promotion International, 15*(20), 143–153.

Chapter 2
Theoretical Grounds and Practical Principles of the Settings-Based Approach

Mark Dooris, Sami Kokko, and Michelle Baybutt

2.1 Introduction

Settings-based health promotion is one of the fundamental approaches in contemporary health promotion (see also Chap. 1). Yet, it has been commonly argued that shared understanding of the basis of the approach and mutual fundamentals—both theoretical and practical—are lacking (Dooris, 2006a; Golden & Earp, 2012; Kok et al., 2008; Kokko et al., 2014; Richard et al., 2011).

The WHO Glossary (1998) defined a 'setting for health' as the social context in which people interact to affect wellbeing and create or solve problems relating to health—it's also clear that most settings are in reality oriented to goals other than health and have pre-existing structures, policies, characteristics and institutional values. It follows that the settings approach involves:

- A focus on structure and agency (and place and people)
- An understanding of a setting not only as a medium for reaching 'captive audiences' but also as a context that directly and indirectly impacts wellbeing
- A commitment to integrating health within the culture, structures and routine life of settings

M. Dooris (✉)
Institute of Citizenship, Society and Change/Healthy and Sustainable Settings Unit, University of Central Lancashire, Preston, Lancashire, UK
e-mail: mtdooris@uclan.ac.uk

S. Kokko
Research Center for Health Promotion, Faculty of Sport and Health Sciences, University of Jyväskylä, Länsi-Suomi, Finland
e-mail: sami.p.kokko@jyu.fi

M. Baybutt
Healthy and Sustainable Settings Unit, School of Community Health and Midwifery, University of Central Lancashire, Preston, Lancashire, UK
e-mail: mbaybutt@uclan.ac.uk

© Springer Nature Switzerland AG 2022
S. Kokko, M. Baybutt (eds.), *Handbook of Settings-Based Health Promotion*,
https://doi.org/10.1007/978-3-030-95856-5_2

The first settings-based initiatives (e.g. cities, schools, hospitals) emerged in the 1980s and were expanded internationally in the 1990s. Subsequent programmes built on this and by the 2000s there was a diversity of settings initiatives globally. While some have worked with comprehensive aims and dynamic means, others have adopted more limited aims and static means, which are fundamentally different. Following the argumentation of Wenzel (1997), the latter can be viewed as 'health promotion in a setting' and the former as 'settings-based health promotion'.

So why use the approach? While the provision of 'health' services is vitally important, our health is largely determined by social, economic, environmental, organizational and cultural circumstances—which directly impact well-being and also have indirect influences through providing more or less supportive contexts within which people make lifestyle choices. It follows that effective health promotion and improvement requires investment in the places and contexts in which people live their lives.

While recognizing that settings vary both within and between different categories, this chapter presents the underlying approaches and theoretical grounds that form the foundations for the settings-based health promotion approach and aims to synthesize conceptualization that can be used to guide effective policy and practice.

2.2   The Emergence of Praxis-Based Theory

The 1990s saw the gradual emergence of theory related to healthy settings. However, as highlighted by Dooris et al. (1998, p. 21), 'attempts to develop settings-related ideas into a defined and conceptually coherent approach have accompanied and grown out of, rather than preceded or necessarily informed, early practice, creating praxis-based theory'. Thus, many of the theorists cited below developed their thinking through active engagement in or with settings-based initiatives.

Building on an article 'Good Planets Are Hard to Find' (Kickbusch, 1989) and a workshop held in Australia in 1990, Chu and Simpson (1994) went beyond the behaviourist-influenced ecological perspective (McLeroy et al., 1988) that had begun to influence health promotion to develop the notion of 'ecological public health'—and suggested that the healthy settings approach represented a key means of building this. They profiled work across a range of settings and—drawing on ecological theory—presented one of the earliest arguments for a 'joined-up' approach, offering a vision of interconnected settings throughout the life course.

Barić (1993, 1994) engaged extensively with the settings approach. Influenced by organization and management theory and drawing particularly on the early experience of Health-Promoting Hospitals, he emphasized the functional relationship between environmental and personal factors within settings, which he suggested should be viewed as systems—each part of a wider interdependent system. Within this, he distinguished between the 'health-promoting health care system' (including health authorities, hospitals and primary care services) and the 'health-promoting community approach' (including cities, schools, workplaces, etc.). Arguing that the shift from a 'problem-based' to a 'settings-based' approach required a shift of emphasis from a medical to an organizational model (Barić, 1994), Barić articulated his understanding of the healthcare setting as a system with an input (clients), a production process (care and treatment) and an output (health gain of clients). His conceptual framework comprising three core elements has provided the basis for many subsequent developments in relation to healthy settings:

• Creating a healthy working and living environment
• Integrating health promotion into the daily activities of the setting
• Reaching out into the community in the form of healthy alliances

Around the same time, Grossman and Scala (1993) wrote *Health Promotion and Organizational Development*, published by the WHO Regional Office for Europe. Subtitled 'Developing Settings for Health', this document drew on the work of systems theorists such as Luhmann and argued the case for the settings approach in terms of intervening in social systems to bring about organizational change. Emphasis was placed on the competencies required for this new health promotion approach, with project management being proposed as the key instrument for introducing and facilitating change.

During the mid- to late-1990s, Kickbusch (1995, 1996, 1997)—one of the key architects of the healthy settings approach (initially at the WHO Regional Office for Europe and subsequently at its Geneva headquarters)—reflected critically on the settings approach. Significantly, she argued that the approach was guided by three premises (Kickbusch, 1997):

The first was *theoretical*, asking the question 'what creates health?'. Influenced by the work of Antonovsky (1985, 1987) in relation to salutogenesis and sense of coherence, this reinforced the importance of creating and sustaining contexts and environments that are supportive to health and highlighted the need to strengthen both sense of place and sense of self.

The second was *public health based*, asking the question 'which investment creates the largest health gain?'. Drawing on the work of Syme (1996), Woodward and Kawachi (2000), and others, this suggested that systems interventions are more efficient than individually oriented prevention programmes, highlighting the importance of investing in the settings of everyday life.

The third was *practical*, asking the question 'how do you foster the health potential within these organizational and geographical settings?'. Influenced by the WHO's existing commitment to community participation and drawing additionally on management and organizational theory, this emphasized the importance of community development and organization development as dual methodologies—and highlighted developments such as systems thinking and the learning organization (Senge, 1990).

Kickbusch's thinking was also significant in that it signalled the need to forge connections between settings and to consider how the approach could be extended to ensure that it promotes equity in health through working in non-traditional, non-institutional settings—a focus also explored by Galbally (1997).

Wenzel (1997) responded to this European-based body of work—and in particular to that of Barić—by questioning its theoretical integrity. He suggested that despite the distinction drawn between 'health promotion in a setting' and 'becoming a health-promoting setting', it presented an understanding of the settings approach that perpetuated the mechanistic view of health promotion as primarily concerned with individual behaviour change:

> The term *setting* is not introduced as a fundamental or strategic characteristic of health promotion but rather as a tactical label representing the direction of measures to be taken by health professionals to improve the health status of selected population groups... Behind this conceptualisation of *setting* lies nothing of different substance than we already know from traditional health education.

Emphasizing the connections between people and their environment and suggesting that settings can be understood in terms of the relationship between context and patterns of action, Wenzel defined settings as 'spatial, temporal and cultural domains of face-to-face interaction in everyday life' that—from the perspective of health promotion—are crucial for the development of lifestyles and living conditions conducive to health. This thinking is echoed in the definition of 'Settings for Health' that later appeared in the WHO Health Promotion Glossary (WHO, 1998, p. 19):

> The place or social context in which people engage in daily activities in which environmental, organisational and personal factors interact to affect health and wellbeing. A setting is also where people actively use and shape the environment and thus create or solve problems relating to health. Settings can normally be identified as having physical boundaries, a range of people with defined roles, and an organisational structure.

While he has been criticized for what was seen as his provocative and unduly harsh stance (Mittelmark, 1997), Wenzel was pioneering in his exploration and articulation of the concept of settings. Significantly, he drew extensively on Bronfenbrenner (1979, 1994), whose work in the field of ecological psychology contends that human development occurs in 'nested' settings within a number of interconnected layers (see Box 2.1 and Fig. 2.1). In doing so, he intimated the importance of moving beyond a simplistic conceptualization of settings as discrete and homogeneous. Instead, he emphasized their interconnectedness and their specificity in terms of socially and culturally defined patterns of interaction and meaning—and highlighted the existence of power relations within and between different settings.

Box 2.1 Bronfenbrenner's Theory of Human Development: Nested Settings

The *microsystem* refers to patterns of activities and relationships within the settings in which a person spends time and develops, such as home, school and locality.

The *mesosystem* is a system of microsystems, comprising linkages and processes between two or more settings. This highlights that a child's

(continued)

Box 2.1   (continued)

development will be influenced not only by individual systems, but also by the interactions between home, school and locality.

The *exosystem* refers to the connections between settings, at least one of which does not contain the developing person but indirectly influences settings in which a person spends time. For example, a child's well-being will be affected by the characteristics of a parent's workplace.

The *macrosystem* refers to the beliefs, laws, norms and values that define the structure and functions of micro-, meso- and exosystems in relation to particular cultures or subcultures.

The *chronosystem* encompasses change or consistency over time, both in the characteristics of the person and in the environment in which that person lives. For example, parental divorce or changes to a locality will influence a child's life and development—and a child's development will in turn affect how it shapes its environment.

(Source: Bronfenbrenner (1994))

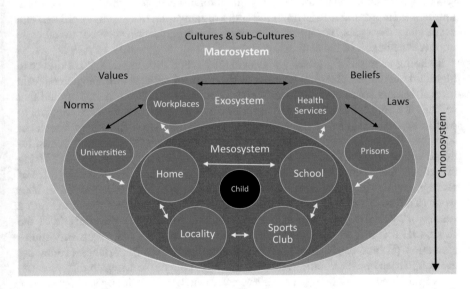

Fig. 2.1 An illustration of settings conceptualized using Bronfenbrenner's theory of human development (Eisenmann et al., 2008) (Adapted from Eisenmann et al. (2008). SWITCH: rationale, design, and implementation of a community, school, and family-based intervention to modify behaviors related to childhood obesity. *BMC Public Health*. 8, 223, Fig. 2.1. Some modifications were made. https://doi.org/10.1186/1471-2458-8-223, licensed under the terms of the Creative Commons Attribution License (http://creativecommons.org/licenses/by/2.0))

Towards the end of the decade, Dooris et al. (1998) attempted to synthesize the ideas of the above theorists to articulate the main characteristics of the settings-based approach—suggesting that the approach is underpinned by principles and perspectives drawn from Health for All, the Ottawa Charter for Health Promotion and Agenda 21; characterized by the use of particular processes and techniques, drawn from organizational, management and systems theory; *and*—drawing on the work of Barić (1994) characterized by creating a healthy working and living environment, integrating health promotion into the daily activities of the setting, and reaching out into the community.

2.3   The Further Conceptualization and Theorization of Healthy Settings and Implications for Policy and Practice

The new millennium also saw advances in the conceptualization of the settings-based approach, which have had implications for policy and practice.

Reflecting on the development and expansion of the settings approach, Kickbusch (2003, p. 386) commented that 'the key intention has been to gain a "political" commitment to improving the health of the entire organization (a systems approach) and developing strategies that allow all parts of the organization to work together to improve the health of the setting'.

Echoing concerns expressed by Wenzel (1997) and drawing on critical theory to highlight the danger of taking an instrumental view of settings as homogeneous and neutral vessels containing target audiences, Green et al. (2000, p. 23) argued that settings are both 'physically bounded space-times in which people come together to perform specific tasks (usually oriented to tasks other than health)' and 'arenas of sustained interaction with pre-existing structures, policies, characteristics, institutional values, and both formal and informal social sanctions on behaviours'. Using this conceptualization, they emphasized variation within and between categories of settings and the importance of context. This theme was further developed in later work (Kontos & Poland, 2009; Poland et al., 2008), with ideas formulated into a framework providing a series of nested questions to facilitate the analysis of the contextual features of particular settings and guide operationalization and implementation (Poland et al., 2009). They also highlighted the importance of viewing the boundaries between settings as permeable (people move between different settings in their everyday lives); the need to acknowledge pre-existing social relations and power structures; and the reciprocal determinism between environment and behaviour, and structure and agency.

Dooris (2004) wrestled further with many of these issues—reflecting on restrictions suggested by the WHO Glossary definition (WHO, 1998) with its seeming focus on organizational rather than area-based and informal settings; highlighting the need for a more sophisticated understanding of settings that acknowledges variation in type and scale; emphasizing the interconnectedness of settings and the need to find ways to coordinate and join up programmes and networks; and proposing a model for articulating and operationalizing healthy settings as a 'whole system' approach that involves holding a number of considerations in tension. Subsequently refined (Dooris et al., 2017), this model highlights the importance of anticipating and responding to both public health and core business drivers; combining long-term organization and/or community development with innovative high-visibility projects; securing top-down leadership while enabling bottom-up engagement and empowerment; and balancing a 'pathogenic' focus on addressing needs and problems with a 'salutogenic' focus on harnessing strengths, assets and potentials to support well-being and flourishing.

Further developing and critically discussing these themes in subsequent research and writing, he synthesized earlier thinking to propose a conceptual framework for healthy settings, built around three key characteristics: an ecological model of health promotion, a systems perspective and a primary focus on whole system development and change (Dooris, 2006a; Dooris et al., 2007; see also end of this chapter for further expansion). Several further models have engaged in more detail with the application of systems theory, organization development and change management within healthy settings practice as a means facilitating the healthy settings approach (Johnson & Paton, 2007; Paton et al., 2005).

Additionally, Dooris (2006b, 2009, 2013) has argued that to be conceptually coherent and practically relevant in the twenty-first century, the settings-based approach must:

- Connect 'within'—mapping and understanding the interrelationships, interactions and synergies with regard to different groups of the population, components of the system and 'health' issues
- Connect 'outwards'—forging links from discrete settings to wider systems (e.g. focusing on the education, healthcare and criminal justice systems rather than just on schools, hospitals and prisons), and between settings programmes and networks to encourage joined-up and integrated approaches within the context of 'place' and place-making
- Connect 'upwards'—ensuring that settings-based work is determinants-focused, combining a local focus with advocacy and action for upstream change
- Connect 'beyond health'—avoiding siloed programmes and instead linking agendas such as health, sustainability and social justice to maximize synergistic change

Prompted by the emergence of Healthy Islands, Galea et al. (2000) also emphasized the need to move beyond the overly simplistic conceptualization of settings as homogeneous and discrete. Highlighting the hierarchical relationship of different settings, they went on to propose a distinction between 'elemental' and 'contextual' settings:

A frame of reference for analysing settings must recognize that they exist in a hierarchy of different levels, with settings, e.g. cities containing others, e.g. schools. In such a frame of reference, it is useful to consider an elemental setting as one which is indivisible for the pur-

pose of organizing meaningful health promotion and health protection programmes…Elemental settings are contained within a broader contextual setting. Thus, a city
may contain important elements, e.g. schools, hospitals and markets. (p. 170)

Within this conceptualization, they recognized that one contextual setting (e.g. a
neighbourhood or city) may be contained within another contextual setting (e.g. a
city or island) and described an elemental setting as having three characteristics: It
is small enough for its members to self-identify as belonging to that setting and to
engender a sense of one entity; it has distinguishing social, cultural, economic and
psychological peculiarities; and it has a recognizable formal or informal administrative structure. Dooris (2009, 2013) has gone further in arguing for the interaction of
elemental and contextual settings to be considered at a range of different levels,
from local through to global. Kokko et al. (2014) reflected on this body of work to
consider relationships and connectivity, focusing on the micro-, meso- and macro-
level interactions between different types of setting at local, national, international
and global levels (Fig. 2.2). Alongside this, Bloch et al. (2014) continued the focus
on the need for an ecological joined-up approach, introducing the notion of the
'supersetting'. This emphasizes a participatory approach and the need for

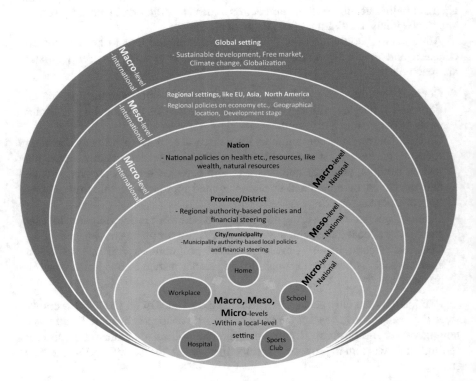

Fig. 2.2 Layers of settings: interaction between settings (Kokko, S., Green, L.W., & Kannas, L. A
review of settings-based health promotion with applications to sports clubs, *Health Promotion
International,* 2014, 29(3), p. 503, by permission of Oxford University Press)

coordinated activities to be carried out in a range of different settings within a local community, with the aim of attaining synergistic and sustainable effects.

Looking back, it is evident that how the settings approach is conceptualized and articulated by policy-level organizations is important in influencing delivery and guiding practice, specifically the extent to which settings programmes have been developed and rolled out in a coherent and joined-up way (Dooris, 2013). The distinction between elemental and contextual settings was made explicit in the policy frameworks and settings-based programmes of certain WHO regions. In the Western Pacific, the Regional Framework for Health Promotion (WHO, 2002a) built on an earlier Regional Action Plan on Healthy Settings (WHO, 1999), which had presented Healthy Cities and Healthy Islands as the natural frameworks for coordinating elemental settings–based programmes such as Health-Promoting Schools, Health-Promoting Hospitals, Healthy Workplaces and Healthy Marketplaces. In Southeast Asia, a technical report on healthy settings (WHO, 2000) conceptualized healthy settings as an approach or process informed by community development— and proposed the development of the Healthy District as the key contextual or umbrella setting, which 'coordinates and encourages the development of a range of healthy settings, including households, schools, hospitals, markets, workplaces, cities, towns, villages' (WHO, 2002b, p. 6). However, in Europe, despite an early focus on looking at the settings-based approach as a whole (Kickbusch, 2003) and initiatives such as Health-Promoting Hospitals and Health-Promoting Universities emerging within the auspices of the WHO European Healthy Cities Project, this integrated model did not last. By the end of the decade and into the new millennium, settings-based programmes within Europe were operating as separate initiatives, led by different divisions within the Regional Office.

Building on conceptual developments and informed by historical review, there have also been important developments that have supported practice by enhancing collaboration across settings and sectors. The International Union for Health Promotion and Education (IUHPE) (2007, p. 4) has been at the forefront of these developments, arguing that 'the reach of settings-based health promotion should be greatly expanded'. It also established a Global Working Group on Healthy Settings, bringing together experts from different settings and different regions of the world. Linked to this has been the establishment of internet portals, with the aim of facilitating information and communication in support of healthy settings.[1,2] The twenty-first century has seen an increased focus on Health in All Policies (WHO, 2013). While there has been little explicit discussion concerning the place of settings in relation to this work, it is clear that the setting-based approach offers the potential to make a tangible contribution through embedding a commitment to health within and across multiple sectors—thinking that was intimated in the Nairobi Call to

---

[1] https://www.who.int/healthpromotion/healthy-settings/en/ (accessed 16 May 2021).

[2] https://www.iuhpe.org/index.php/en/global-working-groups-gwgs/ig-on-healthy-settings (accessed 16 May 2021).

Action (WHO, 2009), which called for leadership by governments for health in all sectors and settings.

Another strand of work has explored the relationship between the settings-based approach and other health promotion perspectives such as topic-based and life-course approaches. For example, Lazenbatt et al. (2009) have proposed a settings approach to domestic violence; Hodgins (2008) has considered how the settings-based approach can be used in relation to bullying in schools and workplaces; Doherty et al. (2011) have applied the settings approach to healthy and sustainable food in universities; and Whitehead (2011) has suggested that it is valuable to map settings against stages of the life span. Reflecting more broadly, Dooris (2009, 2013) has argued that effective action to address complex twenty-first-century public health challenges such as obesity require holistic systems-based responses.

Kokko et al. (2014) found that different settings initiatives have several commonalities, for example: foundation in the Ottawa Charter's five action areas, complexity of the settings emphasizing a need for multilevel actions, focus on organizational change, and the importance of connecting settings-based health promotion to the core business of the setting in question. Differences were found in the year of establishment, target groups, implementation particulars, main activities, range of the settings work, and the quality of evidence. In addition, they noted that different settings reach different populations, which then define and limit the range of potential activities, processes and effects, but also enable population-tailored implementation. As there are differences both within and between settings, it is important to identify the particularities of a given setting—for example, whether a setting is a formal institution within society, like a school or city/municipality, or informally constituted as part of civic society, like many leisure-related and other voluntary associations; and whether there is a formalized programme for health promotion, such as Health Promoting Schools or Healthy Cities, to support development and implementation.

Dooris et al. (2014) drew on a literature review conducted in the field of Healthy Universities to address questions of theorization—their starting point being that while subject to conceptual development, the settings-based approach has lacked a clear and coherent theoretical framework to steer policy, practice and research. Seven theoretical perspectives/conceptual frameworks were identified: the Ottawa Charter, a socioecological approach implicitly drawing on sociological theories concerning structure and agency, salutogenesis, systems thinking, whole system change, organizational development, and the framework previously proposed by Dooris (2006a, 2013). These were used to address interrelated questions on the nature of a setting, how health is created in a setting, why the settings approach is a useful means of promoting health, and how health promotion can be introduced into and embedded within a setting. They concluded by suggesting that further theorization and engagement with theory-driven questions have key roles to play in avoiding the settings-based approach being delivered in a simplistic and instrumental way (i.e. as the implementation of behaviour change interventions within particular contexts); and by drawing attention to other potentially fruitful theoretical perspectives such as complexity, critical realism and public value.

In considering the characteristics of an equity-oriented settings approach, Shareck et al. (2013) also suggest that complexity and critical realism offer promising directions for future theory-driven practice. Having identified four key challenges—a focus on social determinants of health, addressing the needs of marginalized groups, effecting change in a setting's structure, and involving stakeholders—they proposed a conceptual framework that integrates theoretical and methodological approaches with core guiding principles, into a 'settings praxis'.

2.4 Developing Typologies to Classify Settings-Based Practice

Closely linked to advances in the conceptualization, a number of writers have produced typologies of settings-based practice.

Recognizing that despite an emerging theory-based literature, there continued to be significant variation within the field of healthy settings, Whitelaw et al. (2001) identified a range of problems involved in the development and application of settings-based models. These included the 'homogenization' of practice, where divergent activities are unhelpfully brought under a single settings banner; the consequent sense of failure when practice does not live up to the theoretical ideal; and the use of the settings 'label' for traditional health promotion concerned only with individual behaviour change. They responded to these concerns by formulating a typology that distinguishes different forms of settings-based practice. Acknowledging that there are not only different models of health promotion and different analyses of the 'problem' and 'solution' (in terms of individual and organizational focus), but also different organizational contexts with different degrees of opportunity and constraint, they identified five types of practice:

- The *passive model*, where the problem and solution are understood to depend on the individual.
- The *active model*, where the problem is understood to rest with the individual, and the solution is understood to depend on action at the level of both the individual and the setting (i.e. the setting can help shape individual behaviour).
- The *vehicle model*, where the problem is seen to lie primarily within the system, and the solution is understood to be dependent on learning from individually-focused topic-based projects.
- The *organic model*, where the problem is understood to lie within the setting, and the solution is seen to comprise the actions of a collection of individual actions.
- The *comprehensive model*, where the setting is viewed as an entity beyond the individuals within it, and both the problem and the solution are seen to lie within the system.

While, on the one hand, they present what is essentially a representational typology of different models of settings activity and caution against a one-size-fits-all approach, they also go beyond description to argue that 'those who deploy a settings model need to ensure that their work is more than simply a repackaging of traditional individualistic health education in a particular setting' (Whitelaw et al., 2001, p. 348).

This view was reinforced by Johnson and Baum (2001) in relation to work on Health-Promoting Hospitals. Drawing on a review of literature and practice, they proposed a typology based on degree of organizational commitment and types of health promotion activities undertaken—identifying four distinct approaches:

- Doing a health promotion project
- Delegating health promotion to the role of a specific division, department or staff
- Being a health promotion setting
- Being a health promotion setting and improving the health of the community

Suggesting that the latter two forms of practice represent a more comprehensive understanding and application of the healthy settings approach, they concluded by arguing that there is:

> a danger that the rhetoric of reform can be used (in this case labelling an initiative as a healthy setting project whether it be a healthy city, school, workplace or hospital), while in practice the initiative is doing little that is new and certainly not achieving the structural and organizational changes that are foreshadowed by the Ottawa Charter… (Johnson & Baum, 2001, p. 286).

2.5   A Conceptual Framework for Settings-Based Health Promotion

It has been commonly argued that a shared understanding of the theoretical grounds and fundamentals of the settings-based approach, as well as universal framework, are lacking. Many settings initiatives have worked simultaneously, but independently, even though joined-up approaches have long been advocated (Dooris, 2004). While it is important to appreciate the diversity that exists within and between different types of settings (e.g. in relation to scale, structure, formality, focus and context) and acknowledge that, in planning and implementing programmes, 'one size does not fit all', it is also valuable to be able to draw on and apply an overarching conceptualization. Having introduced the theoretical foundations of the settings-based approach as they have emerged over time, we now present the conceptual framework for healthy settings created by Dooris (2006a) and subsequently refined and expanded (Dooris, 2012, 2013).

This argues that to be coherent and effective, the settings-based approach should be underpinned by core values such as equity, partnership, participation, empowerment and sustainability—and comprise five overarching characteristics (Fig. 2.3).

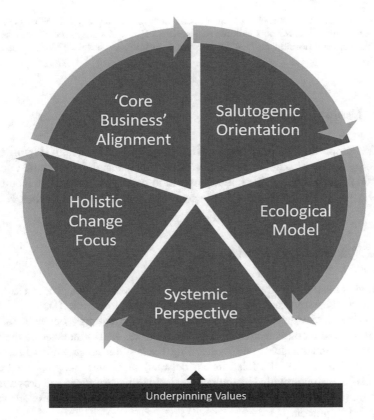

Fig. 2.3 Conceptual framework Settings-based approach conceptual framework for healthy settings

2.5.1 Salutogenic Orientation

First, it represents a shift of focus towards a salutogenic view. Salutogenesis—which taken from the Latin and Greek literally means 'the creation of health'—is concerned with harnessing and releasing the resources for people to be able to flourish. It is thus concerned not only with illness, but with well-being and what makes people thrive—and as Kickbusch (1996, p. 5) argues, this involves fostering health potentials inherent in the social and institutional settings of everyday life:

> The Ottawa Charter starts out from health creation: "where people live, love, work and play" and identifies five action areas which play a significant role in generating health...As a result the "settings approach" became the starting point for WHO's lead health promotion programmes. This meant shifting the focus from the deficit model of disease to the health

potentials inherent in the social and institutional settings of everyday life: What makes a school a healthy place for both children and teachers? How can a hospital create health for both patients and hospital staff? What is a health promotive workplace? What creates a healthy city?

2.5.2 Ecological Model

Second, it adopts an ecological model, which appreciates that health is multilayered and determined by a complex interaction of personal, social, behavioural and environmental factors; focuses on populations within particular contexts; and addresses human health within the framework of ecosystem health (Lang & Rayner, 2012).

2.5.3 Systemic Perspective

Third, it views settings as dynamic complex systems with inputs, processes, outputs and impacts characterized by unpredictability and feedback (Dooris, 2006a); acknowledges and values the interconnectedness and synergy between different components; and recognizes that settings are 'nested', each connected to the world around it. By understanding and harnessing the multidimensional nature of settings—and, within this, the relationship between place and people, between the structural dimension provided by their contexts, facilities, services and programmes, and the human agency within them—it is possible to take a comprehensive and whole system approach.

2.5.4 Holistic Change Focus

Fourth, drawing on learning from organization and community development, it focuses on comprehensive holistic change using whole system thinking and multiple, interconnected interventions to embed health and shift cultures within diverse settings.

2.5.5 'Core Business' Alignment

Fifth, it appreciates that most settings do not have health as their main mission or raîson d'être, and that it is therefore essential to 'translate' arguments into language that resonates with decision-makers, advocating for health, well-being and sustainability in terms of impact on or outflow from the core business of a particular setting.

2.6 From Theoretical Foundations to Principles for Practice: Operationalizing Planning and Implementation

While it is important to engage with and draw on theoretical underpinnings and on the conceptual model presented above, it is also necessary to find ways to translate this into policy and practice. Alongside the context-focused analytic framework for guiding design and implementation referred to above (Poland et al., 2009), it is useful to put in place clear planning, operations and management mechanisms to ensure effective 'on-the ground' delivery.

One way of conceptualizing these is via a cyclical model, proposed by Doherty and Dooris (2006), as shown in Fig. 2.4. This depicts the stages that a programme may go through—including:

- Identifying key entry points and 'windows of opportunity' that exist in a particular context at a particular time
- Securing senior-level commitment, identifying key stakeholders and establishing a steering group to ensure appropriate governance
- Identifying funding and other resources and appointing a coordinator to ensure a whole system joined-up approach, and agreeing on the appropriate grade and location within an organization
- Undertaking stakeholder mapping, needs assessment and audit of what is already in place; agreeing priorities and establishing working groups with appropriate membership and clear accountability to the steering group
- Formulating an action plan that fits with and can link into wider core business strategic and operational planning

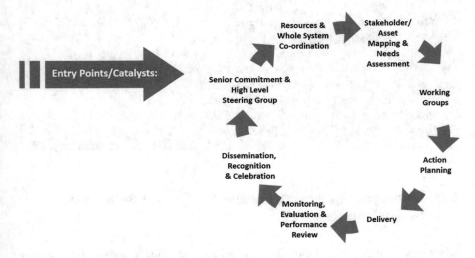

Fig. 2.4 An operational process to guide planning and delivery (adapted from Doherty & Dooris, 2006)

- Ensuring the action plan translates into coherent delivery, with clear allocation of roles and responsibilities
- Putting in place a thought-through monitoring, evaluation and performance review process
- Disseminating achievements and taking time to recognize and celebrate these

Drawing on both this cyclical process model and wider theoretical perspectives considered in this chapter, the following checklist may be helpful in distilling key considerations and guiding practice (Box 2.2).

Box 2.2 A Checklist for Applying the Settings Approach to Practice

- **What kind of setting is it and what are the key contextual factors?** Take stock of the setting you are working with, in terms of focus, size, 'formal' or 'informal' structure and wider environment. Consider what this means for planning and delivering an ecological whole system approach.
- **What is the core business of the setting?** Clarify the setting's key concerns and performance measures. Consider how to connect between this core business and the setting's investment in health promotion – is evidence available? Tailor and translate your health promotion language into language appropriate to the given setting.
- **What is the appetite for settings-based health promotion?** Investigate the motivation and willingness of the setting to start settings-based health promotion work. What are your possible entry points and 'hooks' to get started?
- **How is the settings approach understood and where is the setting 'at'?** Having assessed the situation, start where the setting is and work from there. Tailor programmes and activities to the setting, while applying the foundational principles and concepts of settings-based health promotion.
- **What is the vision?** Hold on to the whole system perspective offered by settings-based health promotion. Develop a plan of action that includes funding, staffing, resources, governance, partnerships, implementation and evaluation (how will you measure success?).
- **What are your achievements?** Celebrate! Build into the action plan activities that acknowledge positive change and the achievement of milestones, recognizing and valuing the people involved.

2.7 Identifying Emerging Themes for Critical Reflection, Debate and Research

As already indicated, the twenty-first century has been characterized by the identification of emerging themes for critical reflection, debate and research. These include the following:

Developing coherent frameworks for healthy settings that recognize interrelationships, strengthen linkages and enhance synergy: As discussed above, developments in the conceptualization of healthy settings have highlighted the practical importance of acknowledging and understanding the interrelationships between different types and scales of settings. Poland et al. (2000) and Dooris (2004, 2006b) have presented a rationale for greater coordination and connectedness based on the fact that people live their lives across a range of settings, that there can be synergistic effects between settings, and that a problem manifest in one setting may have its roots in another. Going one step further, Galea et al. (2000) have proposed the hierarchical categorization of contextual and elemental settings, a consideration that has been further developed by Dooris (2009, 2013), Kokko et al. (2014) and Bloch et al. (2014), and facilitated by the work of IUHPE.

Ensuring that the healthy settings approach tackles inequalities in health and promotes social inclusion: Concern that the healthy settings approach could serve to exacerbate health inequalities and social exclusion was highlighted in the 1990s by Kickbusch (1995, 1997) and Galbally (1997). The challenge has been further discussed during the past two decades, with calls for the approach to be extended to informal and less well-defined settings, to acknowledge and take account of power relations within and between settings, and to work upwards and outwards, influencing organizational policies that really matter and advocating for macrolevel political, economic and social change (Dooris, 2004; Dooris, 2009; Dooris et al., 2007; Dooris & Hunter, 2007; Green et al., 2000). Significantly, the WHO's Commission on Social Determinants of Health (2008) affirmed the effectiveness of the healthy settings approach, but argued for more attention to be given to evaluating its health equity impacts. More recently, Shareck et al. (2013) have argued for an equity-oriented settings approach and Newman et al. (2015) have called for health promotion to shift the focus of settings-based work further upstream and to evaluate programmes for differential equity impacts.

Locating healthy settings in a globalized world: The relationship between healthy settings practice and macro policy has become increasingly important in the context of twenty-first century globalization. Ziglio et al. (2000, p. 149) have convincingly argued the case for the Investment for Health and Development approach, with its shift of focus to strategies 'which maintain and create health equitably and are integral to sustainable social, economic and human development policies'. Highlighting the opportunities and challenges of globalization and the need to make the promotion of health central to the global development agenda, the Bangkok Charter (WHO, 2005) called for all sectors and settings to advocate for health; invest in sustainable policies, action and infrastructure to address the determinants of health; build capacity for health promotion; regulate and legislate for health and well-being; and build partnerships to create sustainable actions. Significantly, Kickbusch has also explored the 'deterritorialization' of health and the implications of globalization for healthy settings (Kickbusch, 2007a, 2007b).

Connecting health, sustainability and social justice agendas: As discussed in Chap. 1, the publication of Agenda 21 strongly influenced the future direction of Healthy Cities. More generally, a number of WHO regions (e.g. Southeast Asia, Americas) have led their healthy settings programmes within the context of their sustainable development work. Growing concern about the health consequences of climate change have further highlighted the imperative of connecting public health and sustainable development within the context of particular settings such as cities, schools and universities (Bentley, 2007; Davis & Cooke, 2007; Orme & Dooris, 2010; Rice & Hancock, 2016). More broadly, there have been strong calls for the settings-based approach to connect agendas by coordinating and integrating action for health, sustainability and social justice, thereby achieving co-benefits across policy domains (Poland & Dooris, 2010; Poland et al., 2011; Dooris, 2012, 2013). At a global level, the Shanghai Declaration on Promoting Health in the 2030 Agenda for Sustainable Development (WHO, 2016) was highly significant in affirming the centrality of health within the Sustainable Development Goals (United Nations, 2015) and in positioning health promotion as a crucial mechanism going forward.

Evaluating healthy settings initiatives and building evidence of effectiveness: Kickbusch (2003, p. 386) reflected that the success of the healthy settings approach does 'not fit easily into an epidemiological framework of "evidence" but needs to be analysed in terms of social and political processes'. In addition to the general difficulties faced by public health and health promotion in responding to the demand for evidence, it has been argued that a number of specific challenges make it difficult to undertake robust evaluation and to build a convincing evidence base for the settings approach. These concern the funding and construction of the evidence base for public health and health promotion; the diversity characterizing both conceptualization and practice; and the complexity of evaluating ecological whole system approaches (Dooris, 2006a; Dooris & Hunter, 2007). Dooris et al. (2007) have explored these challenges and discussed the potential value of critical realism and complexity theory for overcoming the limitations of traditional evaluation models and helping generate evidence of effectiveness (see Chap. 4).

2.8   Summary

This chapter has introduced the theoretical basis and fundamentals of the settings-based approach, complementing Chap. 1, by tracing the evolution of thinking over time. While there have been multiple attempts to establish models, typologies and frameworks for the settings-based approach, a recurring theme has been the absence of a shared understanding of the theoretical foundations of the approach. This chapter has summarized key advances and presented an expanded conceptual framework that can be used to guide future policy and practice.

References

Antonovsky, A. (1985). *Health, stress and coping.* Jossey Bass.

Antonovsky, A. (1987). *Unraveling the mystery of health: How people manage stress and stay well.* Jossey Bass.

Barić, L. (1993). The settings approach – Implications for policy and strategy. *Journal of the Institute of Health Education, 31*(1), 17–24.

Barić, L. (1994). *Health promotion and health education in practice. Module 2: The organisational model.* Barns Publications.

Bentley, M. (2007). Healthy Cities, local environmental action and climate change. *Health Promotion International, 22*(3), 246–253.

Bloch, P., et al. (2014). Revitalizing the setting approach – supersettings for sustainable impact in community health promotion. *International Journal of Behavioral Nutrition and Physical Activity, 11*, 118.

Bronfenbrenner, U. (1979). *The ecology of human development. Experiments by nature and design.* Harvard University Press.

Bronfenbrenner, U. (1994). Ecological models of human development. In T. Husen & T. Postlethwaite (Eds.), *International Encyclopedia of education* (Vol. 3, 2nd ed., pp. 1643–1647). Pergamon Press/Elsevier Science.

Chu, C., & Simpson, R. (Eds.). (1994). *Ecological public health: From vision to practice.* Institute of Applied Environmental Research, Griffith University/Toronto: Centre for Health Promotion, University of Toronto.

Commission on Social Determinants of Health (CSDH). (2008). *Closing the gap in a generation: Health equity through action on the social determinants of health.* Final Report of the Commission on Social Determinants of Health. World Health Organization.

Davis, J., & Cooke, S. (2007). Educating for a healthy, sustainable world: An argument for integrating health promoting schools and sustainable schools. *Health Promotion International, 22*(4), 346–353.

Doherty, S., Cawood, J., & Dooris, M. (2011). Applying the whole system settings approach to food within universities. *Perspectives in Public Health, 131*(5), 217–224.

Doherty, S., & Dooris, M. (2006). The healthy settings approach: The growing interest within colleges and universities. *Education and Health, 24*(3), 42–43.

Dooris, M. (2004). Joining up settings for health: A valuable investment for strategic partnerships? *Critical Public Health, 14*(1), 49–61.

Dooris, M. (2006a). Healthy settings: Challenges to generating evidence of effectiveness. *Health Promotion International, 21*(1), 55–65.

Dooris, M. (2006b). Editorial – healthy settings: Future directions. *Promotion & Education, XIII*(1), 1–5.

Dooris, M. (2009). Holistic and sustainable health improvement: The contribution of the settings-based approach to health promotion. *Perspectives in Public Health, 129*(1), 29–36.

Dooris, M. (2012). The settings approach: An overview – looking back, looking forward. Chapter. In A. Scriven & M. Hodgins (Eds.), *Health promotion settings: Principles and practice.* Sage.

Dooris, M. (2013). Expert voices for change: Bridging the silos – towards healthy and sustainable settings for the 21st century. *Health & Place, 20*, 39–50.

Dooris, M., Doherty, S., & Orme, J. (2017). The application of salutogenesis in universities. In M. B. Mittelmark, S. Sagy, M. Eriksson, et al. (Eds.), *The handbook of salutogenesis [Internet].* Springer; Chapter 23. Available from: https://link.springer.com/book/10.1007%2F978-3-319-04600-6

Dooris, M., Dowding, G., Thompson, J., & Wynne, C. (1998). The settings-based approach to health promotion. In A. Tsouros, G. Dowding, J. Thompson, & M. Dooris (Eds.), *Health promoting universities: Concept, experience and framework for action.* (pp. 18–28 printed version; pp. 21–32 e-version). WHO Regional Office for Europe.

Dooris, M., & Hunter, D. (2007). Organisations and settings for promoting public health. In C. Lloyd, S. Handsley, J. Douglas, S. Earle, & S. Spurr (Eds.), *Policy and practice in promoting public health* (pp. 95–125). Sage/Milton Keynes: Open University.

Dooris, M., Poland, B., Kolbe, L., de Leeuw, E., McCall, D., & Wharf-Higgins, J. (2007). Healthy settings: Building evidence for the effectiveness of whole system health promotion – Challenges and future directions. In D. McQueen & C. Jones (Eds.), *Global perspectives on health promotion effectiveness* (pp. 327–352). Springer Science and Business Media.

Dooris, M., Wills, J., & Newton, J. (2014). Theorising healthy settings: A critical discussion with reference to Healthy Universities. *Scandinavian Journal of Public Health, 42*(Suppl 15), 7–16.

Eisenmann, J. C., Gentile, D. A., Welk, G. J., et al. (2008). SWITCH: Rationale, design, and implementation of a community, school, and family-based intervention to modify behaviors related to childhood obesity. *BMC Public Health, 8*, 223. https://doi.org/10.1186/1471-2458-8-223

Galbally, R. (1997). Health-promoting environments: Who will miss out? *Australian and New Zealand Journal of Public Health, 21*(4), 429–430.

Galea, G., Powis, B., & Tamplin, S. (2000). Healthy islands in the Western Pacific – International settings development. *Health Promotion International, 15*(2), 169–178.

Golden, S. D., & Earp, J. A. (2012). Social ecological approaches to individuals and their contexts: twenty years of *Health Education & Behavior* health promotion interventions. *Health Education & Behavior, 39*, 364–372.

Green, L. W., Poland, B. D., & Rootman, I. (2000). The settings approach to health promotion. In B. D. Poland, L. W. Green, & I. Rootman (Eds.), *Settings for health promotion: Linking theory and practice* (pp. 1–43). Sage.

Grossman, R., & Scala, K. (1993). *Health promotion and organisational development: Developing settings for health*. WHO Regional Office for Europe.

Hodgins, M. (2008). Taking a health promotion approach to the problem of bullying. *International Journal of Psychology and Psychological Therapy, 8*, 13–23.

International Union for Health Promotion and Education (IUHPE) and Canadian Consortium for Health Promotion Research (CCHPR). (2007). *Shaping the future of heath promotion: Priorities for action*. IUHPE.

Johnson, A., & Baum, F. (2001). Health promoting hospitals: a typology of different organizational approaches to health promotion. *Health Promotion International, 16*(3), 281–287.

Johnson, A., & Paton, K. (2007). *Health promotion and health services: Management for change*. Oxford University Press.

Kickbusch, I. (1989). *Good planets are hard to find* (WHO Healthy Cities Papers No. 5). FADL Publishers.

Kickbusch, I. (1995). An overview to the settings-based approach to health promotion. In T. Theaker & J. Thompson (Eds.), *The settings-based approach to health promotion*. Report of an International Working Conference, 17–20 November 1993 (pp. 3–9). Hertfordshire Health Promotion.

Kickbusch, I. (1996). Tribute to Aaron Antonovsky – 'what creates health'? *Health Promotion International, 11*(1), 5–6.

Kickbusch, I. (1997). Health-promoting environments: The next steps. *Australian and New Zealand Journal of Public Health, 21*(4), 431–434.

Kickbusch, I. (2003). The contribution of the World Health Organization to a new public health and health promotion. *American Journal of Public Health, 93*(3), 383–388.

Kickbusch, I. (2007a). Responding to the health society. *Health Promotion International, 22*(2), 89–91.

Kickbusch, I. (2007b). Health governance: The health society. In D. McQueen, I. Kickbusch, L. Potvin, J. Pelikan, L. Balbo, & T. Abel (Eds.), *Health and modernity: The role of theory in health promotion* (pp. 144–161). Springer Science and Business Media.

Kok, G., Gottlieb, N. H., Commers, M., & Smerecnik, C. (2008). The ecological approach in health promotion programs: A decade later. *American Journal of Health Promotion, 22*, 437–442.

Kokko, S., Green, L., & Kannas, L. (2014). A review of settings-based health promotion with applications to sports clubs. *Health Promotion International, 29*, 494–509. https://doi.org/10.1093/heapro/dat046

Kontos, P., & Poland, B. (2009). Mapping new theoretical and methodological terrain for knowledge translation: Contributions from critical realism and the arts. *Implementation Science, 4*(1), 1–10.

Lang, T., & Rayner, G. (2012). Ecological public health: The 21st century's big idea? *BMJ, 345*, 17–20.

Lazenbatt, A., Taylor, J., & Cree, L. (2009). A healthy settings framework: An evaluation and comparison of midwives' responses to addressing domestic violence. *Midwifery, 25*(6), 622–636.

McLeroy, K. R., Bibeau, D., Steckler, A., & Glanz, K. (1988). An ecological perspective on health promotion programs. *Health Education Quarterly, 15*(4), 351–377.

Mittelmark, M. (1997) Editorial: Health promotion settings. *Internet Journal of Health Promotion* (no longer available).

Newman, L., Baum, F., Javanparast, S., O'Rourke, K., & Carlon, L. (2015). Addressing social determinants of health inequities through settings: A rapid review. *Health Promotion International, 30*(S2), ii126–ii143.

Orme, J., & Dooris, M. (2010). Integrating health and sustainability: The higher education sector as a timely catalyst. *Health Education Research, 25*(3), 425–437. https://doi.org/10.1093/her/cyq020

Paton, K., Sengupta, S., & Hassan, L. (2005). Settings, systems and organisation development: The healthy living and working model. *Health Promotion International, 20*(1), 81–89.

Poland, B. & Dooris, M. (2010) A green and healthy future: The settings approach to building health, equity and sustainability. *Critical Public Health, 20*(3), 281–298.

Poland, B., Dooris, M., & Haluza-Delay, R. (2011). Securing 'supportive environments' for health in the face of ecosystem collapse: Meeting the triple threat with a sociology of creative transformation. *Health Promotion International, 26*(S2), ii202–ii215.

Poland, B., Frohlich, K., & Cargo, M. (2008). Context as a fundamental dimension of health promotion program evaluation. In L. Potvin & D. McQueen (Eds.), *Health promotion evaluation practices in the Americas*. Springer Science and Business Media.

Poland, B., Green, L., & Rootman, I. (2000). *Settings for health promotion: Linking theory and practice*. Sage.

Poland, B., Krupa, G, & McCall, D. (2009). Settings for health promotion: An analytic framework to guide intervention design and implementation. *Health Promotion Practice, 10*(4), 505–516.

Rice, M., & Hancock, T. (2016). Equity, sustainability and governance in urban settings. *Global Health Promotion, 23*(S1), 94–97.

Richard, L., Gauvin, L., & Raine, K. (2011). Ecological models revisited: Their uses and evolution in health promotion over two decades. *Annual Review of Public Health, 32*, 7.1-7.20.

Senge, P. (1990). *The fifth discipline: The art and practice of the learning organization*. Random House.

Shareck, M., Frohlick, K., & Poland, B. (2013). Reducing social inequities in health through settings-related interventions — A conceptual framework. *Global Health Promotion, 20*(2), 39–52.

Syme, S. L. (1996). To prevent disease: The need for a new approach. In D. Blane, E. Brunner, & R. Wilkinson (Eds.), *Health and social organisation: Towards a health policy for the 21st century*. Routledge.

United Nations (UN). (2015). *Transforming our World: The 2030 Agenda for sustainable development*. UN.

Wenzel, E. (1997). A comment on settings in health promotion. *Internet Journal of Health Promotion*. Retrieved April 16, 2021, from http://ldb.org/setting.htm

Whitehead, D. (2011). Before the cradle and beyond the grave: A lifespan/settings-based framework for health promotion. *Journal of Clinical Nursing, 20*(15/126), 2183–2194.

Whitelaw, S., Baxendale, A., Bryce, C., Machardy, L., Young, I., & Witney, E. (2001). Settings based health promotion: A review. *Health Promotion International, 16*(4), 339–353.

Woodward, A., & Kawachi, I. (2000). Why reduce health inequalities? *Journal of Epidemiology & Community Health, 54*(12), 923–929.

World Health Organization (WHO). (1998). *Health promotion glossary*. WHO.

World Health Organization (WHO). (1999). *Regional action plan on healthy settings*. WHO Regional Office for the Western Pacific.

World Health Organization (WHO). (2000). *Healthy settings* (Report and documentation of the technical discussions held in conjunction with the 37th Meeting of CCPDM, New Delhi, 31 August 2000). WHO Regional Office for South-East Asia.

World Health Organization (WHO). (2002a). *Regional framework for health promotion 2002-2005*. WHO Regional Office for the Western Pacific.

World Health Organization (WHO). (2002b). *Integrated management of healthy settings at the district level* (Report of an intercountry consultation. Gurgaon, India, 7-11 May 2001). WHO Regional Office for South-East Asia.

World Health Organization (WHO). (2005). *Bangkok charter for health promotion in a globalized world*. World Health Organization.

World Health Organization (WHO). (2009). *Nairobi call to action for closing the implementation gap in health promotion*. World Health Organization.

World Health Organization (WHO). (2013). *Helsinki statement on health in all policies*. World Health Organization.

World Health Organization (WHO). (2016). *Shanghai declaration on promoting health in the 2030 Agenda for sustainable development*. World Health Organization.

Ziglio, E., Hagard, S., & Griffiths, J. (2000). Health promotion development in Europe: Achievements and challenges. *Health Promotion International, 15*(20), 143–153.

Chapter 3
Governance and Policies for Settings-Based Work

Evelyne de Leeuw and Patrick Harris

3.1 Introduction

There is something odd about the concepts of governance and policies in the 'public health mind'. On the one hand virtually anyone that is professionally or academically engaged with health and human development these days embraces the importance and influence of policies, and how these phenomena would influence better outcomes for individuals, groups, communities, and populations. The World Health Organization's Commission on the Social Determinants of Health is a prominent example. The Commission's final report concluded that the 'unequal distribution of health-damaging experiences is not in any sense a "natural" phenomenon but is the result of a toxic combination of poor social policies and programmes, unfair economic arrangements, and bad politics' (p. 1) (World Health Organization, 2008).

On the other hand, there is very little true engagement with understanding how policy happens, and how public health professionals and academics would in fact *shape* governance as a mechanism for creating policy.

In the context of this book, we are arguing that policy (and more precisely—the policy *process*) is a unique setting—for health development, social discourse, and setting the conditions for societies and ecosystems to thrive in support of (planetary) health. Of course this was recognized in the Ottawa Charter under the banner of 'creating healthy public policies', but since then, and particularly in recent years, the idea of creating healthy public policies has necessitated a more sophisticated engagement with the governance of public policy for health. This ought to include

E. de Leeuw (✉) · P. Harris
Centre for Health Equity Training, Research and Evaluation (CHETRE), Part of the UNSW
Australia Research Centre for Primary Health Care and Equity, A Unit of Population Health,
South Western Sydney Local Health District, NSW Health, A Member of the Ingham
Institute, Liverpool Hospital, University of New South Wales, Sydney, NSW, Australia
e-mail: e.deleeuw@unsw.edu.au; patrick.harris@unsw.edu.au

© Springer Nature Switzerland AG 2022
S. Kokko, M. Baybutt (eds.), *Handbook of Settings-Based Health Promotion*,
https://doi.org/10.1007/978-3-030-95856-5_3

a political science perspective in terms of the policy process and the institutions that are the building blocks of healthy public policy governance.

Particularly the notion of 'policy' is colloquially used to mean many different things. '*It is not our policy to admit blonde people*' might be a bouncer's excuse to close the door on someone. '*Opposition policy calls for better funding of public transport*' could be a headline in a newspaper. From their website, we see how two neighbouring universities in Australia share what they call their 'policies' for health:

University of Sydney	University of New South Wales
We believe a healthy university supports healthy people, builds healthy places, develops healthy policies and implements healthy practices to support our students, staff and the broader community. *We aim to develop projects and initiatives in collaboration with students and staff across all levels of the organisation, informed by our five guiding principles and the University's 2016–2020 Strategic Plan.* (The University of Sydney, 2016)	*The University of New South Wales ("UNSW") will provide a world-class campus environment that promotes health and safety and wellbeing. Our objective is that no person will come to harm while working, studying or visiting UNSW. This commitment to health, safety and wellbeing allows the University to teach, conduct research and promote scholarship at the highest international level through the attraction and retention of high quality staff, students and other partners.* *The following values form the basis of achieving the University's health and safety policy objective:* *• We are committed to ensuring the health, safety and wellbeing of everyone in the workplace.* *• Everyone has a responsibility for safety; their own and that of others.* *• Injuries can be prevented and an incident-free working and learning environment is actively pursued.* *• Communication and consultation are central to working together for a safer workplace.* (UNSW Australia, 2016)

'Policy' can variably mean 'the plan'; 'a rule'; 'principles, values and belief systems of organisations'; 'mission statements'; 'guidance'; 'a coherent discourse how the world works and in it, how A shapes B'; 'the expressed commitment to solve a problem by taking accountable decisions on resources, time lines, and capabilities'; and much more. It is no wonder that even its own discipline, political science, has not reached a conclusive consensus about the meaning of the word 'policy'.

Similarly, 'governance' is a term that has started to resonate with many in the health and social development field, but has an equally fuzzy perceived meaning. If the trend identified by Google Ngram viewer (Fig. 3.1) continues, we will be talking about nothing else but governance in a few years. Essentially, and connected to the timeline in Fig. 3.1 around the shift in Western countries towards neoliberalism, governance can be defined as a shift in policymaking from within government to policymaking by many public and private entities in a multilevel, multisectoral world (Stoker, 1998). This is reflected in a governance view as 'the sum of the many ways individuals and institutions, public and private, manage the connections of their common affairs. It is a continuing process through which conflicting or diverse interests may be accommodated and cooperative action may be taken. It includes

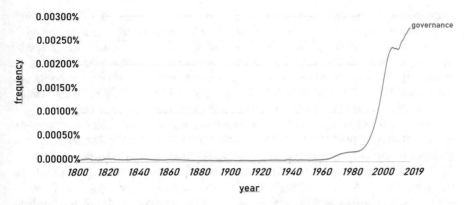

Fig. 3.1 Google Ngram viewer: 'Governance'. The occurrence of the word 'governance' in the corpus of books indexed by Google (generated 11 May 2021) (Source: http://books.google.com/ ngrams, see also Michel et al., 2011)

formal institutions and regimes empowered to enforce compliance, as well as informal arrangements that people and institutions either have agreed to or perceive to be in their interest' (Commission on Global Governance, 1995). This early definition has now morphed into an understanding that governance includes a range of actors and events at many different levels (Jessop, 1998).

Obviously, policy and governance are highly relevant concepts for a settings-based perspective on health and health promotion. We do not intend to produce a 'Readers' Digest' version of the entire political and administrative science literature, but feel compelled to ground this chapter in some core writings and world views from that area of scholarship.

3.2   Politics and Political Science

This 'scholarship' goes by a number of names, depending on the disciplinary flavour and perspective. Fields like sociology and psychology have an interest in policy development and governance. In sociology, the classic Weberian perspective in fact is the cradle of the study of government systems and bureaucracy (Waters & Waters, 2015). Psychologically, people who professionally engage in policy development and political discourse have been described by Lasswell (1931) as suffering from a psychopathology—suggesting that the scholarship of policy and governance is the domain of behaviourist study. The same Lasswell, incidentally, is credited with being the father of the discipline of political science as well as the inventor of political propaganda.

Politics is at the core of the study of policy and governance. Whereas Lasswell, in the 1930s, described politics as '*who gets what, why, where and when*', more recently Adrian Leftwich (2015) said '*Politics comprises all the activities of cooperation, negotiation and conflict, within and between societies, whereby people go about organizing the use, production or distribution of human, natural and other resources in the course of the production and reproduction of their biological and social life'*. Without doubt, politics is about contestation—for scarce resources, or particular world views. Often we see a distinction between *P*olitics and *p*olitics—the capital P version relating to 'official' government, party parliamentarian deliberation, with the lower-case 'p' denoting individual struggle and strategy.

Whether policy is 'a plan' (or something much bigger), and governance 'how we do things around here' (or a more esoteric version), it is clear that arriving at it means a process of engagement, negotiation, and often conflict (Jessop, 1998).

A further definitional point of departure for thinking about settings is to ask the question 'what is a policy setting?' and then to realize that a policy setting is, by its very nature, a form of governance! As we go on to show later in the chapter, reflecting on policy settings through a governance lens, particularly where policy and planning is concerned, has profound implications for the practice of going about 'how we do things around here'. Before getting there, however, it is useful to build the various components of what a policy setting is made up of. For that, we need to think about what policy or political institutions are made up of.

3.3   Institutions

Institutions—not the hardware types like hospitals, but the sociological/political version—lie at the heart of public policy, especially when considering the connection between settings and governance. Focusing on the role of institutions in (for instance) creating policy, shaping cities, and setting social aspirations in a systematic way is called 'institutionalism'. Indeed, some have claimed that up until the 1950s 'institutionalism was political science … the core activity [or which] was description of constitutions, legal systems, and governance structures' (Lowndes, 2009, p. 91). But as the scope of political analysis widened, this deterministic view of policymaking was overtaken by the 'new institutionalism' and, by extension, governance. 'New institutionalism' moves its view beyond classic and inward-looking tools of government, and sees the messiness of society as establishing all sorts of arrangements to make sense of where we go, organize, and set political priorities (Howlett et al., 2009; March & Olsen, 1996). Anyone working in the Health-Promoting Settings will recognize the importance of such a perspective. For instance, very similar schools (in terms of level, curriculum, demographics) can still turn out radically different policies on, for instance, inclusion or sustainability. This happens not just across formal jurisdictions (different Councils or States) but even related to the socio-spatial location of a particular school.

This dynamism was recognized under the banner of 'new institutionalism'. There are four variants of 'new institutionalism'—rational choice, historical, sociological, and discursive. Each was developed independently from each other, but we tend to regard these different types as complementary rather than in competition, and together they establish a complete conceptual toolbox. For governance, the essential differentiation between these types is an emphasis on people or on structures. Behind the institutional dynamics of structure and agency lies the core influence of power on policymaking (Harris et al., 2020). Agentic- or actor-centred theories are broadly conceived as 'instrumentalist' (Fuchs & Lederer, 2007) or 'rational choice' (Hall & Taylor, 1996; March & Olsen, 1996). '*Actors*' are stakeholders and collectives: industry, government and regulators, civil society groups, and local communities. Structuralist approaches emphasize '*Structures*' as overt or implicit (often unrecognized) social and institutional, macro-societal, conditions that act as the famous 'rules of the game' in which policy decisions and choices are made (Arts & Van Tatenhove, 2004). For governance, 'ideas' also powerfully enter the mix as 'core beliefs' driving policy actors and coalitions (Sabatier, 1988) as well as the practices and processes through which ideas are conveyed and communicated (or not communicated) by actors (Carstensen & Schmidt, 2016). In the current international context, the power of ideas on policy and politics plays out over and above any calls for truth or certainty: Elections are won and lost on who can market themselves in populist rhetoric such as 'draining the swamp' as a cover to perpetuate the power of those who have always thrived in the swamp.

Turning back to our goal of understanding the governance behind healthy policy settings, this type of thinking allows a multilevel analysis of governance—whereby different actors bring different values to play into influencing policy choices that are set under specific rules or institutional arrangements—as the basis for strategically engaging to influence the setting under scrutiny to be 'healthy'.

One of us (PH) has been undertaking research in Australia that applies these institutionally focused concepts to progress understanding of how to influence public policy (as a setting) to take on health as an idea (Harris et al., 2015). The research looks at how 'health' was taken up as an idea across the policy system responsible for land-use planning in New South Wales, Australia. The premise behind the research is that the evidence on the links between cities, the built environment, and health are well known. However, there is little knowledge about what land-use planning policy is (as a setting) and, crucially, whether and how that policy system does, does not, or is even able to, take on health-promoting ideas.

Looking at governance using a 'new institutionalist' lens, what we found explains how a mix of actors, ideas, and structures interplayed to open up and close off opportunities to influence land-use planning policy. Ultimately, land-use planning over the life of the research went through various changes that led to health being more acceptable to the system than it had been previously. However, health as an explicit policy driver for land-use planning remains far from institutionalized. This in large part is due to health advocates having trouble keeping up with the core interests of the new governance structures that have been created and continue to operate at differing layers of the system.

Back in 2011 to 2013, for instance, the health agenda had its moment in the sun when pushed as a new 'objective' in a legislative reform process (Harris et al., 2017). The principal actors behind that process of reform were a coalition of government and external supporters of a new system that trumped the purpose of

Fig. 3.2 A model of
human development
(Hancock, T. Health,
human development and
the community ecosystem:
three ecological models,
*Health Promotion
International*, 1993, 8(1),
p. 43, by permission of
Oxford University Press)

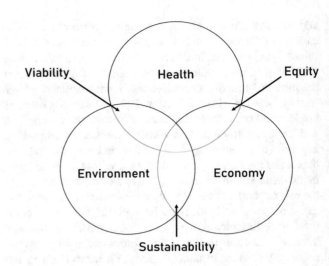

land-use planning to be about economic growth rather than a balance of environmental, social, and economic forces. The health objective almost became acceptable
to the powerful coalition behind the reforms because it fitted both an economic
agenda (a healthy community is a 'richer' community and a 'liveable' community
is one that is easier to market) and was not something that could be seriously challenged as not acceptable. But the inclusion of health in the discourse of those who
held positions of power in the planning system was never seriously considered. The
community push against the reforms, however, was so significant that the whole
process of reform was taken off the table. The loss of inclusion of a health objective
was collateral damage, and the lack of serious consideration meant the idea of health
for the system never recovered its prominence.

The next opportunity came subsequent to the reforms, when a new Planning
Minister was brought in who ushered in a new wave of ideas including depowering
the 'economic growth' agenda to be one of balance between economic growth (now
called 'Productivity'), social (now called 'Liveability'), and environmental sustainability ('Sustainability'). Superficially, such reframing would remind a health promoter of Hancock's Model of Human Development (Fig. 3.2)—but a lesson to be
learnt in policy terms here (and related to the discursive institutionalism model we
described above) is that words are used to frame particular value systems and pol-
icy/governance options. What the NSW Planning Minister meant might not
(entirely) align with Hancock's conceptual perspective—and the health promoters'
belief system.

At the same time, the governance model shifted from being driven centrally to
one that was about negotiation and facilitation across different agencies within government, at different levels including local government, and through a much stronger community engagement process. Alongside this was a strong push to link
strategic planning, which develops a vision for the city, to the planning and delivery
of infrastructure, which are the major investments that allow a city to function. This

would seem to be the perfect opportunity to position a broad view of health as part of the strategic vision for the city, and core to the delivery of infrastructure to improve the health and well-being of the city's inhabitants. However, idea of health as remains underdeveloped as a core concept (Harris et al., 2019). This is for several reasons. The idea of broad connections between a city and the health of its population are not seen as useful framing for policy. Instead, the infrastructure focus, which has tended to emphasize productivity rather than other issues, has defaulted to 'health' becoming about investing in 'hospital precincts', which is essentially how land-use planners have always tended to see 'health'. Liveability is seen as a better alternative, but the connections back to health are not fully developed; the emphasis is enhancing the image of the city rather than reorienting investment in infrastructure to be more equitably distributed to benefit historically disadvantaged parts of the city (McGreevy et al., 2019).

But the reality of policy is that change is slow and incremental, and the activities at that higher level of the land-use planning system have influenced understanding land-use planning systems as a 'setting' for health-focused policy activity. Regional investments in infrastructure to benefit health and equity, like the airport to the traditionally disadvantaged west of the city, are proving fruitful opportunities for a health-focused collaborations and activities. Governance structures are in place to further how that infrastructure can benefit health (and liveability) and health equity. Time, and hopefully more research, will tell whether the benefits of such decisions play out to improve the lives of those living in the region.

Across this research programme has lain the importance of getting the idea of health right as an objective for the planning system. What has been missed in practice, however, is that policy objectives are often developed in concert with the governance structures that are in place to further them (Mossberger & Stoker, 2001; Pierre & Peters, 2012). In urban settings, for instance, governance tends to shore up objectives that promote the economic growth of cities or regions above all else (Brenner, 2019; Scott & Storper, 2015). The positioning of health as an idea for public policy and the governance that goes behind this needs to be better articulated and governance strategies developed to progress that objective. This is what we will argue in the remainder of this chapter.

3.4 Policy for Health

For the argument in this chapter it makes sense to establish a more or less stable definition of 'policy'. Richards and Smith (2008) say that *'"Policy" is a general term used to describe a formal decision or plan of action adopted by an actor … to achieve a particular goal… 'Public policy' is a more specific term applied to a formal decision or a plan of action that has been taken by, or has involved, a state organisation'*. de Leeuw et al. (2014) claim a more instrumental governmental definition that distinguishes between the policy issue, its resolution, and the tools or policy instruments that should be dedicated to attaining that resolution. Public policy, to them, is '*the expressed intent of government to allocate resources and capacities to resolve an expressly identified issue within a certain timeframe*'.

Carpenter (2012) explains how public policy around health adds an altogether different level of complexity to the political process of policymaking. 'Health' is an issue that is personal, value-laden, in which ownership is distributed and contested between a wide variety of claimants of its territory—hospitals, professionals, pharmaceutical industries and biomedical equipment companies, insurance businesses, governments at every level, 'consumers' (or 'patients'), communities, and, yes, even infrastructure developers. The boundaries between these stakeholders aren't always clear and their influence often opaque. Batt, for instance, using a health policy example, debunks the romantic notion that patient/consumer groups freely advocate for a voice in decisions on clinical procedures and government policies. Instead, Batt shows how their actions are often 'bought' by industry such as Big Pharma (Batt, 2017). In similar vein, others have explained that the oft-vaunted notion of the engaged consumer voice in policy development may, in fact, be too romantic (de Leeuw, 2020).

Many authors seem to be rather careless in using the 'health policy' terminology. It is our estimate that the vast majority of pronouncements on 'health policy' actually refer to 'public policy for healthcare'. Considering the foundations of the settings-based health promotion effort this is an important observation. Many learnings from the literature on 'health policy' would not be applicable to settings-based health promotion: Settings are rarely healthcare establishments (with the exception of *health-promoting hospitals and health services*) or have a remit to shape healthcare priorities (a study by Green (1998) for the European Office of the World Health Organization showed that only a minuscule group of European countries' local governments is directly charged with planning and maintaining healthcare facilities, and of those, most aim to develop primary care facilities—we assume that this is the same around the globe but information on this is fragmented—see also Chap. 5, Healthy Cities). However, all settings may well have the prerogative to make policies for health: they do have a—moral—responsibility to address the wider determinants of health.

This is not just wordplay. Putland et al. (2011) have identified policy opacity as the main barrier to the constructive development of true policy for health (rather than disease, care, etc.). Precision in language is essential to the (political and social) processes that shape policy—and deliberate obfuscation might be an appropriate strategy in shaping policy agendas (Stone, 1997). Further, Laumann and Knoke (1987) show in their policy domain network analysis that mastery of the frames that define policy issues and domains allows for entry into the discourse of new policy players. A 'policy domain' therefore, becomes constructed purely by those actors and actants (cf. Latour's and Callon's Actor Network Theory—see Bilodeau & Potvin, 2018) that have framed it, for instance, whether deliberately or accidentally opaquely as 'health' policy when the object of the policy may in fact be the resourcing of 'clinical services in intensive care'.

3.5 Healthy Public Policy and Health in All Policy

When introducing 'policy' as a setting for health, we must address two essential health promotion notions. They both find their foundations in the WHO-sponsored international/global health promotion conferences—Ottawa (1986) for 'Healthy Public Policy', and Helsinki (2013) for 'Health in All Policies' (Tang et al., 2014).

Based on pronouncements by nursing and community political scientist Professor Nancy Milio and public health activist, futurist and co-founder of the Canadian Greens Party Professor Trevor Hancock in the early 1980s, the Ottawa Charter for Health Promotion included a call to build 'Healthy Public Policy'. Both thinkers recognized that virtually any public policy impacted on the health potential and outcomes of individuals, groups, and societies. They also profoundly saw this as an equity issue. Policies drive the (re)distribution of resources and therefore inherently reduce or exacerbate social and health equity. Whether it is at the agriculture–food–nutrition nexus (Milio, 1990), transport and mobility (Green et al., 2015), welfare payments and income equality (Lynch et al., 2004), housing (WHO, 2011), or more obvious determinant areas like education and health services access (de Leeuw, 2017), policy choice in each of these areas will influence whether individuals and communities can pursue and fully attain their health potential. Milio (1981) and Hancock (1985) both called on governments to integrate health considerations across all government policy sectors. The second international health promotion conference Adelaide (1988) concluded that such a policy view is critical for the further development of (settings-based) health promotion.

The Adelaide Statement was a bit opaque on the issue of *who* was to develop such 'Healthy Public Policies' and at what level of government. Soon a small body of evidence started to emerge, demonstrating (or at least suggesting) that at the level of the nation-state such policies are extremely hard to design, let alone to be implemented (e.g. de Leeuw & Polman, 1995). At that level of governance (see below) and government, systems, stakeholders, and structures are very hard to reorient towards (what the political and administrative science literature has declared) 'the holy grail of policy making': joined-up, whole-of-government, integral and/or horizontal policy (Peters, 1998). Added to this mix is recognizing 'the power of the State' as a blurring of public, private, and civil governance engagement in public policy. The idea of joined-up policy for health, however, never disappeared entirely off the health promotion radar—in fact, it was reinvigorated by two diametrically antipodean partners, the governments of Finland and South Australia. In the early 2000s, they both started government programmes that aimed at including health in all policy (de Leeuw, 2017), leading to the idea of Health in All Policy (HiAP). For the Fins, this coincided with their presidency of the European Union, and for the South Australians with the presence of a 'Thinker in Residence'—Ilona Kickbusch. There were differences in emphasis and approach, but the HiAP idea advocated unequivocally that social and political engagement would enable policy actors across sectors to consider the health dimension in their priorities (WHO, 2015). In South Australia this was enhanced, for instance, by a strong academic and boundary-spanning support system that continues to work with a vast diversity of stakeholders and the application of a 'health lens' at the executive level of government (the Premier) rather than the healthcare ministry and bureaucracy. This was supported institutionally by the inclusion of HiAP in the South Australian Strategic Plan—mandates indeed matter. History matters too: In Finland the creation of institutional accountabilities between sectors is one of the key approaches to developing HiAP, grounded in the Finnish track record of health promotion innovation that started in North Karelia (Puska & Ståhl, 2010; Willingham, 2018).

That said, the major challenge to HiAP that is currently emerging is whether or not it is an approach that subsumes or is subsumed by the original idea of Healthy Public Policy. Our view, supported by recent commentators in South Australia (Lawless et al., 2017), is that HiAP is best viewed as a strategy to achieve healthy public policy (HPP). This is because there is simply no getting away from the fact that the object of attention is Public Policy, with 'Health' of lesser import (Harris et al., 2012). This revelation not only connects up HPP activities, including HiAP, to Public Policy and whole of government activity (a la Milio and Hancock), but usefully centres attention on the known dimensions of public policy that have been around since the middle of the last century. That body of knowledge explains several core points for health advocates. First, and crucially without an ideational framing that centres on the core dimension of the object of attention—Public Policy—the idea of 'health' will remain abstract at best, or at worst 'health imperialism' (while 'health(care)' already sucks up policy budgets). Second, without knowledge of the rules that govern the often siloed nature of policymaking, very little progress can be achieved. Third, without recognizing that values, often driven by those rules, shape policy choices, very little progress can be achieved. Fourth, that constellations of actors and networks form around those values, rules, and ideas, with more or less power to influence policy at different points in time. And finally, that different policy actors and institutions use particular procedures to develop policies, which often have nothing to do with positioning health as a policy issue. These are all the hurdles that need to be addressed to make public policy a healthy setting.

Perhaps a helpful analogy to think about the various framings of the relation between health(care), policy, the public, and public sector perspectives is Fig. 3.3—various stacks of pancakes. '**Health policy**' is all policy (public and private) aimed at resolving issues related to the prevention and promotion of health, prolonging life, treating health threats, disease and infirmity, managing the people, professionals, services, and technologies. When policy is made to enable individuals, groups, and communities to assume the fullest possible control over the determinants of their individual, social, and ecological health and ability, and enacted by the public sector (governments at all levels from local to global), and not necessarily the health sector, we would call this '**healthy public policy**' (HPP). Policies exist within HPP that are driven by public policy sectors outside the traditional health bureaucracy (i.e. ministries and departments of health, which should more appropriately be called ministries of public health and healthcare delivery in the majority of instances). However, two particular sets of policies are grown within the traditional health bureaucracy: **public health policy** and **healthcare policy**. 'Healthcare

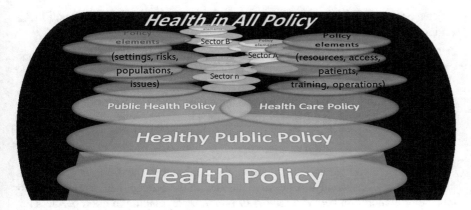

Fig. 3.3 The policy pancakes

policy' tends to address policy elements around the allocation and distribution of resources, access, and operations for healthcare delivery through the traditional institutions of the healthcare sector (hospitals, primary care clinics, service delivery professionals) and focus on their appropriate training in addition to regulating technologies for healthcare (including pharmaceuticals) so that patients may receive the highest possible level of care and care within acceptable social parameters of the particular system. **'Public health policy'** must be seen as 'public health' policy (policy for population health) rather than being conflated with public sector 'health policy' stemming from the traditional health bureaucracy. Public health is also, institutionally, the point in the health bureaucracy that tends to look 'outward' and therefore to see the relevance of public policy for health.

The policy elements for 'public health policy' are qualitatively different from those of the 'healthcare policy' domain. Where healthcare policy typically deals with the allocation of (scarce) resources (admittedly under a veil of 'evidence-based medicine' and 'patient-centred care'), public health policy looks at values of coverage and access for populations and settings, dealing with particular population health issues more than operations of a system. Other policy domains (sectors) have similar pancake stacks of elements, and depending on the nature of the domain and its discourse those elements may take on more contentious or more technological characteristics, depending on historical and cultural attributes of policy systems. For instance, the welfare policy discourse in nation-states that have been classified as Liberal (Esping-Andersen, 2013) is more contentious and in flux than the same domain in Corporatist-Statist or Social Democratic states; the infrastructure portfolio might be seen as more contentious in the Social Democratic, and as a mere technological policy domain in the Liberal context.

Such differences also explain why the formation of Health in All Policies Policy as a strategy to achieve healthy public policy is unique to each nation and setting. In Fig. 3.3, reaching out from either (public/health/care) policy to other sectors and their priorities is a political process that requires cunning vision and the mastery of many different perspectives (Baker et al., 2018; Lawless et al., 2018).

Two critical differences between Healthy Public Policy (HPP) and Health in All Policy (HiAP) are as follows:

- HPP emphasizes the many and varied connections between public policy and health, and aims to influence public policy to be 'healthy' from an institutional perspective and not necessarily driven by health advocates.
- HiAP is a sub-strategy of HPP, most often led by health advocates but emphasizing collaboration with other sectors, that aims to work across sectors from whatever leverage point that makes it possible to include 'health' in any policy at any level for any organisation or community.

In different countries and jurisdictions, the emphases of the different dimensions of HiAP vary. Consistently, values associated with the concept centre on the importance of collaboration between sectors of public policymaking in good partnership. Other aspects where less coherence exists between the different jurisdictions include health equity, the attainment of synergy, HiAP leading to or driven by accountability, the character of innovation, ways of integration and the very nature of policy, for example (Rudolph et al., 2013):

> *Health in All Policies is a collaborative approach that integrates and articulates health considerations into policy making across sectors, and at all levels, to improve the health of all communities and people.* (US Association of State and Territorial Health Officers [ASTHO])

> *Health in All Policies is a collaborative approach to improving the health of all people by incorporating health considerations into decision-making across sectors and policy areas.* (California Health in All Policies Task Force)

> *Health in All Policies is the policy practice of including, integrating or internalizing health in other policies that shape or influence the [Social Determinants of Health (SDoH)] ... Health in All Policies is a policy practice adopted by leaders and policy makers to integrate consideration of health, well-being and equity during the development, implementation and evaluation of policies.* (European Observatory on Health Systems and Policies)

> *Health in All Policies is an innovative, systems change approach to the processes through which policies are created and implemented.* (National Association of County and City Health Officials)

How such policies are formulated, applied, monitored, and implemented (and—an issue we tend to forget—are terminated) depends on implicit and explicit rules—rules that have institutionalized how we prefer our societies to be shaped and run. This is the domain of 'governance'.

3.6 Governance

Like 'policy', 'governance' is a term that is easily used (sometimes by people that wish to impress—saying 'governance' rather than 'government' as the latter may seem so bland) but consequently has a range of definitions that often don't fully align (see, for instance, Barbazza & Tello, 2014; Bevir, 2013). In popular colloquialism it may mean 'the act of governing', corrupted by some into 'the art of government'. Yet, the essence of governance can be described as 'the systematic, patterned way in which decisions are made and implemented' (Greer et al., 2016). Colloquially, it is 'how things are done around here'.

(Intersectoral) governance can be defined as

> the sum of the many ways individuals and institutions, public and private, manage the connections of their common affairs. It is a continuing process through which conflicting or diverse interests may be accommodated and cooperative action may be taken. It includes formal institutions and regimes empowered to enforce compliance, as well as informal arrangements that people and institutions either have agreed to or perceive to be in their interest. (Commission on Global Governance, 1995)

In the European Region of the WHO, from the early stages of the Healthy Cities programme, an institutional commitment to inter-sectoral governance has been a criterion for designation as a Healthy City. Implicitly or explicitly this commitment has extended to other settings for health. From phase II onwards, European Healthy Cities needed to submit evidence that they had established an inter-sectoral steering committee (ISC) that would oversee policy and intervention development (Heritage & Green, 2013; Lipp et al., 2013). There are no specific requirements to the design or architecture of such ISCs, as they are often driven by unique local contexts and requirements. Whether cities lived up to the expectation beyond their formal application commitments was ascertained via annual reporting templates. Virtually all members of the network reported that they did establish an ISC, although the frequency with which this body met was variable. In some cities it met only once a year, in others more regularly, up to monthly. In cities where the ISC met annually, the role of the body was more at a systems and regulatory level, such as driving and approving policy development and monitoring of inter-sectoral deliverables; ISCs that met more regularly tended to engage more directly in the operational aspects of partnership development, such as allocation of resources and direct supervision of working relationships.

Both the strategic and the operational aspects of inter-sectoral governance are important. In their multiple governance framework, Hill and Hupe (2006) show these different dimensions of governance as complementary requirements for effective and transparent policy development and implementation (Fig. 3.4). Inter-sectoral governance moves between, and encompasses, an architecture in which implicit and explicit rules at a systems level ('institutional design' in Fig. 3.4) explicitly connect to the way in which individuals in collaborative processes manage their contacts.

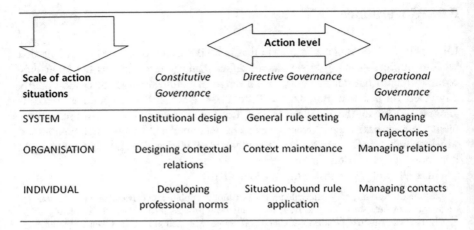

Fig. 3.4 Multiple governance framework (Source: Hill & Hupe, 2006)

Hill and Hupe see the interrelated dimensions and trajectories of systems-, orga-
nizations-, and individuals-driven actions as explanatory and predictive pathways
for accountable policy development—not just for governments (at any level), but
also in coming to grips with the ways in which organizations and their individual
stakeholders relate to each other and make sense of the world. Well-wrought governance, they demonstrate (Hill & Hupe, 2002), enables efficient policy and administrative pathways. It combines high-value rule setting ('constitutive governance')
with regulatory parameters ('directive governance') and their applications ('operational governance').

Values do play a role in and for governance (Kickbusch & Gleicher, 2012; Zürn
et al., 2010). One can differentiate between the descriptive account (how something
is governed) and the normative account (how something ought to be governed)
(Barbazza & Tello, 2014). Values are often formulated to show the direction in
which governance ought to lead. Barbazza and Tello (2014) mention core values of
governance: control of corruption, democracy, human rights, ethics and integrity,
conflict prevention, public good, rule of law. Additional dimensions of governance
also reflect values: accountability, participation and consensus, transparency, effectiveness, efficiency, equity, sustainability, improved health. These are all attributes
of Hill & Hupe's multiple governance framework.

3.7   Governance for Settings-Based Health Promotion

How does this apply to arguments for settings-based health promotion?

McQueen and colleagues reviewed the different ways in which governments
around the world have applied the various dimensions (in our perspective, of the
Hill & Hupe approach) of governance for integration of health in all policies. In

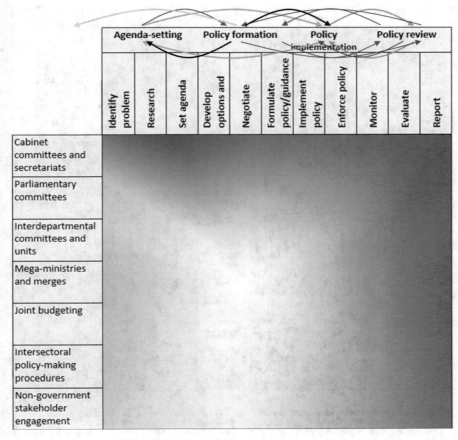

Fig. 3.5 An adaptation of the work by McQueen as reproduced in the *WHO HiAP Manual* with additional columns highlighting equivalent 'settings' arrangements and examples

Figs. 3.5 and 3.6 we reproduce (from the *WHO HiAP Manual*) their inventory. We hope to show that their idea of the stages heuristics for policymaking and implementation (i.e. discrete and sequential steps that have to be taken in the policy process) is, in fact, more fuzzy and full of feedback loops. Also we show that the institutional arrangements for making (HiAP) governance work have a multi-agentic and interconnected nature that especially across different settings in the same spatial domain (cf. the Island of Rondraperina in Fig. 3.7) must be recognized.

Obviously, there is a significant difference in policy and governance perspectives, depending on whether the particular setting is dominated by a public sector 'flavour' or not. Territorially and jurisdictionally, cities and islands tend to align with a public policy and public sector governance perspective, although both Australian veteran Healthy Cities (Kiama/Illawarra and Noarlunga/Onkaparinga) are run by and through community-based non-governmental organizations.

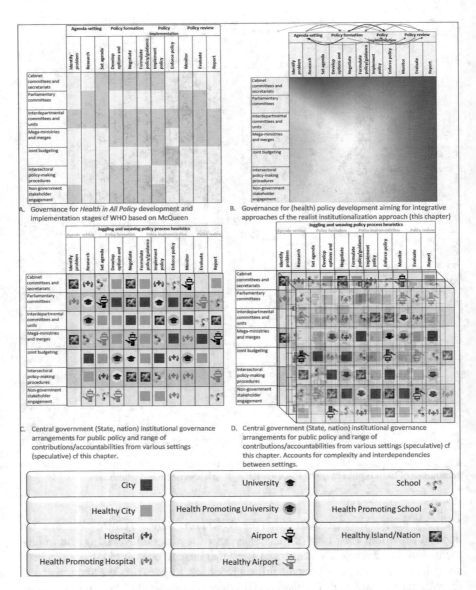

Fig. 3.6 Adding complexities and overlaying health settings based on HiAP governance (Fig. 3.5) and the Island of Rondraperina

Workplaces tend to be private, corporate entities – however, many workplaces (like public hospitals) are under the direct control and accountability of a government – at local, district, provincial, national, or even federal levels.

What Figs. 3.5 and 3.6 show is that the various governance perspectives for policy development apply equally well to a range of settings. We just may need to be more analytical in our review of public sector responsibilities and approaches.

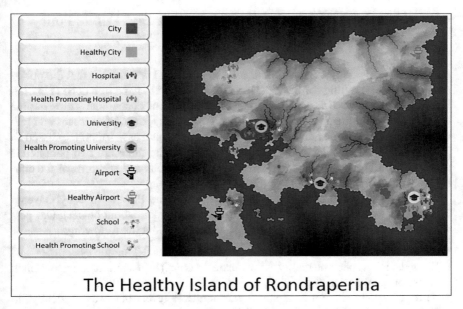

The Healthy Island of Rondraperina

Fig. 3.7 Aligned and non-aligned health settings on a Healthy Island (map created in PolygonMap Generator https://www.redblobgames.com/maps/mapgen2/)

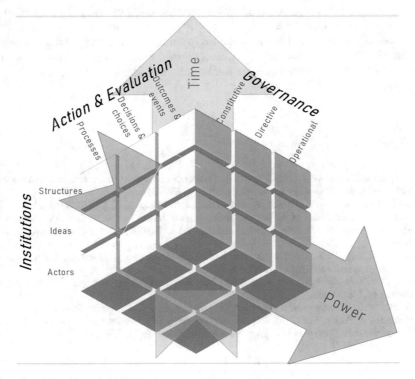

Fig. 3.8 The policy cube (Harris & de Leeuw, 2020)

3.8   A Final Proposition to Consider: 'Healthy' Public Policy as a Setting

At this near end point, it is worth returning to our initial proposition that the policy environment is a setting for health. This setting takes the shape of a cube (Fig. 3.8, Harris & de Leeuw, 2020). We interleaved the different conceptual gazes outline above into three dimensions (the institutional approach; governance issues and levels; and views on stages and iterations of the policy process—often expressed in policy actions and evaluations), and then identified that there are two parameters that consistently and dynamically shift the configurations and relations of the constituent parts: time, and power.

The concept of the policy cube was inspired by the Power Cube by Gaventa (2006, whose cube also was inspired by a great many ideas about power). Our policy cube similarly invites reflection and engagement about the following:

- How power in policy systems interacts with health as a dynamic system.
- How decisions become reality at the upstream point (be it supranational, national, state. or local policies).
- How they then are implemented (again multiple levels but usually locally) to then have effects or impacts on health and health equity over time.

In this way, 'healthy' public policy can be seen as an attribute of a larger policy system, based on the pragmatic assumption that not all policies aim to be healthy, but some do. A 'healthy' public policy setting is one that is self-reflective, and can self-correct over time in response to changes in the programmes or populations that it aims to impact. This, necessarily, emphasizes processes and the range of governance actors and the institutions and ideas that make up policy as a setting.

References

Arts, B., & Van Tatenhove, J. (2004). Policy and power: A conceptual framework between the 'old' and 'new' policy idioms. *Policy Sciences, 37*(3–4), 339–356.

Baker, P., Friel, S., Kay, A., Baum, F., Strazdins, L., & Mackean, T. (2018). What enables and constrains the inclusion of the social determinants of health inequities in government policy agendas? A narrative review. *International Journal of Health Policy and Management, 7*(2), 101–111.

Barbazza, E., & Tello, J. E. (2014). A review of health governance: Definitions, dimensions and tools to govern. *Health Policy, 116*(1), 1–11.

Batt, S. (2017). *Health Advocacy, Inc.: How pharmaceutical funding changed the breast cancer movement*. UBC Press.

Bevir, M. (2013). *Governance: A very short introduction*. Oxford University Press.

Bilodeau, A., & Potvin, L. (2018). Unpacking complexity in public health interventions with the Actor–Network Theory. *Health Promotion International, 33*(1), 173–181.

Brenner, N. (2019). *New Urban spaces: Urban theory and the scale question.* Oxford University Press.

Carpenter, D. (2012). Is health politics different? *Annual Review of Political Science, 15,* 287–311.

Carstensen, M. B., & Schmidt, V. A. (2016). Power through, over and in ideas: Conceptualizing ideational power in discursive institutionalism. *Journal of European Public Policy, 23*(3), 318–337.

Commission on Global Governance. (1995). *Our global neighbourhood: The report.* Oxford University Press.

de Leeuw, E. (2017). Engagement of sectors other than health in integrated health governance, policy, and action. *Annual Review of Public Health, 38,* 329–349.

de Leeuw, E. (2020). The rise of the consucrat. *International Journal of Health Policy and Management.* https://doi.org/10.34172/ijhpm.2020.36

de Leeuw, E., Clavier, C., & Breton, E. (2014). Health policy–why research it and how: Health political science. *Health Research Policy and Systems, 12*(1), 55.

de Leeuw, E., & Polman, L. (1995). Health policy making: the Dutch experience. *Social Science & Medicine, 40*(3), 331–338.

Esping-Andersen, G. (2013). *The three worlds of welfare capitalism.* John Wiley & Sons.

Fuchs, D., & Lederer, M. M. (2007). The power of business. *Business and Politics, 9*(3), 1–17.

Gaventa, J. (2006). Finding the spaces for change: A power analysis. *IDS Bulletin, 37,* 23–33.

Green, G. (1998). Health and governance in European cities: A compendium of trends and responsibilities for public health in 46 member states of the WHO European Region. *European Hospital Management Journal.*

Green, J., Roberts, H., Petticrew, M., Steinbach, R., Goodman, A., Jones, A., & Edwards, P. (2015). Integrating quasi-experimental and inductive designs in evaluation: A case study of the impact of free bus travel on public health. *Evaluation, 21*(4), 391–406.

Greer, S. L., Wismar, M., & Figueras, J. (2016). Introduction: Strengthening governance amidst changing governance. In S. L. Greer, M. Wismar, & J. Figueras (Eds.), *Strengthening health system governance: Better policies, stronger performance* (pp. 3–52). Open University Press.

Hall, P. A., & Taylor, R. C. R. (1996). Political science and the three new institutionalisms. *Political Studies, 44*(5), 936.

Hancock, T. (1985). Beyond health care: From public health policy to healthy public policy. *Canadian Journal of Public Health/Revue canadienne de sante publique, 76,* 9–11.

Hancock, T. (1993). Health, human development and the community ecosystem: Three ecological models. *Health Promotion International, 8*(1), 41–47.

Harris, P., Baum, F., Friel, S., Mackean, T., Schram, A., & Townsend, B. (2020). A glossary of theories for understanding power and policy for health equity. *Journal of Epidemiology and Community Health.* jech-2019-213692.

Harris, P., & de Leeuw, E. (2020). *Unpacking the black of policy, with a cube! Blog, Centre for Health Equity Training, Research and Evaluation CHETRE, at SWSLHD.* Ingham Institute and UNSW. Retrieved May 11, 2021, from https://chetre.org/2020/08/unpacking-the-black-box-of-policy-with-a-cube/

Harris, P., Friel, S., & Wilson, A. (2015). 'Including health in systems responsible for urban planning': A realist policy analysis research programme. *BMJ Open, 5*(7), e008822.

Harris, P., Kent, J., Sainsbury, P., Marie-Thow, A., Baum, F., Friel, S., & McCue, P. (2017). Creating 'healthy built environment' legislation in Australia; A policy analysis. *Health Promotion International.* dax055-dax055.

Harris, P., Kent, J., Sainsbury, P., Riley, E., Sharma, N., & Harris, E. (2019). *Healthy urban planning: An institutional policy analysis of strategic planning in Sydney.* Australia.

Harris, P. J., Kemp, L. A., & Sainsbury, P. (2012). The essential elements of health impact assessment and healthy public policy: A qualitative study of practitioner perspectives. *BMJ open, 2*(6), e001245.

Heritage, Z., & Green, G. (2013). European National Healthy City Networks: The impact of an elite epistemic community. *Journal of Urban Health, 90*(1), 154–166.

Hill, M., & Hupe, P. (2002). *Implementing public policy: Governance in theory and in practice*. Sage.

Hill, M., & Hupe, P. (2006). Analysing policy processes as multiple governance: Accountability in social policy. *Policy and Politics, 34*(3), 557–573.

Howlett, M., Ramesh, M., & Perl, A. (2009). *Studying public policy: Policy cycles and policy subsystems* (3rd ed.). Oxford University Press.

Jessop, B. (1998). The rise of governance and the risks of failure: The case of economic development. *International Social Science Journal, 50*(155), 29–45.

Kickbusch, I., & Gleicher, D. (2012). *Governance for health in the 21st century*. WHO Europe.

Kickbusch, I., Macdonald, H., & King, R. (1988). *Healthy public policy: Report on the Adelaide Conference: 2nd International Conference on Health Promotion, April 5-9, 1988, Adelaide, South Australia*. Commonwealth Department of Community Services and Health and World Health Organization, Adelaide South Australia.

Lasswell, H. D. (1931). Psychopathology and politics. *The Journal of Nervous and Mental Disease, 74*(5), 676.

Laumann, E. O., & Knoke, D. (1987). *The organizational state: Social choice in national policy domains*. Univ of Wisconsin Press.

Lawless, A. P., Baum, F., Delany, T., MacDougall, C. J., Williams, C., McDermott, D. R., & van Eyk, H. C. (2017). Developing a framework for a program theory-based approach to evaluating policy processes and outcomes: Health in all policies in South Australia. *International Journal of Health Policy and Management*.

Lawless, A. P., Baum, F., Delany, T., MacDougall, C. J., Williams, C., McDermott, D. R., & van Eyk, H. C. (2018). Developing a framework for a program theory-based approach to evaluating policy processes and outcomes: Health in all policies in South Australia. *International Journal of Health Policy and Management, 7*(6), 510–521.

Leftwich, A. (2015). *What is politics? The activity and its study*. John Wiley & Sons.

Lipp, A., Winters, T., & de Leeuw, E. (2013). Evaluation of partnership working in cities in phase IV of the WHO Healthy Cities Network. *Journal of Urban Health, 90*(1), 37–51.

Lowndes, V. (2009). New institutionalism and urban politics. In J. S. Davies & D. L. Imbroscio (Eds.), *Theories of urban politics* (pp. 91–105). Sage.

Lynch, J., Smith, G. D., Harper, S. A., Hillemeier, M., Ross, N., Kaplan, G. A., & Wolfson, M. (2004). Is income inequality a determinant of population health? Part 1. A systematic review. *The Milbank Quarterly, 82*(1), 5–99.

March, J. G., & Olsen, J. P. (1996). Institutional perspectives on political institutions. *Governance, 9*(3), 247–264.

McGreevy, M., Harris, P., Delany-Crowe, T., Fisher, M., Sainsbury, P., & Baum, F. (2019). Can health and health equity be advanced by urban planning strategies designed to advance global competitiveness? Lessons from two Australian case studies. *Social Science & Medicine, 242*, 112594.

Michel, J.-B., Shen, Y. K., Aiden, A. P., Veres, A., Gray, M. K., Brockman, W., The Google Books Team, Pickett, J. P., Hoiberg, D., Clancy, D., Norvig, P., Orwant, J., Pinker, S., Nowak, M. A., & Aiden, E. L. (2011). Quantitative analysis of culture using millions of digitized books. *Science, 331*(6014), 176–182. https://doi.org/10.1126/science.1199644

Milio, N. (1981). *Promoting health through public policy*. F.A. Davis Co.

Milio, N. (1990). *Nutrition policy for food-rich countries: A strategic analysis*. Johns Hopkins University Press.

Mossberger, K., & Stoker, G. (2001). The evolution of urban regime theory: The challenge of conceptualization. *Urban Affairs Review, 36*(6), 810–835.

Peters, B. G. (1998). Managing horizontal government: The politics of co-ordination. *Public Administration, 76*(2), 295–311.

Pierre, J., & Peters, B. G. (2012). Urban governance. In *The Oxford handbook of urban politics*. Oxford University Press.

Puska, P., & Ståhl, T. (2010). Health in all policies—The Finnish initiative: Background, principles, and current issues. *Annual Review of Public Health, 31*, 315–328.

Putland, C., Baum, F. E., & Ziersch, A. M. (2011). From causes to solutions-insights from lay knowledge about health inequalities. *BMC Public Health, 11*(1), 67.

Richards, D., & Smith, M. J. (2008). *Governance and public policy in the United Kingdom*. Oxford University Press.

Rudolph, L., Caplan, J., Ben-Moshe, K., & Dillon, L. (2013). *Health in all policies: A guide for state and local governments*. American Public Health Association and Public Health Institute.

Sabatier, P. A. (1988). An advocacy coalition framework of policy change and the role of policy-oriented learning therein. *Policy Sciences, 21*(2), 129–168.

Scott, A. J., & Storper, M. (2015). The nature of cities: The scope and limits of Urban theory. *International Journal of Urban and Regional Research, 39*(1), 1–15.

Stoker, G. (1998). Governance as theory: Five propositions. *International Social Science Journal, 50*(155), 17–28.

Stone, D. A. (1997). *Policy paradox: The art of political decision making*. WW Norton.

Tang, K. C., Ståhl, T., Bettcher, D., & De Leeuw, E. (2014). The Eighth global conference on health promotion: Health in all policies: From rhetoric to action. *Health Promotion International, 29*(Suppl_1), i1–i8.

University of Sydney. (2016). *Health and wellbeing checklist. For university decision-making*. Healthy Sydney University. Retrieved May 4, 2018, from https://sydney.edu.au/content/dam/corporate/documents/about-us/values-and-visions/Healthy-Sydney-University-checklist.pdf

UNSW Australia. (2016). *Health and safety policy*. University of New South Wales. Retrieved May 4, 2018, from https://www.gs.unsw.edu.au/policy/documents/ohspolicy.pdf

Waters, T., & Waters, D. (Eds.). (2015). *Weber's rationalism and modern society* (Vol. 240, p. 79). Palgrave Macmillan.

WHO. (2011). *Housing: Shared interests in health and development*. World Health Organization.

WHO. (2015). *Health in all policies training manual*. WHO. Retrieved May 17, 2018, from http://apps.who.int/iris/bitstream/10665/151788/1/9789241507981_eng.pdf?ua=1

Willingham, E. (2018). Finland's bold push to change the heart health of a nation. *Knowable Magazine*. Retrieved May 17, 2018, from https://www.knowablemagazine.org/article/health-disease/2018/finlands-bold-push-change-heart-health-nation

World Health Organization (2008). *Closing the gap in a generation: Health equity through action on the social determinants of health*. Final Report of the Commission on Social Determinants of Health. World Health Organization.

Zürn, M., Wälti, S., & Enderlein, H. (2010). Introduction. In H. Enderlein, S. Wälti, & M. Zürn (Eds.), *Handbook of multi-level governance* (pp. 1–13). Edward Elgar Publishing.

Chapter 4
Assessment for and Evaluation of Healthy Settings

Marilyn E. Rice

4.1 Introduction

There is no common agreement as to what comprises a healthy setting. Some would say that a healthy setting is a place that strives to incorporate health promotion and sustainable development into comprehensive strategies that improve conditions that facilitate creating and maintaining the health and well-being of the population. There are many types of settings on which health promotion can build, but it represents a place where people actively use and shape the environment; thus, it is also where people create or solve problems relating to health. A healthy setting supports the processes that make it possible for its members to take control over their own health and quality of life, and to participate in the development and sustainability of that setting being healthy. Others would say that to create and maintain a healthy setting, interlocking systems need to synergistically be nested to work together to ensure a sustained healthy environment. Healthy settings are characterized by an ecological model of health promotion, a systems perspective, and a primary focus on whole system development and change (Dooris, 2006; Dooris et al., 2007). Accordingly, a sound and appropriate evaluation of a healthy setting must focus both on the component projects within a settings program, as well as on the interconnected "whole" and the value this adds.

For purposes of this handbook, it is important to understand the differences between assessment, evaluation, and research within the healthy settings context. Assessment refers to appraising the situations, conditions, interventions, and/or players at distinct times during the life of a setting. It is meant to take a snapshot to describe the setting at a particular moment in time and identify contributing and inhibiting factors that affect the status of the setting and its population. Evaluation is more focused on objectively measuring the processes, impacts, and outcomes of

M. E. Rice (✉)
Consulting International, LLC (merci), Fairfax, VA, USA

© Springer Nature Switzerland AG 2022
S. Kokko, M. Baybutt (eds.), *Handbook of Settings-Based Health Promotion*,
https://doi.org/10.1007/978-3-030-95856-5_4

what takes place in the settings over time. And research is an objective and calculated way of comparing and contrasting the effects of interventions on modifying or sustaining situations and conditions within a particular setting. This chapter is focused on presenting some practical guidance on how these approaches can be applied to various specific settings.

Since the movement to promote healthy settings developed independently for each setting, they each had a different approach in their respective visions and approaches, which in turn implies different approaches to evaluation. For example, in the ideally nested systems approach advocated by Mark Dooris for health-promoting schools, the movement is driven by creating the social, cultural, and environmental conditions for promoting healthy behaviors in schoolchildren. Accordingly, they have an epidemiological focus to their evaluation efforts. However, there are few studies that evaluate both the process and outcomes. Yet, process, intermediate, contextual, and outcome data are necessary in order to establish the effectiveness of health-promoting schools. Experimental designs, for example, may be most appropriate for measuring changes in school context, policy, and practice, as well as knowledge, behavior, and attitudinal outcomes. Qualitative approaches, on the other hand, may be utilized in evaluating the implementation process as well as obtaining more in-depth information on the efficacy of the intervention. Rather than try to evaluate all aspects of the intervention using a single methodology, researchers should employ triangulation of the most appropriate methods for answering the evaluation questions for each area of the intervention. This maximizes the strengths of each approach. Implementation of health promoting schools is a multilevel, multi-strategy undertaking, and the evaluation is equally complicated. In developing an evaluation framework for health-promoting schools, quantitative and qualitative methodologies that comprehensively evaluate the process, intermediate, and long-term outcomes should be employed. The challenge lies in achieving a balance between scientific rigor and considerations of practical possibilities and needs (Mukoma & Flisher, 2004).

The workplace health promotion movement is driven by productivity considerations with the idea that healthy workers are more productive workers. In this case, the desired outcome measures are focused on the quantity and quality of the products produced, though in some cases there is a focus on creating healthy working conditions for the workers. The healthy cities and communities movement took a more systems approach, using a sociological–organizational perspective to look at how structured urban planning could lead to creating healthier environments to support healthy living conditions for people to more easily make healthier choices. In the case of healthy markets, the movement focused on creating sanitary conditions for the marketplace and for the people using it, as well as ensuring sanitary control of the foods sold. For healthy islands, notably in the Pacific, the rationale was quite straightforward: small island developing states (SIDS) are extremely contained environments in a vast expanse of water which sustains and threatens livelihoods (de Leeuw et al., 2018).

It turns out then that the need for evaluation of the different approaches and settings might be the only common ground. In a world where demands to address the determinants of health are being placed on multiple systems, it is more important than ever for decision makers to know how best to invest their time, resources, and energies. When it comes to a question of promoting health and not just treating diseases and illnesses, the result of decisions will have direct and indirect impacts on the quality and duration of life of current and future generations. Therefore, monitoring and evaluating healthy settings initiatives will be critical in helping to determine where it is most appropriate to invest efforts and resources.

Assessing and monitoring the success and effect of healthy settings ideally can be done at two different moments in time. Assessing the situations in which healthy settings will be developed and the potential effects of their implementation should be conducted before the planning and implementation of an initiative is done. It should identify potential obstacles and maximize participatory efforts. A Health Impact Assessment conducted prior to the planning process for initiation of the healthy setting initiative will help to identify potential obstacles and maximize potential positive effects. When a healthy setting has been in place for some time, evaluation of different aspects of its effects can be done to see what has been learned and achieved.

Evaluation is the systematic collection, analysis, and reporting of information about an initiative, program, or group of programs. The information collected should be used to facilitate and inform decision-making and, to be effective, it should contribute to taking appropriate and effective remedial actions. There are many reasons for evaluation, including:

- **Establishing accountability and good governance**: Collect evidence of a program's effectiveness or impact, including the role played by health promotion; influence decision makers and policy makers by showing them evidence of an initiative's benefit; support advocacy for health promotion and healthy settings; ensure that the people for whom the program exists are receiving tangible, real benefits.
- **Improving communication**: Create opportunities for exchange of ideas and opinions among multi-sectoral partners; strengthen participatory efforts; share what works and what doesn't work with others; develop networks, alliances, and contacts among different settings-based processes.
- **Strengthening good management**: Assess the needs of individuals, groups, communities; improve the usefulness of materials used and activities conducted; determine what works, what doesn't, in what contexts and conditions, with what populations, and why; better understand staffing patterns and the delivery of programs from a management perspective; plan for revisions and adjustments.
- **Ensuring financial sustainability**: Show various contributors that their social investment is working, that there is a positive return on investment; be accountable to funders, volunteers, staff, and boards; prove that the program is worthy of the public trust and the resources given because of that trust; ensure funding over the long term.

In this chapter, there will be a focus on a few approaches to evaluation as examples of what is useful. It is not intended to be a comprehensive cookbook of all that is possible—there are substantial methodology handbooks out there that should guide you. Although a number of different assessment and evaluation methods are mentioned here, it is recognized that a realist synthesis methodology, driven by a wide range of qualitative and quantitative methods, is the most appropriate perspective to address the wide geopolitical, demographic, population, and health diversities in different settings. It provides explanations for why interventions may or may not work, in what contexts, how and under what circumstances, and for what populations (de Leeuw, 2011). Asking the right questions is critical; they need to be appropriate, relevant, and appreciative of the unique situational context of the setting. It is important to determine the strengths and weaknesses of particular actions in specific environments. The most desirable assessments and evaluations will address the unique systems determinants that impact on good governance of health and well-being, assessing changes in the social, political, and economic context that have enabled or prevented the initiatives from achieving the goals established for the programs.

This chapter reviews two approaches to conducting an assessment of a healthy setting, basic elements to include in a healthy settings evaluation, some of the most common and effective evaluation types and tools, a few examples of monitoring and evaluation, some of the challenges faced in monitoring and evaluating healthy settings, and overall conclusions.

4.2 The Assessment

Before an effective evaluation can be conducted, it is wise to have a baseline of information and data against which changes can be measured. It is also effective to have done an assessment of the situation, assets, and resources, as well as perceptions and desires on which healthy settings initiatives can be developed. This section of the chapter describes two assessment instruments—Health Impact Assessment and Urban HEART—that are examples of what can be done to develop a baseline view of a setting before new interventions are developed.

4.2.1 Health Impact Assessment

Health Impact Assessment (HIA) is a combination of methods and research tools by which policies, programs, or projects can be assessed to identify their potential effects on the health of populations, and the distribution of those effects within populations. The tool is used during the planning process, **before** policies, programs, or projects are carried out. The purpose of HIA is to develop evidence-informed recommendations to advise decision makers about actions to increase the positive and reduce the negative impacts on health of their plans, projects, or policies. It aims to ensure that the potential health benefits are maximized, that possible health inequities that might emerge from their implementation are identified and addressed, and that the potential negative health consequences and health risks are minimized.

HIA is a structured process by which evidence is gathered and stakeholders are engaged. It uses a broad range of evidence from public health, social sciences, biophysical sciences, and political science to assess plans, programs, projects, or policies with stakeholders and affected communities or populations. The steps used in HIA are as follows:

- **Screening**: Determine whether an HIA is appropriate or required.
- **Scoping**: Set the parameters or the terms of reference for the HI.
- **Assessment**: Assess potential positive and negative impacts of the proposed program on human health.
- **Recommendations**: Develop actions to enhance health and minimize harms.
- **Follow-up and Evaluation**: Follow up with monitoring and use of a health management plan; evaluate the processes involved in the HIA and their impact (IUHPE, 2017)

4.2.2   Urban HEART

A good example of combining the **assessment** with the appropriate **response** is the Urban Health Equity Assessment and Response Tool (Urban HEART) (WHO, 2008). Created by the WHO Centre for Health Development in Kobe, Japan, Urban HEART was developed to conduct an assessment and corresponding response to addressing local conditions within a city context. Unfortunately, given the concentrated amount of data collection required to use this instrument, unless the situation analysis and response are updated on a regular basis, it might be a more static look at the local situation. Although this tool was designed to be applied to an urban setting, the principles might well be appropriately applied to other settings as well. Its objectives are as follows:

- To help policymakers and key stakeholders achieve a better understanding of the social determinants and risk factors, and the associated health outcomes faced specifically by the urban poor and other vulnerable groups.
- To assist program managers and staff in the development of better communication strategies dealing with the various determinants of health, particularly those affecting the urban poor and other vulnerable groups.
- To stimulate policymakers, program managers, and key stakeholders to make strategic decisions and take specific actions that are sensitive to the needs of the urban poor and other vulnerable groups.
- To help communities to more objectively understand the difference between reality and perception in their own locations. Better information on conditions and trends relative to their areas in a city, or among cities, will assist in achieving political consensus in setting priorities for problem-solving.

4.2.2.1 The Assessment Component

The assessment component is designed to measure the city or urban area performance in different policy domains according to various program indicators. Two monitors are used:

1. The City Health Equity Performance Monitor, which provides a broad assessment of the city's performance on a specific indicator through both internal and external benchmarking and using an equity yardstick.
2. The National Urban Health Equity Monitor, which presents a summary and broad comparison of performance among cities or urban areas and a broad determination of effectiveness among policy fields and programs.

The assessment component includes the following:

Policy Domain Indicators—a cluster of indicators referring to or indicative of a broad policy field that is generally considered a major determinant of health. In this tool, the indicators are grouped into four major policy domains: (1) physical environment and infrastructure, (2) social and human development, (3) economics, and (4) governance and politics. The degree of performance or accomplishments in each policy domain eventually leads to a certain level of improvement in health outcomes as indicated by the major vital health indices, which have been grouped separately from the indicators under the four policy domains.

Aggregate Health Outcome Indicators—indicators denoting a national or city average (e.g., infant mortality rate, maternal mortality ratio, etc.).

Equity Indicators—indicators denoting a range of differences between or among population groups or geographic areas (data disaggregated by population group or geographic area, such as male versus female infant mortality rate or the difference in maternal mortality ratio between mothers in poor communities and mothers in nonpoor communities, etc.). The distinction between "poor" and "non-poor" localities is used throughout the tool to denote differences in living conditions that cover a wider range of deprived living conditions (e.g., the homeless, transients, people who live in tents) rather than using "slum" and "non-slum."

4.2.2.2 Response Component

The response component of the tool contains a menu of evidence-based interventions that have been described in both gray and published literature. It is envisioned that the matrix will be adapted at regional or national level to highlight context-specific interventions that work and are most relevant to local needs and priorities. Five prototypes of response packages are provided with a list of potential areas for action. Entry points include: incorporate health into slum-upgrading, target urban poor through urban primary healthcare, strengthen health equity focus on healthy cities and settings, put health equity on the agenda of local governments and urban planning authorities, and pursue a national policy and decision-making process that support healthy urban settings.

4.3 The Evaluation: Steps and Considerations

An effective healthy settings **evaluation** should consider the following **elements**:

- **Scope.** When possible, the entire process of establishing and maintaining a setting as a healthy one should be included, especially the process of building local capacity. The evaluation should go beyond just documenting the outcome or end result.
- **Context.** The political, economic, social, and cultural circumstances of the setting should be taken into consideration for the evaluation.
- **Use of multiple methods.** The best results will come from using an appropriate mix of evaluation methods, techniques, and tools, combining both quantitative and qualitative information.
- **Participation.** Key stakeholders and those who have a genuine interest in the healthy setting initiative should be involved in ways that build upon their assets and strengths.
- **Value.** Local experience and knowledge should be respected and valued. Where possible, it is helpful to uncover ideological and political assumptions and power relations.
- **Individual and collective empowerment.** The evaluation should be based upon the strengths of the members of the setting and promote ownership.
- **Usefulness.** The evaluation should strive to indicate whether the healthy settings initiative is working toward positive change.
- **Integrate the evaluation process.** Ideally, the evaluation should be used from the beginning of the healthy settings process, though it can be introduced at any time along the way.

Most evaluation processes follow a similar pattern which might include these **steps and considerations**:

- Develop evaluation questions (what it is you want to find out—outputs, results, impacts).
- Select the most appropriate methods and information sources.
- Prepare the evaluation work plan.
- Collect the information.
- Analyze, interpret, and reflect upon the information collected.
- Communicate the results to the most appropriate audiences, tailoring them respectively.
- Act on the results.
- Establish a continuous process of monitoring, data collection, reflection, and action.

Some basic elements to include in the development of an indicator for measuring a healthy setting

The indicator should include the following features:

- Be observable and measurable

- Specify or qualify who and what is being measured
- Be time specific

Elements to consider when evaluating the sustainability of a healthy setting might include:

- Maintenance of the "benefits" achieved through the initiative
- Level of institutionalization of the initiative
- Measures of capacity building
- Continuity of the initiative's activities
- Use of multiple strategies
- Mobilization of existing social capital
- Commitment of national and local authorities
- Shared leadership
- Building consensus among multiple stakeholders

4.4   Evaluation Types and Tools

Depending upon what you hope to achieve through your evaluation, this will determine the type of evaluation and methodology you will pick and the process you will use in your evaluation. For the results to be most effective in sustaining or modifying initiatives based upon what is learned from the evaluation, the findings should link policy with practice. Given the multidimensional nature of issues addressed in healthy settings initiatives, a multilevel set of interconnected and often innovative assessment, monitoring, and evaluation methods are needed to address the complex nature of evaluating healthy settings. Additionally, since there are essential values inherent in establishing healthy settings (such as sustainability, equity, community participation, and empowerment), it will be as important to evaluate the effectiveness of specific interventions as it is to assess how the adoption of this value system would generate new and enhanced options for the actual implementation of such interventions (de Leeuw, 2009). Below is a description of some of the most common and effective evaluation types and tools.

In **participatory evaluation**, the key stakeholders are involved in all phases of the evaluation process. It involves active participation of the members of the setting in research and actions that result in improvements in health and quality of life (PAHO, 2011). It involves participation of key stakeholders in all phases of the process, negotiation and consensus building, continuous learning, and flexibility. To be effective, it should be a continuous process of data collection, learning from experience, and incorporating changes into the strategies used as the healthy setting process continues over time. This method is built on trust and equity, and it is characterized by working with community partners and citizens in all aspects, from community assessment to evaluation.

Economic evaluation is a very structured approach. It includes the following eight actions: a description of the decision context and the perspective from which the analysis will take place; specification of the question being addressed; description of the alternatives (the options) that will be considered; identification, measurement, and evaluation of the costs of each alternative; identification, measurement, and valuation of the consequences of each alternative; a technical step where costs and consequences are adjusted for differences in their timing (called discounting); an extensive sensitivity analysis to assess the importance of uncertainties arising from missing information; and interpretation of the results of the evaluation and proposal of recommendations (PAHO, 2007).

Process evaluation involves analyzing **how** program activities are delivered, looking at their implementation process, and seeking to answer these central questions: Who delivers the program and how often? To what extent was the program implemented as planned? How is the program received by the target group and program staff? What are barriers to program delivery? What problems were encountered (sufficient resources, well managed, staff and participants trained adequately)? Was the data used to make program improvements/refinements? If so, what changes were made? These questions enable practitioners to also assess the quality of implementation, which is critical to maximizing the program's intended benefits and demonstrating strategy effectiveness. Process evaluation also provides the information needed to adjust strategy implementation to strengthen effectiveness (SAMHSA, 2019).

Outcome evaluation looks at **results** and the **effectiveness** of a program in producing change. It measures the direct effects of program activities on targeted recipients, such as the degree to which a program increased knowledge about how to promote health or create conditions supportive of healthy behaviors within a particular setting. However, it does not take process evaluation into consideration, without which the evaluation will not provide information about why a program did or did not work.

Impact evaluation often serves an **accountability** purpose to determine if and how well a program worked, and it can determine which, among several alternatives, is the most effective approach, through a cause-and-effect analysis. It uses an experimental or quasi-experimental design, employing an alternate control group generated by random selection in the case of experimental designs or a comparison group which is not randomized in the case of a quasi-experimental design, to show what happened in the communities or settings where the initiatives were realized compared to places where they were not.

The Logic Model is a visual framework that facilitates the identification of the outcomes, activities, and areas that might be included in the evaluation by setting goals (that can be problem oriented or positive outcome oriented), then formulating outcomes that will lead to them, and finally identifying the most appropriate and feasible activities that can be carried out based upon resources that are available.

4.5   Examples of Monitoring and Evaluations

4.5.1   Monitoring, Accountability, Reporting, and Impact (MARI) Research Framework

This methodology was developed to evaluate the status of and results from cities participating in the European Healthy Cities Network (Tsouros & Green, 2009). This evaluation approach values and celebrates the unique contributions of each city.

The model shows a pathway linking prerequisites (leadership, vision and strategy, structures and processes, networks) through activities (policies, programs, projects) which should "make a difference" to city status in the areas of determinants of health, lifestyles, and health outcomes. These elements all form part of the formal process through which interested local governments become designated as "Healthy Cities." To be designated as a "Healthy City" in each phase, city administrations take an official position and express commitment to attributes of local action for health such as governance, equity, working in partnership, assuming leadership for health, engaging all stakeholders and communities to participate in health, and moving toward sustainable policy development for health. None of these attributes exist in isolation, and they are found in different mixes and balances, stages of evolution, implementation, and configurations in the designated Healthy Cities (de Leeuw et al., 2015).

The MARI tool grounds its perspectives in the sets of designation criteria to which European Healthy Cities sign up in each "Phase" of the WHO/EURO movement. It acknowledges that designation in itself is a pivotal stage in the success of Healthy Cities (de Leeuw & Skovgaard, 2005), as it requires a political decision to commit to key principles for urban health development. MARI recognizes, however, that maintaining political and social momentum over the life cycle of a designation period may be variable and applies a dynamic lens, asking for initial conditions; political, social, and demographic changes; and stakeholder support for being a Healthy City and delivering the actions and outputs required. In the full MARI concept, Healthy City administrators and politicians were asked over 400 questions. MARI also morphed into a much simpler format for accountability purposes, with responding to the Annual Reporting Template (ART) that asked 12 high-level questions (de Leeuw, 2009) each year and submitting an ART annually, being part of the designation requirement of each member city.

The MARI conceptual methodology and ART rollout was supplemented by **case study** submissions as key data sources for the evaluation of the entire (5 year) phase.

A second data collection tool consisted of a **General Evaluation Questionnaire (GEQ)**—both for city level and for National Networks of Healthy Cities. The conceptual approach again followed the logic of information requested in the case studies and asked for self-assessment on prerequisites, activities, and city status for 3 years (2009, 2014, and 2019). It allowed for a dynamic response to issues that may have emerged during the lifetime of the project. GEQ also required the provision of information on political and organizational changes in the local Healthy City environment, the level of commitment and support (e.g., through council statements and decisions), resourcing (budget size, numbers of full-time paid staff, volunteer staff), and efforts at capacity-building focused on professional development and community agency.

The case studies and GEQ were further complemented by compiling information from **existing data**. This is very much a feature of a Realist Synthesis methodology. For many phenomena, data and evidence already exist, and they simply need to be "plugged in" to the program logic of a new evaluation project. Such a "logic of method" had been successfully developed and implemented by the DECiPHEr (Developing an evidence-based approach to city public health planning and investment in Europe) Program (Whitfield et al., 2013). In the case of the European Healthy Cities evaluation, additional existing data were integrated from sources such as local City Health Profiles, Healthy City designation files, earlier attempts at establishing comprehensive sets of indicators (de Leeuw & Webster, 2018), and existing data at city-level from, for instance, Eurostat.

In the evaluation effort, the team also established groupings to identify particular patterns within the nearly 100 designated Healthy Cities across Europe. These included distinctions between veteran cities in the movement and novice ones, city size in population, and geopolitical groupings (East–West–North–South, OECD–non-OECD, EU–non-EU, Welfare State typology) (Esping-Andersen, 2013).

4.5.2 The Complementary Use of Total Quality Management and the Balanced Scorecard approach Within Health-Promoting Hospitals

The complementary use of **Total Quality Management** and the **Balanced Scorecard** approach within Health-Promoting Hospitals offers significant promise (Brandt et al., 2005). This approach was applied as a pilot project at Immanuel Diakonie Group (Baptist Group of healthcare centers in Berlin and Brandenburg, Germany).

The general mission of a **Health-Promoting Hospital** (HPH) is to promote the health of patients and staff, to improve the health promotion potential of the hospital organization, and to provide health promotion services for the community they serve.

The **European Foundation for Quality Management** (EFQM) Model is based on nine criteria (leadership, people, policy and strategy, partnership and resources, processes, people results, customer results, society results, and key performance results), which in turn embrace 32 sub-criteria. The models' basis is that excellent results relating to performance, customers, employees, and society will be achieved by management that places a high value on policy and strategy, employees, partnerships, resources, and processes (Groene et al., 2009).

EFQM terminology was found to be strange in the hospital context, difficult for employees to understand why the self-assessment had to be done according to these procedures, and what value the hospital expected from the exercise. Moreover, there was fear that besides creating more work, the whole project could bring with it unpleasant changes for the working context. In the case of combining HPH and EFQM, difficult concepts and terminology, such as health promotion and empowerment, had to be dealt with. The fact that a critical view of their own institution was called for in the self-assessments (because only an honest analysis can provide a safe basis for the future improvement process) contradicted the common hierarchical structure of hospitals, which often requires employees to perform and deliver what is expected "from above." This "problem" in the long term and for each institution offering EFQM, could create an unexpected potential of informed and involved employees, since it succeeds in making positive use of their critical ability and competence instead of devaluing them.

The organization and time requirement for an EFQM analysis is considerable. Consequently, a strong central project management is required that can overcome the daily business of hospital organization, and so directors should be involved in the EFQM teamwork to reduce possible problems with the hospital hierarchy. Training requirements for the employees are high, but worthwhile because their competence and organizational knowledge are considerably increased by their work in the project.

In the self-assessment result, potentials for improvement are communicated and prioritized. They are the basis for the ongoing improvement process for middle- and long-term planning of measures, initiatives, and projects in the "operative business." HPH projects that derive from such self-assessments are thus incorporated with goal direction into the relevant hospital's Quality Management.

The **Balanced Scorecard** (BSC) has developed into a management instrument that was designed to solve problems, and it has achieved worldwide recognition in matters of strategy implementation. At its center are the selection and presentation of strategic objectives, since these control behaviors in the strategy direction. The BSC transforms the strategy into an integrated system made up of four basic business perspectives: the finance, the customer, the process, and the innovation perspectives. Implementation of a Balanced Scorecard consists of five phases: create the organizational framework for its preparation, clarify the strategic bases, develop the BSC itself, manage the rollout, and finally assure the continuous implementation of the BSC. The goal of the five phases is to develop a business into a "strategy-focused organization" in which the Balanced Scorecard is firmly rooted in the management system. As part of the implementation process, every perspective is allocated several objectives, measurement strategies, target values, and improvement initiatives. The resulting archive of measurements paired with strategy-borne cause-and-effect relationships builds up to a powerful toolkit to facilitate the implementation of health promotion strategies in hospital settings.

As a rule, for every objective (which can also be formulated as a standard), a measurement, a target value (or several target values for different periods), and a strategic initiative (measure, project) are defined, for which objectives need to be achieved. If these objectives correspond to the HPH concept and the strategic initiatives are aimed at its realization, a hospital develops automatically into an "HPH strategy-focused organization," with the implementation of a BSC oriented to HPH proposals.

Considered as an interim result of the pilot project, the Balanced Scorecard is thought to be very appropriate for the implementation of the HPH concept when the leaders of the institution who are involved in the BSC core team keep the HPH proposals in mind and are influenced by them when developing the strategy of the business.

The Balanced Scorecard, in combination with the EFQM Model, is a useful tool to guide strategy development and implementation in healthcare organizations. Its strength is the combination of generic business perspectives with internally identified key themes for strategic development. These are illustrated in a strategy map and summarized in the scorecard. As for other quality improvement and management tools not specifically developed for healthcare organizations, some adaptations are required to improve acceptability among professionals.

4.5.3 Health-Promoting Schools

For schools to be effective in improving health, education, and other social outcomes, it would require the integrated efforts of students, families, staff, and public, not-for-profit, and private-sector agencies in and out of school hours. While such an approach is being advanced by the Health-Promoting Schools movement, relatively few schools plan, implement, and evaluate such actions in an integrated manner (Dooris et al., 2007). Rather, they usually offer fragmented efforts to meet urgent health problems and fail to build mutual trust, enjoyment, commitment, and collaboration. Furthermore, schools infrequently help young people to build assets such as caring for others, connectedness, or civic engagement (Institute of Medicine, 2002; Moore & Lippman, 2004).

A major theme in debates on the Health-Promoting School (HPS) is the search for indicators (Denman et al., 2002; Pattenden, 1998; Stears et al., 2000). It is argued that through the development of indicators, the ideal of the school as a health-promoting setting could be achieved. To be defined as a Health-Promoting School, the school must portray certain features, which will be judged by the requirements and the implications of the broader concept of health promotion. On the biophysical level, indicators for an HPS would show, for example, that children are physically well and have good nutrition, that a school has a working relationship with local health services, and that the school nurse is a regular visitor to the school. On a psychosocial level, indicators for an HPS would show, for example, that peer group support is in place, learners are socially supported, and families are involved in school activities. A characteristic of indicators is that they can measure visible things—like features, and invisible things—like characteristics. As schools are complex phenomena, a set of indicators should be developed to measure the distinct components of the system implied by the HPS concept. A set of indicators will also provide information about how the individual components work together to produce the overall effect; facilitate strategic planning, policy development, management, and decision-making (Voljoen et al., 2005); and can motivate people to take action, indicate direction and speed of change, help in the identification of priorities, stimulate action, challenge assumptions about strategies and targets, and encourage policy-makers and managers to rethink appropriate strategies (Corvalan et al., 1997; WHO, 1981).

A systematic review was conducted of the effectiveness of **health-promoting schools** in improving health-related outcomes, in determining whether health-promoting schools are more effective than other ways of delivering health-promoting interventions, and in identifying the relative costs associated with individual changes in self-esteem, health-related knowledge and/or attitudes, self-reported behavior (eating habits, physical activity, leisure activities, smoking, drinking, drug use), physical fitness, and risk behavior. Also reviewed were whether school-wide evaluation elements included provision and quality of school lunches, staff training and involvement of students, aspects of health-related behavior such as dietary intake (assessed by self-report, observed choices, plate waste, uptake of school meals, school lunch content analysis), cardiovascular risk factors (assessed by a variety of physiological measures), physical fitness, dental health (plaque, gingivitis, and caries assessed by clinical examinations), pregnancy rates, self-reports of self-esteem, experience of bullying and aggression, associated knowledge and attitudes, substance abuse, and exposure to the sun. The conclusions from this systematic review were that the optimum method of evaluation of health-promoting schools is currently under debate but that programs to promote mental and social well-being would be likely to improve overall effectiveness, that the impact of staff health and well-being needs more consideration, and that development of measures of mental and social well-being is important for future evaluation (Lister-Sharp et al., 1999). **The Global School-based Student Health Survey** (GSHS) was developed by the World Health Organization (WHO) in collaboration with UNICEF, UNESCO, and UNAIDS; and with technical assistance from the United States Centers for Disease Control and Prevention (CDC) and its school-based survey conducted primarily among students aged 13–17 years. This survey is designed to help countries develop priorities, establish programs, and advocate for resources for school health and youth health programs and policies; allow international agencies, countries, and others to make comparisons across countries regarding the prevalence of health behaviors and protective factors; and establish trends in the prevalence of health behaviors and protective factors for use by each country in evaluation of school health and youth health promotion programs. It measures health behaviors and protective factors among students, covering the areas of alcohol use; dietary behaviors; tobacco and other drug use; hygiene; mental health; physical activity; protective factors; sexual behaviors related to HIV infection, other sexually transmitted infections, and unintended pregnancy; tobacco use; and violence and unintentional injury (CDC, 2019).

Evaluation of school-based health promotion should measure the outcomes of the different levels of intervention from the perspective of resources (developers, i.e., The US Center for Health Education and Health Promotion, The Chinese

Table 4.1 Intervention mapping analysis of HPS (Courtesy of Albert Lee)

Resource system	Intermediate user system	End user system
Developer: CHEP-CUHK system: – Professional development for school health educators – System of accreditation and self-evaluation system –Student health surveillance system – Thematic Network of HPS	**Implementers: Schools, community system:** – Identification of strength and weakness based on school health profile and student health profile for systematic planning – Using framework of HPS to handle health crisis, i.e., SARS, obesity, emotional problems, violence, and accidents – Creating a platform of sharing and networking	**Program participants: Students, parents, and staff system:** – Parental education through "Parent College of Health" mobilizing community resources – Improvement of health literacy of students via improvement of the key areas of HPS – Improvement of staff health via school healthcare and promotion services, healthy working environment and healthy school policies

University of Hong Kong—CUHK-CHEP), the intermediate users (implementers, i.e., schools), and the end users (program participants, i.e., students and staff). Linkages can also be identified through interventional mapping (Bartholomew et al., 1998). Table 4.1 provides examples of evaluation from the three systems.

The indicators of the school health profile and student health profile utilized by The Hong Kong Health School Award Scheme (HKHSA) provides the structured framework of incorporating the four types of outcome indicators, inputs, process, impact, and outcomes as suggested by Nutbeam (1996) to measure the success of health promotion (Lee et al., 2005) (Table 4.2). Those outcomes can also describe health status of students including life satisfaction and emotional health, health behaviors, school environment (physical and social), healthy policies, pedagogy on health training, and organizational practices.

4.5.4 Participatory Action Research (PAR) in Health Promotion as a Methodological Approach

The participatory action research process means collaboration throughout the whole research process between those acting in the school community and the research professionals. During the research process, an emphasis is placed on collaboration, discussion, reflection, cooperative ways of working, and empowerment. Through the results produced by the subjects of the school community in their school environment during the participatory action research process, the personnel and the researchers together try to develop new understanding of health promotion, and thereby to renew the health instruction and health learning by the pupils and the school staff with the aim of finding a reflective way of examining the customary practices in a new light. When this approach was applied in Finland, it was found to have a very positive influence on the sense of participation of the school community

Table 4.2 Summary of how the different types of outcomes are measured (Lee et al., 2019)

Types of outcomes	Indicators to be measured	Measuring instrument
Health and social outcomes	Depressive symptoms, life satisfaction, perceived health status, perceived academic achievement	Validated questionnaires: Satisfaction with Life Scale (LIFE), Depression Self-Rating Scale (DSRS), Youth Risk Behavior Survey (YRBS)
Intermediate outcomes	Attitudes, lifestyles and risk behaviors School environment and school ethos School health services	Questionnaires to students and schools, school observation, documentary review, interviews
Health promotion outcomes	Health skills and knowledge, and self-efficacy School health policies Networking with parents, the local community and other schools to launch health programs	Questionnaires to students and schools, curriculum review, documentary review, individual or focus group interviews, participant observation
Health promotion actions	School timetable for health education activities (formal and extra-curricular) PTA and community involvement	Documentary review

Reprinted from Lee, A., Lo, A.S.C., Keung, M.W., et al. (Lee et al., 2019). Effective health promoting school for better health of children and adolescents: indicators for success. *BMC Public Health*. 19, 1088, Table 4.1. https://doi.org/10.1186/s12889-019-7425-6, licensed under the terms of the Creative Commons Attribution 4.0 International License (http://creativecommons.org/licenses/by/4.0/)

and its individual members. Motivation increased, and people had positive experiences of success and collaborative action. This enhanced their sense of ownership and promoted them to take time to develop a sense of mission-motivated loyalty, commitment, and confidence in the school community. Empowerment, participation, and control over things were essential aspects of health promotion. Empowerment enabled equal participation of the participants in the health promotion process. Health promotion had been adopted into both the written and the implemented curricula of the participating schools, and the schools seemed to have positive attitudes toward accomplishing successful health promotion in schools and communities. However, the building and development of a health-promoting curriculum was one of the most crucial tasks in developing multi-professional and multidisciplinary health promotion in Finnish schools. To be successful, it was found that the principal's duty would be to make sure that a written action plan was made and discussed thoroughly with the staff, pupils, and parents, and then supervised to ensure that it was appropriately carried out in the school community. This should be done in a collaborative school environment, with harmonization of the professional educational autonomy of the teachers with the managerial authority of the principal (Clift and Bruun Jensen, 2005).

4.5.5   Evaluating a Healthy University

A Healthy University aspires to create a learning environment and organizational culture that enhances health, well-being, and sustainability of its community, and enables people to achieve their full potential.

Levels of Evaluation

Within the context of a Healthy University, evaluation is likely to be focused at two levels:

Component Activities and Projects: A Healthy University Initiative is usually comprised of a range of different activities, interventions, and projects (e.g., a green/active travel plan, a peer education project on drugs and sexual health, campaigns on mental health and stigma, healthy and sustainable food procurement procedures). It is important to evaluate these individual elements, assessing whether they achieved their stated objectives and exploring the implementation process to understand what worked well, what did not, and why.

Overall "Whole System" Approach: While evaluation of these individual components is a crucial part of assessing the worth of a Healthy University Initiative, it does not by itself provide feedback on the effectiveness of the overall whole-system Healthy University approach. For evaluation to capture the possible "added value" of a whole system that is working and help generate and build evidence of effectiveness, it must adopt nonlinear approaches, looking at the whole and mapping and understanding the interrelationships, interactions, and synergies – with regard to different population subgroups, different components of the system, and different health issues. This is clearly a much more challenging endeavor than evaluating component activities and projects.

The UK Healthy Universities Network Self-Review Tool provides a useful resource. It provides a mechanism to review and reflect on progress in embedding a whole-system approach to health and well-being into core business and culture. The Self-Review Tool is an online questionnaire structured under five headings: Leadership and Governance; Service Provision; Facilities and Environment; Communication, Information and Marketing; and Academic, Personal, Social, and Professional Development. Once a university has completed the questionnaire, a graphic "traffic light" representation (red, amber, green) of progress will be generated, highlighting areas where the university is achieving progress and those areas where additional input is needed (UK Healthy Universities Network, 2020).

4.5.6   Evaluating Complex Whole System Initiatives

Focusing on this higher level of evaluation, there is no simple "how to" guide to evaluating complex whole system initiatives—although it becomes even more important to utilize multi-method approaches (in order to deal with complexity more effectively) and to integrate outcomes and indicators that relate to both "health" and the core business of the setting (e.g. for a school or university it might include student experience, retention, and achievement; staff performance and productivity; corporate social responsibility).

The literature also suggests that there is a growing appreciation of the value of theory-based approaches, examples being **Realist and Theory of Change Evaluation**. Realist evaluation (Pawson & Tilley, 1997) does not seek to factor out context in the way that experimentation or randomized controlled trials tend to. Instead, it seeks to understand how causal mechanisms work within specific contexts, thereby leading to outcomes. It thus looks inside what is often referred to as the "black box" of evaluation, addressing process and outcome evaluation at the same time, and moving from the traditional question "does this work?" to ask "what works, for whom, in what circumstances, and why?"

The Theory of Change Approach (Connell & Kubisch, 1998) serves as both a planning/development and evaluation framework. In exploring links between activities, outcomes, and contexts, it argues that it is necessary to make explicit the chain of assumptions and hypotheses on which an initiative is based. The approach draws on and combines insights from both realist evaluation and logic modelling, and has been developed as a means of evaluating complex community initiatives—with a number of stages: identify long-term goals and assumptions behind them, carry out backward mapping to reveal the necessary preconditions to achieve these goals, identify the interventions that will be undertaken as a means of achieving the required changes, develop outcome indicators to enable the initiative to be assessed, and then write a narrative to explain the logic of the initiative. In this way, it explores both process and outcomes, tracking the stages that make up overall programs, mapping the links between the programs that comprise a larger initiative, and enabling a more sophisticated and utility-focused understanding not only of whether something works, but also of why and how it works or does not work in particular situations.

4.6   Challenges of Monitoring and Evaluating Healthy Settings

Many evaluation efforts are focused on vertical interventions that are narrowly oriented toward limited circumscribed changes rather than looking at changes in the whole system of the setting in which the initiatives take place. Programs that mainly focus on risk factor interventions or specific diseases or problems will fail to take into consideration the complexity of multiple interventions aimed at strengthening the support system within a particular setting. To look comprehensively at how a setting might be influential in promoting or maintaining health, it is necessary to look at the complexity of relationships, structures, and processes; and to examine the connections among systems, environments, people, and behaviors. This requires the use of multiple approaches and methods for evaluation and addressing different evaluation questions focusing on a whole health promotion system, characterized by synergies and integration. It means looking at where the interaction of two or more influences creates an effect greater than the sum of their individual effects.

Politicians may want to know whether their policies provide a return on investment and whether their political agendas are being advanced through a healthy-settings initiative (Dooris et al., 2007). This might be very difficult to demonstrate concretely. Also, the time frame in which politicians and other funders might want to see changes and the reality of time it takes to produce those changes may not coincide. For this reason, it is important to demonstrate results that might appear long before the harder-to-reach outcomes are achieved, so that information can be used to positively contribute to informed decision-making.

Since settings-based health promotion seeks to address issues of equity and power relations, within, outside, and across settings, assessment and evaluation efforts must address these issues as well. The effectiveness of healthy settings initiatives must also be judged in terms of their focus on organizational structures, policies, and practices that redress inequalities, and their successful advocacy for macro-level social, economic, and political change. This requires the forming of partnerships among a diversity of stakeholders from multiple sectors, and this collaboration and construction and maintenance of networks must be part of what is evaluated as part of enabling or inhibiting successful healthy settings experiences. The patterns of relationships that make up systems are essentially qualitative and, to be understood, must be mapped.

Most funding for evaluation is for issue-based rather than settings-based initiatives; and most research designed to evaluate complex, ecological programs does not qualify for inclusion within systematic reviews and meta-analyses (Dooris et al., 2007). And clearly it is easier to evaluate a system-wide change in a smaller setting over a larger and more complex one.

In order to document what works, it will be important to take into consideration the context in which initiatives are conducted—how and under what circumstances activities are carried out, and what works better, for whom, and under what circumstances. And in terms of effectiveness, it may be easier to demonstrate whole-system change within a small setting such as a primary school than in a large multilayered setting such as a university, or indeed, a city (Dooris et al., 2007).

Additionally, since creating a healthy setting implies creating a well-functioning system, its evaluation must focus on interrelationships and seeing patterns of change over time, rather than taking a snapshot of a situation at just one moment or one point in a process. The interaction of the various components of the system needs to be taken into consideration as a whole process, along with the interaction and synergies with other settings. The evaluation must look at the whole and attempt to map and understand these interrelationships, interactions, and synergies within and between settings – with regard to different groups of the population, components of the system, and "health" issues (Dooris, 2006).

Harnessing and applying thinking from critical realism and complexity theory offers potential for overcoming the limitations of traditional evaluation models and helping generate evidence of effectiveness for ecological, whole-system settings-based health promotion. Critical realism looks at the interaction between context, events, and people, and what are the effects of certain interventions that are implemented in specific times and places and with certain populations. Evaluation then would be looking at unpacking the complex components of programs to identify how and why programs work. A chain reaction of events may get triggered by healthy settings interventions and changes that will trigger different outcomes depending upon the conditions and actions that take place over time.

In contrast, complexity theory looks at the autonomy of people whose actions are interconnected with others working and living in the healthy setting, and whose actions might change over time based upon experience gained and lessons learned. It means that evaluation should focus on the identification of new ways to harness the creativity and knowledge of frontline staff, by stimulating and supporting ways for them to share experiences and learn from each other (Dooris et al., 2007).

4.7   Conclusions

Monitoring and evaluation of healthy settings can only be meaningfully tackled through adopting holistic and comprehensive approaches within the places where people are born, live, play, work, and study throughout their lives. This means combining several assessment and evaluation methods to explore links among activities, outcomes, and contexts, taking into account the relationships between people and their environments. Effective healthy settings initiatives begin with a vision and strategic goals, but they also include accounting for context in terms of needs and assets of the population, along with the identification of a rationale for the chosen range of "interventions," expected consequences, and performance indicators. The monitoring and evaluation components will examine how a whole system is working, as well as assessing the effectiveness of individual programs and projects. This will include measuring both process and outcomes, tracking the stages that make up overall programs, mapping the links between and among different programs that comprise an entire healthy settings initiative, and including an understanding not only of whether something works, but why and how it works or does not work in particular situations.

Acknowledgments The author would like to express a special thanks to the following people for their valuable contributions to the content of this chapter: Albert Lee, Evelyne de Leeuw, and Mark Dooris, and to Cynthia J. Berg for helping with edits and organization of this chapter.

References

Bartholomew, L. K., Parcel, G. S., & Kok, G. (1998). Intervention mapping: A process for developing theory- and evidence-based health education programs. *Health Education & Behavior, 25*(5), 545–563.

Brandt, E., Schmidt, W., Dziewas, R., & Groene, O. (2005). Implementing the health promoting hospitals strategy through a combined application of the EFQM excellence model and the balanced scorecard. In O. Groene & M. Garcia-Barbero (Eds.), *Health promotion in hospitals: Evidence and quality management*. WHO Regional Office for Europe.

Centers for Disease Control and Prevention (CDC). (2019). https://www.cdc.gov/gshs/index.htm

Clift, S., Bruun Jensen, B., & The Health Promoting School: International Advances in Theory, Evaluation and Practice. (2005). *Research programme for environmental and health Education at the Danish University of Education*. Danish University of Education Press.

Connell, J. P., & Kubisch, A. C. (1998). Applying a theory of change approach to the evaluation of comprehensive community initiatives: Progress, prospects, and problems. In K. Fulbright-Anderson, A. C. Kubisch, & J. P. Connell (Eds.), *New approaches to evaluating community initiatives. Volume 2: Theory, measurement, and analysis* (pp. 15–44). The Aspen Institute.

Corvalan, C., Briggs, D., & Kjellstrom, T. (1997). Development of environmental health indicators. In D. Briggs, C. Corvalan, & M. Nurminen (Eds.) *Linkage methods for environment and health analysis: General guidelines*, A report of the Health and Environment Analysis for Decision Making Project (HEADLAMP).

de Leeuw, E. (2009). Evidence for Healthy Cities: reflections on practice, method and theory. *Health Promotion International, 24*(Suppl_1), i19–i36.

de Leeuw, E. (2011). Do Healthy Cities work? A logic of method for assessing impact and outcome of healthy cities. *Journal of Urban Health: Bulletin of the New York Academy of Medicine, 89*(2). https://doi.org/10.1007/s11524-011-9617-y. The New York Academy of Medicine.

de Leeuw, E., Green, G., Dyakova, M., Spanswick, L., & Palmer, N. (2015). European Healthy Cities evaluation: Conceptual framework and methodology. *Health Promotion International, 30*(S1), i8–i17. https://doi.org/10.1093/heapro/dav036

de Leeuw, E., Martin, E., & Waqanivalu, T. (2018). Healthy Islands. In M. Van den Bosch & W. Bird (Eds.), *Oxford textbook of nature and public health: The role of nature in improving the health of a population* (p. 285). Oxford University Press.

de Leeuw, E., & Skovgaard, T. (2005). Utility-driven evidence for healthy cities: Problems with evidence generation and application. *Social Science and Medicine, 61*, 1331–1341.

de Leeuw, E., & Webster, P. (2018). *The healthy settings approach: Healthy Cities and environmental health Indicators. 8.6 in Oxford Textbook of Nature and Public Health: The role of nature in improving the health of a population*. OUP.

Denman, S., Moon, A., Parsons, C., & Stears, D. F. (2002). *The health promoting school: Policy, research and practice*. Routledge/Falmer.

Dooris, M. (2006). Healthy settings: Challenges to generating evidence of effectiveness. *Health Promotion International, 21*(1), 55–65.

Dooris, M., Poland, B., Kolbe, L., de Leeuw, E., McCall, D., & Wharf-Higgins, J. (2007). Healthy settings: Building evidence for the effectiveness of whole system health promotion – Challenges & future directions. In D. V. McQueen & C. M. Jones (Eds.), *Global perspectives on health promotion effectiveness* (pp. 327–352). Springer Science & Business Media. ISBN: 9780387709734.

Esping-Andersen, G. (2013). *The three worlds of welfare capitalism*. John Wiley & Sons.

Groene, O., Brandt, E., Schnmidt, W., & Moeller, J. (2009). The balanced scorecard of acute settings: Development process, definition of 20 strategic objectives and implementation. *International Journal for Quality in Health Care, 21*(4), 259–271. https://doi.org/10.1093/intqhc/mzp024

Institute of Medicine. (2002). *Community programs to promote youth development*. National Academy of Sciences.

International Union for Health Promotion and Education (IUHPE). (2017, June). *IUHPE Position Paper on Health Impact Assessment*.

Lee, A., Cheng, F. F. K., & St. Leger, L.H. (2005). Evaluating health promoting schools in Hong Kong: the development of a framework. *Health Promotion International, 20*(2), 177–186.

Lee, A., Lo, A. S. C., Keung, M. W., et al. (2019). Effective health promoting school for better health of children and adolescents: indicators for success. *BMC Public Health, 19*, 1088. https://doi.org/10.1186/s12889-019-7425-6

Lister-Sharp, L., Chapman, S., Stewart-Brown, S., & Sowden, A. (1999). *Health promoting schools and health promotion in schools: two systematic reviews. Database of Abstracts of Reviews of Effects (DARE): Quality-assessed Reviews [Internet]*. University of York.

Moore, K., & Lippman, L. (2004). *What do children need to flourish? Conceptualizing and measuring indicators of positive development*. Springer.

Mukoma, W., & Flisher, A. (2004). Evaluations of health promoting schools: A review of nine studies. *Health Promotion International, 19*(3), 357–358. https://doi.org/10.1093/heapro/dah309

Nutbeam, D. (1996). Health outcomes and health promotion-defining success in health promotion. *Health Promotion Journal of Australia, 6*(2), 58–60.

Pan American Health Organization (PAHO). (2007). *Guide to economic evaluation in health promotion*. Washington, DC.

Pan American Health Organization (PAHO). (2011). *Guide to participatory evaluation of healthy municipalities, cities and communities*. Washington, DC.

Pattenden, J. (1998). Indicators for the health promoting school. In *First workshop on practice of evaluation of the health promoting school – Models, experience and perspectives* (pp. 39–41). World Health Organization.

Pawson, R., & Tilley, N. (1997). *Realistic evaluation*. Sage.

Stears, D., Holland, J., & Parsons, C. (2000). *Healthy schools assessment tool: An instrument for monitoring and recording health promotion assets in schools*. The National Assembly of Wales.

Substance Abuse and Mental Health Services Administration (SAMHSA). Retrieved March 5, 2019., from http://zone.msn.com/en/mssolitairecollection/default.htm?intgid=hp_card_1

Tsouros, A., & Green, G. (2009). Special supplement on European Healthy Cities. *Health Promotion International, 24*(Suppl. 1), 1–107.

UK Healthy Universities Network. *Evaluating Healthy Universities*. Retrieved January 7, 2020., from https://healthyuniversities.ac.uk/research-development-evaluation/evaluating-healthy-universities/

Voljoen, C. J., Kirsten, T. G. J., Haglund, B., & Tillgren, P. (2005). Towards the development of indicators for health promoting schools. In S. Clift & B. B. Jensen (Eds.), *The health promoting school: International advances in theory, evaluation and practice*. Danish University Press.

Whitfield, M., Machaczek, K., & Green, G. (2013). Developing a model to estimate the potential impact of municipal investment on city health. *Journal of Urban Health, 90*(1), 62–73.

World Health Organization. (1981). *Development of indicators for monitoring progress towards health for all by the year 2000, health for all series, No. 4*. World Health Organization.

World Health Organization (WHO). (2008). *Urban HEART: Urban health equity assessment and response tool*. Kobe.

Part II
Applying the Settings-Based Approach to Key Settings

Chapter 5
Healthy Cities

Evelyne de Leeuw

5.1 Introduction

'Healthy Cities' are often considered the mothership of the healthy settings perspective. Indeed, if we take 'healthy settings' as originating from the adoption of the Ottawa Charter for Health Promotion in November 1986, Healthy Cities were the first setting considered as a demonstration effort of the Charter.

In this chapter, Healthy Cities will be positioned and contextualized in both in the modern health promotion movement, and in the urban world that we have come to live in. In placing this setting in history, a very narrow and dogmatic approach to defining Healthy Cities is framed on the one hand, and an eclectic much broader view on the other. Following this the future of health in cities is identified and the chapter ends with connecting the Healthy City story with the other Theme Cities we will encounter on the way.

5.2 Healthy Cities: A Brief History

There has always been a connection between urban growth, urban planning and public health. In the early great cities of the Levant and the Indus Valley, up to ten millennia ago, designs and regulations were developed and implemented (and a legacy left in the archaeological record) that sanitation, safe food storage, and access to facilities pertinent to health were a key concern of city dwellers and their rulers. Aqueducts and waste disposal management systems were features of cities of Western antiquity (the Greek civilization and Roman empire), but have also been

E. de Leeuw (✉)
Centre for Health Equity Training, Research and Evaluation (CHETRE), UNSW, Sydney, NSW, Australia
e-mail: e.deleeuw@unsw.edu.au

© Springer Nature Switzerland AG 2022
S. Kokko, M. Baybutt (eds.), *Handbook of Settings-Based Health Promotion*,
https://doi.org/10.1007/978-3-030-95856-5_5

found in the urban environments of the past great empires of the Americas, Africa and East Asia.

In later centuries, cities were the places that were literally the pivots of the great epidemic scourges of the world, including the bubonic plague that ravaged the world, traveling along the centres of trade along the urban centres along the Silk Road. The Black Death came from East China and ended up in north-west Europe in the summers of the middle of the fourteenth century. This global epidemic led to urban health responses that are still deployed today, such as quarantine, originally designed to protect cities from the arrival of infectious disease (Venice, cf. Crawshaw, 2016). 'Reverse quarantine', that is, expelling citizens from city living to pest houses outside the walls was also invented in these days. In some urban environments the concern for health went further than in others. In Germany, the 'Medizinische Polizey' (medical police) became a branch of government to maintain sanitation standards in the seventeenth century.

When Baron Hausmann famously was charged with redesigning Paris in the nineteenth century he took into account many considerations for his modern city, including efficiency, military purposes, airiness, and sanitation. Grounding his idea partially in the accomplishments of the French hygienist and early sociologist Louis-René Villermé (instrumental in the French *'mouvement hygiéniste'* to legislate for the 'Première Loi sur l'urbanisme interdisant la location des logements insalubres' in 1850: the 'First Urban Planning Act Prohibiting the Rent of Substandard Housing'), George Eugene Haussmann (1809–1891) set out to *'aérer, unifier, et embellir'* (provide air, unify, and beautify) the great city. The grand boulevards radiating through the city have become emblematic for Parisian charm, but Haussmann clearly had health in mind in designing the infrastructure; in his memoirs he wrote: *'The underground galleries are an organ of the great city, functioning like an organ of the human body, without seeing the light of day; clean and fresh water, light and heat circulate like the various fluids whose movement and maintenance serves the life of the body; the secretions are taken away mysteriously and don't disturb the good functioning of the city and without spoiling its beautiful exterior'* (De Moncan & Heurteux, 2002).

Similar sentiments could be identified later in the nineteenth century in more nature-based programmes of work such as the oeuvre of Frederick Law Olmsted (designing, among many others, Central Park in New York and Mont Royal in Montreal as the lungs of the city) and Ebenezer Howard (the father of the Garden City movement in the British Empire—in response to the obviously filthy cities of the Industrial Revolution).

But the absolutely essential role of cities in the birth of modern public health is generally identified with a bunch of British medical doctors, lawyers and engineers in the second half of the nineteenth century who went down in history as 'the Hygienists'. Famously it was 'royal physician' John Snow who identified water as a source of an infectious agent causing cholera in inner-city London, taking the handle off the Broad Street pump and thereby creating the first 'modern' public health intervention.

In summary, from the Neolithic Demographic Transition (where humanity moved from hunter-gatherer to settler status—de Leeuw, 2017), urbanisation and health have been connected intimately in social, cultural, spatial and economic ways. Where and how we live creates opportunities and challenges to health and well-being, and urban living exacerbates both. It is therefore no surprise that the emergence of modern public health, through its evolutionary waves, is profoundly interwoven with processes of statehood, industrialization and urbanization. Analytical accounts of the evolution of 'modern' public health (since the early 1800s) distinguish five waves that, rather than superseding each other, have built joint momentum to find ourselves, in the early 2000s, in a 'health society' (Fig. 5.1, de Leeuw, 2020). Davies et al. (2014) and Kickbusch (2007) also describe that each of these 'waves' are inherently political, even the 'technical' structural, biomedical and clinical waves, each of which has been perhaps more socio-political than technical (see, for instance, Hommels et al., 2014).

The different waves in public health all build on and reinforce each other, rather than supersede previous stages. An early adopter of the social and cultural waves at the interface of (public) health and urban development was Professor Leonard Duhl—as the first Director of the 'Long-Range Planning' unit of the US National Institute of Mental Health, he convened a group of highly interdisciplinary thinkers to explore the linkages between mental health and urbanization—these 'Space Cadets' contributed to the volume we find to be the foundation of the modern

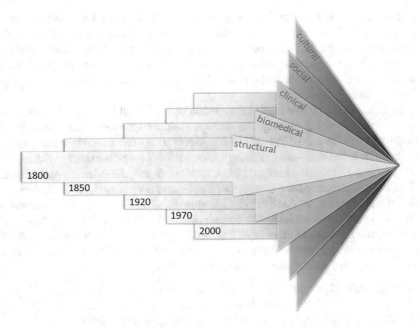

Fig. 5.1 Five waves of modern public health (de Leeuw (2020). Health promotion. In J. Firth, C. Conlon & T. Cox, eds., *Oxford Textbook of Medicine, 6th Edition*. Copyright © Oxford University Press, 2020. Reproduced with permission of the Licensor through PLSclear)

Healthy Cities movement. Contributors of this '*The Urban Condition – People and Policy in the Metropolis*' (Duhl, 1963) discuss health, housing, ethology, violence, mental health, pathology, planning and matters that have only re-emerged since the turn of the twenty-first century: climate change, systems thinking and complexity in the urban environment. Duhl teamed up in the mid-1980s with one Trevor Hancock, who was the Chief Medical Officer of the City of Toronto in 1984—the year that saw the tenth anniversary of the landmark Lalonde Report in which a government (Canada) for the first time in history committed to what we would now call the 'social determinants of health'. Hancock, Duhl and the WHO European office representatives met at the celebrations of the Toronto event where the ambition for that city to be the first 'Healthy City' was firmed up. For Ilona Kickbusch this was a serendipitous occasion. She had been crafting a future for health promotion with a range of colleagues and agencies that were at the cutting edge of systems thinking for health (de Leeuw & Harris-Roxas, 2016). One of them, John Ashton, was Chief Medical Officer for Liverpool—a town that in many ways already was seeking to be a 'Healthy City' (Ashton, 1992). Ashton became a driving force behind European emancipatory urban health programmes.

5.3   The Ottawa Charter, Healthy Cities, and a Movement

The critical year for settings and health promotion became 1986. Based on her encounter with Duhl and Hancock, and the ongoing European health promotion developments, Kickbusch organized an exploratory meeting with a small number of European city governments in the spring of 1986. The enthusiasm and potential for 'Healthy Cities' turned out to be many times greater than anticipated in anyone's wildest dreams.

The Ottawa Charter for Health Promotion was adopted in November 1986, and its signatories (meeting participants and institutional sponsors—the WHO, Health Canada and the Canadian Public Health Association) felt strongly empowered to take the vision forward—and Healthy Cities kick off enthusiastically with a group of cities from European member states, support from public health agencies and their leaders (including June Crown in London and Slobodan Lang in Zagreb, and Leo Kaprio as well as Jo Asvall, WHO Europe Regional Directors) and substantial enthusiasm from local social health entrepreneurs. Hancock and Duhl (1986), at the request of the European Office of WHO, did a systematic and brief review of what was known to create health in the urban context 'Ottawa style'. They accumulated eleven qualities a Healthy City should strive to attain:

- A clean, safe, high quality physical environment (including housing quality).
- An ecosystem which is stable now and sustainable in the long term.
- A strong, mutually supportive and non-exploitative community.
- A high degree of public participation in and control over the decisions affecting one's life, health and well-being.

- The meeting of basic needs (food, water, shelter, income, safety, work) for all the city's people.
- Access to a wide variety of experiences and resources with the possibility of multiple contacts, interaction and communication.
- A diverse, vital and innovative city economy.
- Encouragement of connectedness with the past, with the cultural and biological heritage and with other groups and individuals.
- A city form that is compatible with and enhances the above parameters and behaviours.
- An optimum level of appropriate public health and sick care services accessible to all.
- High health status (both high positive health status and low disease status).

A handful of European cities signed up to this experiment in Lisbon (April 1986) and Dusseldorf (June 1987) meetings. According to Baum and Brown (1989), the participants agreed that

- Health is a social rather than medical matter.
- Health is the responsibility of all city services.
- Health should be monitored by physical, social, aesthetic and environmental indicators of well-being.
- Health is an outcome of collaboration between community members, planners and providers of public and private sector services.
- The city should be a cradle of good health and not merely a survival unit.

This was a radically different mindset from what had been an influential 'urban health' perspective that was driven by epidemiologists attempting to measure and correlate health parameters against city indicators (see also Kim et al., 2020). Initially European, but soon to follow Canadian, Australian and New Zealand, and Japanese networks of Healthy Cities quickly departed from existing traditions in that area. In many places around the world (and notably in the English-speaking global North) centres and institutes had emerged since the 1950s that predominantly looked at the intriguing epidemiology of cities and their health patterns. The differences between urban and rural, the sometimes enormous inequities between neighbourhoods, and industrial/occupational issues involving risk management, etc., were driving these establishments. The legacy of this work continues, for instance, in the impressive 'urban liveability' number crunching by experts like Billie Giles-Corti and her team (Higgs et al., 2019).

Healthy Cities were different. Invariably championed by engaged and visionary connectors, they explicitly embraced a value-based perspective on what a city might be and become. As Hancock and Duhl (1986) stated in their foundation document, a Healthy City is a place…

> …that is continually creating and improving those physical and social environments and expanding those community resources which enable people to mutually support each other in performing all the functions of life and in developing to their maximum potential.

So, Healthy Cities are a process and a journey, much more than an exercise in epidemiology and local government management. The fast growth and excitement around the world, however, was sometimes at the detriment of sound science. Healthy Cities, in their decades of evolution, have demonstrated that community activism and entrepreneurial spirit must always be coupled with a sound foundation in data.

In managing the unexpected enthusiasm for Healthy Cities in Europe, WHO decided on a process in which cities could apply and be designated to be an 'official' Healthy City. In a series of approximately 5-year phases, the WHO, in cooperation with cities, set objectives for each Phase. Apart from some standard requirements (e.g. the express political commitment to Healthy Cities values and principles; the obligation to resource personnel, office, and networking; the existence of an intersectoral steering group) each phase set specific goals Cities should pursue. In response to the lack of a sound numerical evidence base, these included a *Healthy City Development Plan* and commitments to data collection and processing. Also, specific themes were to be pursued, including tobacco-free cities, active transport and health equity.

Cities outside Europe developed along substantively diverging patterns. Other regional offices of the WHO provided guidance and support in different ways. On two occasions 'Healthy Cities' were the subject of the annual World Health Days—in 1996 and in 2010 (Fig. 5.2). World Health Days are coordinated by the Geneva headquarters of the WHO; in 1996 a dedicated professional (Dr Greg Goldstein) enthusiastically sponsored the global rollout of the World Health Day, celebrated by thousands of cities and organizations around the world. In 2010 the world had changed, and there was a WHO institution expressly dedicated to urban health: the WHO Kobe Centre (WKC). WKC led the development of *Urban HEART* (Urban Health Equity Assessment and Response Tool; Prasad, 2018)—which sits

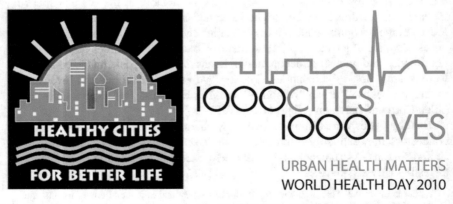

Fig. 5.2 World Health Day 'Healthy City' logos: 1996 (left) and 2010 (right). (Reproduced from World Health Day, World Health Organization, Copyright 1996; 2010, https://www.who.int/docstore/world-health-day/en/documents1996/yellowi.pdf;   https://www.who.int/world-health-day/2010/WHDtoolkit2010_en_full.pdf?ua=1. Accessed on 6 October 2021)

somewhere between the classical epidemiology–driven urban health paradigm and the community-led value-based Healthy Cities perspective.

Healthy Cities networks in different parts of the world expanded and evolved to meet unique local needs based on distinct sociopolitical and geospatial histories. They all embrace human values rather than an epidemiological risk paradigm as their foundations, and most—at least rhetorically—recognize that the pursuit of health is an intersectoral journey and that health is not the result of urban development but a critical driver of it. As Curitiba mayor Jaime Lerner once said: '*Cities are not the problems, cities are the solutions*' (de Leeuw, 2018).

By a recent account, the smallest self-declared Healthy Community is '*l'Isle-Aux-Grues*' (less than 200 souls on an island in the mouth of the Quebec St. Lawrence River) and the largest is Shanghai (over 24 million, China Statistical Yearbook, 2018). Although it is hard to gauge the global number of value-based Healthy Cities (as there are only two formal accounts—the WHO/EURO-designated Healthy Cities and accredited networks, and the membership of the Alliance for Healthy Cities—see www.alliance-healthycities.com), we estimate that there are over 15,000 formally and self-declared Healthy Cities following the original 1980s principles (de Leeuw & Simos, 2017). Necessarily, their foci are dramatically different. Some cities struggle with basic sanitation, while others face enormous challenges in air pollution. Some cities are already confronted with the consequences of climate change, such as rising sea levels (e.g. Tarawa, the capital of Pacific nation Kiribati—one of the most densely populated cities in the world; de Leeuw et al., 2018), whereas others face other climate change–related challenges (e.g. urban heat islands).

Some Healthy Cities have endured and sustained themselves since the mid-1980s, including two original Australian pilot sites (Kiama/Illawarra and Noarlunga/Onkaparinga), initiatives across Canada (including the thriving *Réseau québécois de villes et villages en santé*), veterans in Europe like Rennes, Pécs and Horsens and early adopters across Japan and South Korea.

Healthy City initiatives have become increasingly sophisticated in their approaches of health equity and social determinants of health, but at the same time the value propositions that drive systems change are constantly challenged and (re) discovered by local governments and well-meaning global individual and institutional players. Especially in what has now become known as 'the urban century', the city has become a flashpoint for evolutionary change, stagnation as well as entrepreneurship.

5.4 Health-Promoting Cities or Health Promotion in Cities?

When Healthy Cities kicked off in the mid-1980s, they quickly became a movement, as alluded to in the first European account of its rapid growth (Tsouros, 1991). They were among the first of a series of international networks that brought together local governments for global action. Others included, for instance, efforts in environmental health, stimulated by the 1992 Rio de Janeiro Earth Summit (e.g. Elander & Lidskog, 2000). But in subsequent decades we have witnessed a proliferation of 'Theme Cities' (so dubbed by Davies, 2015). To sample this smorgasbord, these now include international networks around Just Cities, Green Towns and Cities, Sustainable Cities, Transition Towns and EcoDistricts, Winter Cities, Resilient Cities, Creative Cities, Knowledge Cities, Safe Cities and Communities, Festive Cities, Slow Cities, Happy Cities, Smart Cities, Child-Friendly Cities, Age-Friendly Cities, and Inclusive Cities. In fact, since 2016 there are two distinct networks of Healthy Cities: One grounding itself in the original value system established by the European office of the WHO in the 1980s, and another one sponsored by American philanthropist Michael Bloomberg and the Geneva Headquarters of the WHO ('*The Partnership for Healthy Cities is a prestigious global network of cities committed to saving lives by preventing noncommunicable diseases (NCDs) and injuries*'; Partnership for Healthy Cities, 2018). Forbat et al. (2018) sought to assess a dozen of 'Theme Cities' against parameters that would demonstrate a commitment to health equity, health and sustainable development, and systems approaches to upstream (distal) determinants health (in some circles called 'Health in All Policies'; cf. de Leeuw, 2017).

Such an analysis aligns with addressing the question whether 'Healthy Cities' deal with health promotion in urban contexts, or see the urban environment in its broadest sense as a health-promoting platform. The preferred evolution of insight in the settings for health heuristic seems to argue that the setting as such is a system for health promotion. The question can be addressed in two ways—normatively and empirically. Forbat et al. (2018) took the former course of action (Table 5.1).

They produced a systematic inventory for 12 Theme Cities and sought to document each of these global networks' credentials. These included the identification of a foundation document; a definition; operational and/or ideological principles that have been endorsed by a sponsor or membership representative body; the availability of critical appraisal in the peer-reviewed international scholarly literature; membership or sponsorship governance arrangements; the presence of explicit commitments to human development, health, equity and sustainability principles; and international 'reach' in terms of the number of local government members and estimated total population reached. In Table 5.1, some of the findings are summarized. These suggest that Sustainable Cities and Transition Towns score highest on their potential to address health, politics and equity on a systems level, and that 'Ottawa Charter'–style Healthy Cities, Resilient Cities, Inclusive Cities, and Age-Friendly Cities are runners-up. However, the evidence must generally be contextualized. For instance, in the Resilient Cities Network cities set their own key priorities—and these may not always resonate with a strongly political agenda for equity and sustainability. The City of New York identifies equity as a key challenge for its resilience and seeks to design and implement durable policies and infrastructures to embed equity in its work. Other cities will not have identified such priorities and would therefore not qualify as systems-driven urban environments for health.

To provide an assessment of the degree to which (Healthy) cities have moved towards the 'health promoting settings' end of the scale is a much more difficult

Table 5.1 A comparison of the health equity dimensions of selected Theme Cities (Forbat et al., 2018)

	Statement of principles and operations?	Number of citations in the literature (Nov 2018)?	Sponsor public / private	People reached (*N* cities, *N* people estimate)	Assessment: politics & equity (1 [not] to 5 [explicit]) – estimates
Healthy Cities	Yes; Ottawa Charter 1986, 'yellow booklets'	150	WHO	10,000 At least 0.5B	4
Healthy Cities (Bloomberg)	No; website commitment to NCDs and injuries	335	WHO / Bloomberg	50 Around 0.5B	1
Smart Cities	No, although some national government policies (India)	1062	Smart Cities	~1000 ?	1
Cittaslow	Yes, based on Slow Food (Greve, Chianti, 1999)	102	Cities	238 ?	2
Resilient Cities	Yes; Rockefeller Foundation 100 Resilient Cities 2013	754	Rockefeller	100 Around 1B	4
Transition Towns	Yes, but meshed with community and sustainability ideals	90	Communities	1200 ?	5
Happy Cities	Montgomery book 2013	140	Consultancy	? ?	2
Creative Cities	Yes, two sources from creative industries 2006, 2012	3054	Creative Cities	116 ?	2
Inclusive Cities	Yes, Habitat and World Bank, early 2000s	234	World Bank	? ?	4
Sustainable Cities	Yes, Aalborg and Basque Declarations 1994/2016	906	EU/Aalborg/ Basque	479 Around 1B	5
Child-Friendly Cities	Yes, UNICEF and Habitat 1996	111	UNICEF	? ?	3
Age-friendly Cities	Yes, WHO from early 2000s, in EURO and EU formally AFEE, 2007	673	WHO	500 115M	4

question. Anecdotally, de Leeuw and Simos (2017) see the full spectrum in each of the world's geographic regions they cover (Africa, both Francophone and Anglophone—Lusophone missing; Eastern Mediterranean; Latin America; North America; Europe; Asia and Far East; Oceania; it should be noted that they identify a dearth of Healthy Cities initiatives in the Indian subcontinent).

There are few comprehensive evaluation efforts with the exception of efforts throughout the phases of the European project. In the most recent assessment (de Leeuw, Green, Dyakova, et al., 2015; de Leeuw, Green, Spanswick, & Palmer, 2015; de Leeuw, Green, Tsouros, et al., 2015; de Leeuw, Kickbusch, Palmer, & Spanswick, 2015; Farrington et al., 2015; Grant, 2015; Green et al., 2015; Jackisch et al., 2015; Ritsatakis et al., 2015; Simos et al., 2015; Tsouros, 2015; and Tsouros et al., 2015) the network of European Healthy Cities demonstrated that upstream, systems-based and sustainable policymaking within accountable governance systems can be attributed to adopting the value system that this network has been advocating for 30 years.

5.5 The Future

The Healthy Cities vision that started in the mid-1980s (and was grounded in urban planning efforts starting as far back as the dawn of human civilization in Mesopotamia) has endured for more than three decades. It clearly resonates with strongly felt value systems at the local level.

In mid-February 2018, the World Health Organization European Regional Office convened a strategic session with leaders of local government where hundreds of Mayors committed to better, more equitable and sustainable cities for all.

Their Copenhagen Consensus is based on eight key pillars:

1. We commit to take action together to improve the health and well-being of all who live, love, learn, work and play in our cities.
2. A healthy city leads by example, by emphasizing a human focus in societal development and by prioritizing investment in people to improve equity and inclusion through enhanced empowerment.
3. A healthy city leads by example, with the social, physical and cultural environments aligned to create a place that is actively inclusive, and facilitates the pursuit of health and well-being for all.
4. A healthy city leads by example, by ensuring the participation of all individuals and communities in the decisions that affect them and the places in which they live, work, love and play.
5. A healthy city leads by example, by striving for enhanced community prosperity and strengthened assets through values-based governance of common goods and services.
6. A healthy city leads by example, by promoting peace through inclusive societies that focus on places, participation, prosperity and the planet, while putting people at the centre of all policies and actions.

7. A healthy city leads by example, by ensuring that the protection of the planet is at the heart of all city policies, both internal and external.
8. We commit to act collectively with other cities in both the WHO European Region and globally, through a focus on people, participation, prosperity, planet, places and peace, for the health and well-being of all, to meet the urgent and transformative demands of the 2030 Agenda.

These commitments reflect recent insights around the world that change happens locally, and often trickles up rather than down. Tobacco control has been championed by local communities and professionals first before it entered national and international policy agendas. When President Donald Trump renounced the US commitment to the Kyoto Protocol and Paris Climate Accord within the United Nations Framework Convention on Climate Change (UNFCCC), it took only days for hundreds of US cities (and states) to commit to the internationally agreed goals, and sometimes even surpass them, a political feat not (yet) seen in Australian state, territory or local government—it appears here we do not want to rock the boat too much and engage in a friendly, perhaps somewhat technocratic, and certainly politically invisible 'Cities Power Partnership'.

Such 'policy transfer', according to the theory, may happen horizontally (between similar levels of governance, e.g., State–State or municipality–municipality) but also vertically (from local to higher levels of governance and government). Horizontal policy transfer could be characterized by the term 'scaling wide', whereas vertical policy transfer is a case of 'scaling up'. Popularly, however, 'scaling up' is taken to mean both. Policy transfer (i.e., the adoption of—policy—approaches by larger groups of institutional actors; this may include non-state agents such as communities and industry) is dependent on networking and communication. Such networking and communication, however, must not be 'random' but cunningly policy relevant and bespoke to particular governance level and personal characteristics. Good policy transfer is enabled by strong evidence foundations, but must also be 'quick and dirty' as Paul Cairney (2016) has demonstrated.

So, what is different at the local level? And how can we use the local uniqueness to engage more comprehensively and sustainably in creating health, health promotion and health policy that is not only relevant for 'ordinary' people but will have an effect on larger and higher systems levels? As Benjamin Barber says in 'If Mayors Rule the World' (2013): Cities collect the garbage. Local government sees and engages with issues and communities—in different places around the world not necessarily always with great accountability or responsiveness, but the local is the level of government and governance where things happen.

In most local government areas around the world the governance and accountability lines between affected communities and individuals and elected representatives have the potential to be short and responsive. Whether local government is actually empowered to influence decisions that directly affect the lives of their communities is not always clear. For instance, in the Australian state of New South Wales, local government has little or no planning authority over larger infrastructural developments, leaving the City of Liverpool with a major international airport development in its footprint (and very little influence over its shape; cf. Crimeen et al., 2018). With the growth of interest in health political science, the evidence base for capacity building programmes is also firming up.

But this is not the only, and possibly not even the most important, reason why investment in local health policy development is so essential. The rhetoric that we are living in a global village that has been seen around since the 1960s and the publications out of the Club of Rome is ever more a reality. The fact that local meets global is integral to the Sustainable Development Goals (the SDGs) and the New Urban Agenda—one of the first concrete glocal commitments to making a better world.

Interestingly, not every jurisdiction seems to embrace the SDGs as enthusiastically. This may well be at their own detriment. The SDGs were formulated after extensive consultation rounds with states, civil society and industry, and are a shared global pledge. Yes, this involves collaboration and solidarity between all stakeholders, but it also strives to motivate communities and organizations locally and nationally in each and every country.

The pursuit of and commitment to the SDGs is very much a mainstream concern in most OECD countries. Some of the SDGs—and the associated more specific sets of targets and indicators—are of course less relevant to some parts of the world than they are to others.

There is an important question, then, when it comes to the future of settings for health in local governance arenas. Local governments see their global responsibilities—whether it comes to the consequences of climate change, control of NCDs like obesity that drive global life expectancies downward, or an infectious disease like COVID-19 that requires governments at any level to deliver health measures. But traditionally, local governments have not created a global voice.

Different 'theme city' networks are changing this, some more politically conscious than others. 'Healthy Cities' have been the first, and continue to present themselves as a significant voice. But importantly, other networks are (re)emerging. For instance, ICLEI—Local Governments for Sustainability, United Cities and Local Governments (UCLG), Metropolis.org and the United Nations Advisory Committee of Local Authorities (UNACLA) all connect and advocate for global connectedness and unity. It is clear that health, and Healthy Cities, must have a place at these tables.

References

Ashton, J. (1992). *Healthy Cities*. Open University Press.
Barber, B. R. (2013). *If mayors ruled the world: Dysfunctional nations, rising cities*. Yale University Press.
Baum, F., & Brown, V. A. (1989). Healthy Cities (Australia) Project: Issues of evaluation for the new public health. *Community Health Studies, 13*(2), 140–149.
Cairney, P. (2016). *The politics of evidence-based policy making*. Springer.

China Statistical Yearbook. (2018). *Table 2.6, Population at Year-end by Region*. http://www.stats. gov.cn/tjsj/ndsj/2018/indexeh.htm

Crawshaw, J. L. S. (2016). *Plague hospitals: Public health for the city in early modern Venice*. Routledge.

Crimeen, A., de Leeuw, E., & Freestone, R. (2018). Towards a health promotion paradigm for airport development. *Cities & Health, 2*(2), 134–142.

Davies, S. C., Winpenny, E., Ball, S., Fowler, T., Rubin, J., & Nolte, E. (2014). For debate: a new wave in public health improvement. *The Lancet, 384*(9957), 1889–1895.

Davies, W. K. (Ed.). (2015). *Theme cities: Solutions for urban problems*. Springer.

de Leeuw, E. (2017). Engagement of sectors other than health in integrated health governance, policy, and action. *Annual Review of Public Health, 38*, 329–349.

de Leeuw, E. (2018). Global health disruptors: The urban planet. *BMJ Opinion*, November 30, 2018, https://blogs.bmj.com/bmj/2018/11/30/global-health-disruptors-the-urban-planet/

de Leeuw, E. (2020). Health promotion. Chapter 2.13. In J. Firth, C. Conlon, & T. Cox (Eds.), *Oxford textbook of medicine* (6th ed.). https://doi.org/10.1093/med/9780198746690.003.0019

de Leeuw, E., Green, G., Dyakova, M., Spanswick, L., & Palmer, N. (2015). European healthy cities evaluation: Conceptual framework and methodology. *Health promotion international, 30*(Suppl_1), i8–i17.

de Leeuw, E., Green, G., Spanswick, L., & Palmer, N. (2015). Policymaking in European healthy cities. *Health Promotion International, 30*(Suppl_1), i18–i31.

de Leeuw, E., Green, G., Tsouros, A., Dyakova, M., Farrington, J., Faskunger, J., Grant, M., Ison, E., Jackisch, J., Janss Lafond, L., Lease, H., Mackiewicz, K., Östergren, P.-O., Palmer, N., Ritsatakis, A., Simos, J., Spanswick, L., Webster, P., Zamaro, G., … , on behalf of the World Health Organization European Healthy Cities Network. (2015). Healthy Cities Phase V evaluation: further synthesizing realism. Health Promotion International. In E. de Leeuw, A. Tsouros, & G. Green, (Eds.), *Intersectoral governance for health and equity in European Cities - Healthy Cities in Europe, Supplement, 30*(Suppl1), i118–i124

de Leeuw, E., & Harris-Roxas, B. (2016). Crafting health promotion: From Ottawa to beyond Shanghai. *Environnement, Risques & Santé, 15*(6), 461–464.

de Leeuw, E., Kickbusch, I., Palmer, N., & Spanswick, L. (2015). European Healthy Cities come to terms with health network governance. *Health Promotion International, 30*(Suppl_1), i32–i44.

De Leeuw, E., & Simos, J., (2017). *Healthy cities – The theory, policy, and practice of value-based urban planning*. Springer, New York.

de Leeuw, E., Martin, E., & Waqanivalu, T. (2018). Healthy Islands. In M. Van den Bosch & W. Bird (Eds.), *Oxford textbook of nature and public health: The role of nature in improving the health of a population*. Oxford University Press.

De Moncan, P., & Heurteux, C. (2002). *Le Paris d'Haussmann*. Les éditions du Mécène.

Duhl, L. J. (Ed.). (1963). *The Urban condition – people and policy in the metropolis*. Basic Books.

Elander, I., & Lidskog, R. (2000). *The Rio Declaration and subsequent global initiatives. Consuming cities: The Urban environment in the global economy after the Rio Declaration* (pp. 30–53). Routledge.

Farrington, J. L., Faskunger, J., & Mackiewicz, K. (2015). Evaluation of risk factor reduction in a European City Network. *Health Promotion International, 30*(Suppl_1), i86–i98.

Forbat, J. Simos, J., Cantoreggi, N., & de Leeuw, E. (2018) *Theme cities: A survival guide*. Abstract No 164, WHO International Healthy Cities Conference 'Changing cities to change the world. Celebrating thirty years of the Healthy Cities Movement'. Belfast, Northern Ireland, 1-4 October 2018.

Grant, M. (2015). European healthy city network phase V: Patterns emerging for healthy urban planning. *Health Promotion International, 30*(Suppl_1), i54–i70.

Green, G., Jackisch, J., & Zamaro, G. (2015). Healthy cities as catalysts for caring and supportive environments. *Health Promotion International, 30*(Suppl_1), i99–i107.

Hancock, T., & Duhl, L. (1986). *Promoting health in the Urban Context*. (WHO Healthy Cities Papers No. 1). FADL Publishers.

Higgs, C., Badland, H., Simons, K., Knibbs, L. D., & Giles-Corti, B. (2019). The Urban liveability index: Developing a policy-relevant urban liveability composite measure and evaluating associations with transport mode choice. *International Journal of Health Geographics, 18*(1), 14.

Hommels, A., Mesman, J., & Bijker, W. E. (2014). *Vulnerability in technological cultures: New directions in research and governance.* MIT Press, Boston.

Jackisch, J., Zamaro, G., Green, G., & Huber, M. (2015). Is a healthy city also an age-friendly city? *Health Promotion International, 30*(Suppl_1), i108–i117.

Kickbusch, I. (2007). The move towards a new public health. *Promotion & Education, 14*(2_suppl), 9–9.

Kim, J., de Leeuw, E., Harris-Roxas, B., & Sainsbury, P. (2020). The three paradigms on urban health. *European Journal of Public Health, 30*(Supplement_5), ckaa166-155. See also Retrieved February 26, 2021, from https://chetre.org/2020/11/urban-health-paradigms/

Partnership for Healthy Cities. (2018). *A global network of cities committed to saving lives by preventing noncommunicable diseases and injuries.* Retrieved December 20, 2021, from https://partnershipforhealthycities.bloomberg.org/about/

Prasad, A. (2018). The Urban health equity assessment and response tool (HEART)—A decade of development and implementation. *Journal of Urban Health, 95*(5), 609–609.

Ritsatakis, A., Ostergren, P. O., & Webster, P. (2015). Tackling the social determinants of inequalities in health during phase V of the healthy cities project in Europe. *Health Promotion International, 30*(Suppl_1), i45–i53.

Simos, J., Spanswick, L., Palmer, N., & Christie, D. (2015). The role of health impact assessment in phase V of the healthy cities European network. *Health Promotion International, 30*(Suppl_1), i71–i85.

Tsouros, A., de Leeuw, E., & Green, G. (2015). Evaluation of the Fifth Phase (2009–2013) of the WHO European Healthy Cities Network: Further sophistication and challenges. *Health Promotion International, 30*(Suppl_1), i1–i2.

Tsouros, A. D. (1991). *World Health Organization Health Cities Project: A project becomes a movement. Review of progress 1987 to 1990.* World Health Organization/Sogess.

Tsouros, A. D. (2015). Twenty-seven years of the WHO European Healthy Cities movement: A sustainable movement for change and innovation at the local level. *Health Promotion International, 30*(Suppl_1), i3–i7.

Chapter 6
Health-Promoting Schools

Lawrence St. Leger, Goof Buijs, Nastaran Keshavarz Mohammadi, and Albert Lee

6.1 Introduction

Lawrence St. Leger

The model of the Health-Promoting School (HPS) has existed for over three decades. Its origins can be traced to the development of the Ottawa Charter for Health Promotion that sought to identify those action areas that promoted the health and well-being in populations in the settings where they 'live, work and play'. Using the 1986 Ottawa Charter as a framework, The European Office of the World Health Organization (WHO), working with its Collaborating Centre in Scotland, first used the term in the title of a conference in May 1986 at Peebles in Scotland attended by 28 of 32 member states in the European Region at that time. The early version of this model soon spread and evolved globally, and the WHO (Western Pacific

---

Authorship is ordered by appearance of section in the chapter.

L. St. Leger (✉)
Faculty of Health, Deakin University, Melbourne, VIC, Australia
e-mail: lstleger@bigpond.com

G. Buijs
UNESCO Chair Global Health and Education, Paris, France
e-mail: goof.buijs@unescochair-ghe.org

N. Keshavarz Mohammadi
Shahid Beheshti University of Medical Sciences, Tehran, Iran
e-mail: n_keshavars@yahoo.com

A. Lee
Centre for Health Education and Health Promotion, Lek Yuen Health Centre, Shatin, NT, Hong Kong
e-mail: alee@cuhk.edu.hk

© Springer Nature Switzerland AG 2022
S. Kokko, M. Baybutt (eds.), *Handbook of Settings-Based Health Promotion*,
https://doi.org/10.1007/978-3-030-95856-5_6

Regional Office) developed a framework for HPS in the 32 member states in the region in the mid-1990s (WHO, 2009). Comprehensive guidelines were developed for action by school communities with an accompanying set of indicators of progress. An award system based on the Olympic Games—gold, silver and bronze medals—was part of the package to enable schools to aspire to continue their efforts over a number of years and to be rewarded with the accolade of gold, silver and bronze when they met certain criteria. Evidence-based guidelines such as these were very successful in motivating schools to take action when their governments and other agencies provided substantial financial support over 5–7 years and linked the schools with universities and other research institutes which collected data and analysed the effectiveness of the various HPS initiatives.

Meanwhile research that examined specific health topic areas (e.g. physical activity, healthy eating, etc.) generated considerable evidence about how to build better health outcomes of young people within the school setting. The International Union for Health Promotion and Education (IUHPE), with the financial support from the Centers for Disease Control and Prevention (CDC) in the USA, created two documents that provided schools, education and health sectors with an evidence-based summary of what worked and what did not work (IUHPE, 2009). The documents also provided the education and health sectors with evidence-based guidelines about how to design, implement and sustain HPS initiatives. Also included was the evidence at the time about the effectiveness of programmes directed at specific health issues such as healthy eating, mental health, physical activity, drug education, etc. These documents were promoted internationally and were available in 11 languages.

I argue that HPS initiatives are effective when they follow evidence-based guidelines in the following scenarios: (a) Financial resources and encouragement are provided by governments and national and international agencies such as WHO, CDC, IUHPE; (b) country-based or region-based bodies such as Schools for Health (SHE) in Europe and the Hong Kong HPS; and (c) there is clear leadership from individuals and small groups in these countries and regions.

But the momentum of the first two decades of HPS has diminished. This is because the three factors identified above have either ceased to exist or been reduced because of ongoing financial issues. Also the emergence of competing priorities for school time and commitment, such as an increased focus on improving literacy and numeracy, and the appearance of external lobby groups, such as those from the environmental community, have diluted the focus on HPS.

However, in the last few years there has been a strong focus on a new health area, which has become a priority for schools. This time it is driven by the education sector and not the health sector as HPS was for the last two decades. The health area is described in various ways such as Social and Emotional Well-Being (SEWB), Social and Emotional Learning (SEL) and School Connectedness (SC).

HPS stands for Health Promoting Schools communities and why it provides a stronger and more relevant focus for schools to commit to HPS, it is worthwhile to briefly examine the building blocks of health.

I argue that while mental health and social health were acknowledged in the early constructs of health in the late 1980s, when the HPS was emerging, the main emphases were often based around physical health. Recently I examined the literature about how health is portrayed in the context of people's lives.

It is argued that health for the whole population is made up of six components. These are (not in any particular order) as follows:

- Physical health: When the body is functioning as it was designed to function.
- Emotional health: Self-esteem, security, self-actualization and the expression of emotions in assertive and respectful ways.
- Social health: The relationships and interactions an individual has with others and with social institutions.
- Spiritual health: The way individuals seek and express meaning and purpose and the way they experience their connectedness to the moment, to self, to others, to nature, and to the significant or sacred.
- Environmental health: The components of the natural and built environments (physical, chemical, biological) affecting individual behaviours and physical states.
- Intellectual health: The cognitive capacities, particularly the ability to access knowledge, understand it, analyse the information, synthesize the facts, evaluate the applications of the knowledge and create new ideas and solutions.

It is all these six components of health on which we need to focus when we promote and nurture the health of young people (St.Leger, 2015).

There is a wealth of strong evidence that shows if schools focus on building the health assets of young people in the areas of SEWB, SEL and SC then there will be significant improvements in educational outcomes (Clarke et al., 2015; Weare, 2015). Educational achievements are the core business of schools. Also providing opportunities for students to engage much more with the creative arts, particularly music, will also improve learning outcomes and commitment to education (Vaughan et al., 2017).

This is probably the first time I have seen a very comprehensive commitment by schools to a particular health issue, which is to enhancing the SEWB of students. It is simply because addressing this issue with evidence-based strategies will actually improve educational outcomes which is how schools are mainly judged by parents, their communities and government authorities. Many schools have actually reduced their formal teaching time to engage in quality initiatives that overtly address the first five components from the above six components of health. Schools always addressed intellectual health but now place more emphasis on the higher orders of learning, for example, creativity, and now see this component as being integral to the overall health status of a young person.

This strong emphasis on SEWB, SEL and SC has provided educational authorities and schools with new ways of thinking about what is offered to students and how students are partners in the educational experiences. I believe it provides the foundation for at least two decades of new energy in HPS. But it is different. It will not always be about health being defined and practised in the physical health domain. It will largely be about using research which shows us how schools themselves influence two interrelated outcomes—enhanced educational achievements and the acquisition of lifelong health assets, particularly in SEWB.

There have been a number of outstanding initiatives of HPS around the world over the last 20 years. What follows are three perspectives from three diverse regions—Asia (Hong Kong, in particular), Europe and the Middle East. The three authors, who are the leaders of these initiatives in HPS, reflect on what happened in their region and offer insights into why it worked, or did not work. They also provide some ideas for the future of HPS.

6.2   Europe

Goof Buijs

During the last three decades in the European region, school health promotion has evolved from innovative projects trying to link the new concept of health promotion into a more structural whole school to health and well-being in countries. In most of these countries it was common in schools to have lessons about health, going back to the nineteenth century. The focus was on discipline and knowledge, paying attention to issues such as regular eating, hygiene and enough sleep. From the 1960s health education about topics such as smoking, safety and even sex became fashionable. The health-promoting school concept was introduced in the late 1980s, applying whole school thinking and regarding schools as a setting to reach children and young children. In 1992 the European Network of Health Promoting Schools was created by six European countries. It started as an initiative to set up national pilot projects on health-promoting schools and work together under the umbrella of three international organizations: the WHO, the European Commission and the Council of Europe. The whole school approach to health was taken as a starting point. Joint initiatives in these pilot countries from both the Ministry of Health and the Ministry of Education resulted in the development of activities to help schools to better understand how health and well-being could be integrated into the school plan. This was a step beyond doing projects on relevant health topics, which traditionally are more focused on knowledge and classroom activities, instead of involving the school environment, the members of the school community and policies. The approach focuses on promoting health and well-being through increased health literacy, on promoting healthy lifestyles and living conditions. Therefore, the focus shifted from the prevention of specific diseases, mostly related to lifestyles (noncommunicable diseases) to the promotion on of health and well-being of the children and to create a healthy environment.

The European network gradually evolved with participation from a growing number of countries. A marking point in its history was the creation a set of common values at the first European conference on health-promoting schools in 1997 (Barnekow & Rivett, 2000). Relevant concepts included empowerment, active participation of students, democracy and equality. In some former Soviet Union countries in Central and Eastern Europe, the introduction of health-promoting schools coincided with democratization of the society. The 'Health-Promoting School' concept became an entry point for educational reform. Currently the Schools for Health in Europe (SHE) network counts around 40 countries and regions in Europe participating. In the European region, HPS are considered as a main entry point for promoting children's health and for school improvement.

However, the broad whole school focus does not always reflect the daily practice of health education in schools, where knowledge about specific diseases is still often emphasized. A key issue is the intersectoral nature of school health promotion. Health professionals regard schools as a relevant entry point to reach children and young people with health messages. Schools, on the other hand, regard health as one of the many relevant themes that society imposes on their curriculum. In many political debates it is often concluded that the root cause of many social 'problems' in our societies should be made obligatory in schools. Schools often feel overloaded with an already full curriculum; therefore, health competes with the more traditional subjects taught in a school. The health and social sectors also deal with all the aspects outside school in the local community that impact children's health and well-being. The health, education and social sectors do not speak the same language; are organized as separate silos in our societies; and have their own structures and funding mechanisms. They are part of the common goods in our society, which are more and more under pressure of the 'free' market–oriented economy.

On the other hand, the need to take effective action to promote children and young people's health is increasing. One of the challenges in the twenty-first century is the global burden of non-communicable diseases. It particularly affects people from lower socioeconomic backgrounds and in emergency situations.

Because education and health are inextricably linked, schools are considered an ideal setting for both health education and health promotion initiatives targeted at children and young people. In addition, there is a growing body of evidence that shows the close relationship between health; physical, mental and cognitive development; school participation; and educational achievement. Schools are especially important settings for health promotion reaching children from all socioeconomic and cultural backgrounds, who spend 40% of their time in school.

Actions in a school will be more effective when school activities are embedded in the local community, which will provide synergistic effects. This has been elaborated in the 'supersetting' approach (Bloch et al., 2014) that summarizes sustainable approaches to optimized health, well-being and quality of life, and involves mobilizing the local community. Also the active involvement and participation of students in the creation of healthy school policies and practices is required to create ownership. The same is true for their parents/carers and teachers.

In the European region, the 2016 WHO high-level conference on improving the health of the future generation emphasized the importance of intersectoral and interagency working among the health, education and social sectors. The conference was organized jointly with the UNESCO and the UNICEF, for the first time working together on this level. The 'Paris Declaration' (WHO, 2016) resulting from this conference, stresses the importance of inclusive and equitable high-quality education, including preschool education as a key determinant of the health and well-being of children and adolescents. Governments are called to put this issue high on their political agendas, including adequate budgets and financing. School health promotion is part of sustainable development and fits very well in the Sustainable Development Goals (SDG) agenda, in particular SDG 3 (Ensure healthy lives and promote well-being for all at all ages) and SDG 4 (Ensure inclusive and quality education for all and promote lifelong learning).

There is a need to develop new research strategies that focus on both programme content and on the implementation process of HPS, which is needed to demonstrate effectiveness and impact on both health and learning outcomes. The most promising focus for future research would be on supporting the living conditions of children and young people that have a direct impact on health, realizing direct and easy access to educational and health services and educating children and young people to get the means to take care of their own health in an autonomous and responsible way.

6.3 Eastern Mediterranean

Nastaran Keshavarz Mohammadi

Adoption of health-promoting schools (HPS) programme has not been similar within and between countries in this region. While Europe and Australia were pioneering its implementation in the 1990s, it diffused about a decade later in regions such as the Middle East (WHO, 2006). The first regional consultation on HPS in Eastern Mediterranean Regional Office of the World Health Organization (EMRO) in 2005 led to development of a regional implementation framework significantly based on a comprehensive school health approach with a set of implementation and evaluation criteria shaped mainly by health education and health services at schools but with limited reference to school policies. The first regional conference on HPS in EMRO took place in 2007 followed by establishing a regional network of HPS (WHO/EMRO, 2007). A number of schools were chosen to be HPS, after the implementation of a set of indicators, and also establishing an award system by external evaluation. This was similar in many countries in the region. Often HPS was a joint initiative by ministries of education and health.

6.3.1 School Health in Iran

Iran was among the first countries in the EMRO region where the government established a department for school health within the Ministry of Education in 1935. This department conducted routine physical examination and health education for students by allocating doctors and supervisors for school health (Nouri, 2006). In 2010, Iran adopted the concept of HPS starting with assigning 72 schools in 5 provinces and then increasing to more than 2000 schools in all provinces by 2017 (Yazdi-Feyzabadi et al., 2018). The Iranian Ministry of Health and Medical Education in collaboration with the Ministry of Education moved towards a model for Iranian Health Promoting Schools (IHPS) very similar to the EMRO framework of HPS. This consisted of eight components of comprehensive school health programmes. The development of healthy school policies was not an explicit component except for healthy canteen policies.

There has been little research conducted on HPS in Iran. Few qualitative studies have explored the current understanding of the concept among stakeholders as well as barriers to its implementation (Fathi et al., 2014; Yazdi-Feyzabadi et al., 2018; Zarei et al., 2017). These limited research studies showed that HPS has not been understood as a whole school approach and that the national HPS framework lacked an adequate system approach to school health. It also showed that most schools ignored the importance of school health policies except in the area of mental health. There are also contextual, structural, capacity and resource barriers inhibiting the effective implementation of HPS. Two evaluation studies looked at the impact of HPS on some aspects of students' health, including students' mental health (Kochaki et al., 2011) and the nutritional status and behaviour of students (Zarei et al., 2017). It claimed that there was no difference between HPS and schools not so identified.

There have been similar findings in some other countries. For example, in Australia, as an earlier adopter of the HPS approach, there have been reported different understandings and implementation methods among schools identified as HPS (Keshavarz Mohammadi et al., 2010). This is not limited to HPS concept as similar findings have been reported regarding health-promoting hospitals (Johnson & Baum, 2001) and health-promoting workplaces (Motalebi et al., 2017). It might be argued that shifting reductionist mindsets of health professionals to whole systems in order to embrace the settings approach to health has not been as easy as expected.

6.3.2   The Need for a Systems Approach to School Health

I argue that there are a number of explanations about why it has been difficult to bridge the gap between the health-promoting school concepts and their implementations. Complexity is frequently identified. Not only is health a complex and multifactorial phenomenon, but also individuals and organizations are complex systems, which to varying degrees adapt to the continuous changes in their environments. Hence, promoting a complex phenomenon in complex systems is of greater complexity and uncertainty. Despite the increased use of terminologies such as 'systems' or 'complexities', there is little adoption from system science in school health research. I believe the failures in achieving whole system changes can be attributed to a simplistic reductionism approach to health. There now needs to be new thinking and a holistic approach to promoting health in settings such as schools (Keshavarz et al., 2010).

Twenty-five years back Baric argued for a rethink about how school health is approached (Baric, 1994). Building upon the historical changes in the way schools have been understood, from convenient settings to educational and social organizations, and more recently as systems, some researchers suggest that schools need to be understood as complex adaptive systems (Keshavarz et al., 2010). They are nested systems composed of diverse autonomous agents and components interacting within a network structure based on their knowledge, values and the school rules (Keshavarz et al., 2010). Literature from nearly 30 years ago suggested schools as complex adaptive systems are not fully predictable as their system-level change emerges from a process of self-organization rather than being designed and controlled externally or by a centralized body (Zimmerman et al., 1998). Lack of central control in addition to non-linearity, the dynamic nature and unpredictability of complex adaptive systems, seriously limits the ability to fully control complex adaptive systems such as schools (Seel, 2000). I believe this means that HPS cannot be introduced as an external project where schools have limited capacity to shape the HPS. Our challenge in the future is to redefine the barriers and enablers to a sustainable and whole system implementation of HPS.

The survival of complex adaptive systems such as HPS depends on adaptability. Facilitating the adaptation of health-promoting schools for schools requires strategies such as

- Establish mechanisms which provide easy access and exchange of information and experiences about HPS among schools, and also parents.
- Develop supportive rules/policies at multiple levels of education sector and health sector for HPS.
- Develop mechanisms to attribute more credit or value to becoming a HPS such as shown in the research literature about the Hong Kong HPS.
- Establish interactive networks and communication strategies among schools and health sector.
- Acknowledge the value and importance of diversity and the unique context of schools from the stages of planning to evaluation of schools.

6.4   Hong Kong

Albert Lee

There have been increasing concerns by the public and parents regarding the health and wellbeing of students in Hong Kong beginning about three decades ago. Curriculum reform at the turn of last century highlighted five essential learning experiences namely '*ethics, intellect, physique, social skills and aesthetics*' for whole person development (Curriculum Development Council, 2001). In order to maximize the opportunity to drive education policy with a greater focus on school health education, the Centre for Health Education and Health Promotion of the Chinese University of Hong Kong (CHEP) led by me initiated the HPS movement to facilitate education reform in health education by adopting a bottom-up policy with a school and community focus. Since late 1990, we have developed strategies facilitating the implementation of HPS by addressing the issues of professional development, policy implementation, the provision of adequate funding, community network development and school health research for the HPS programme in Hong Kong.

The early initiatives in capacity building was in the form of University Professional Diploma programme that included teachers' training, health curriculum development, community participation, changing policies and practices related to health, and school health research. We had managed to create a paradigm shift from a conventional health education approach emphasizing individuals and narrow aspects of health issues at the micro level, to a broader perspective of health with a macro view on health and society (Lee et al., 2003). This aligned very closely with the top priority of the education reform for twenty-first-century Hong Kong, which was aimed to promote the concept of lifelong learning experiences among educators and the society at large, and to mobilize existing resources to provide room and support to learning activities beyond the confines of the classroom. It was the first step to enable the concept of HPS to be translated into practice. It closely followed initiatives by the WHO that moved beyond individual behavioural change to consider organizational structural change such as improving the school's physical and social environments, its curricula, and teaching and learning methods (WHO, 1996). However, the WHO HPS framework is a guiding framework and much of the work still needs to be done to develop a robust model to fit into the context of the school setting in respective countries. Because of its comprehensive nature it appears very few schools have been able to implement HPS in its entirety (Adamowitsch et al., 2017; Joyce et al., 2017).

Our step-by-step approach in Hong Kong started with building the capacities of key stakeholders in addition to comprehensive needs assessment of each school, leading to the development of a system of evaluation and monitoring and the subsequent establishment of the 'Hong Kong Healthy School Award' system (HKHSA) from the late 1990s (Lee et al., 2014). Schools in Hong Kong are now able to measure their own performance against the six key HPS areas as identified by the WHO. The HKHSA has provided data identifying the potential markers of success, associated with the process of implementation as means of supporting schools and teachers. Inchley et al. (2006) called for the development of indicators highlighting the ways in which schools are able to adopt HPS principles successfully and the conditions to be in place for the HPS concept to flourish. The orthodox biomedical approach, for example, Randomized Controlled Trials (RCTs) in evaluating the effects of HPS, leads to missing out on the richness of school health activities by evaluating a narrow set of predetermined outcomes. The statistical assumptions underpinning RCT are not valid reflecting organizational or structural change. It is important to find out what constitutes successful outcomes and to involve increased inputs from students, teachers and parents.

The HKHSA has enabled CHEP to establish a system of monitoring and evaluation of HPS, and data monitoring which would motivate change (Joyce et al., 2017). The HKHSA is similar to the Wessex Healthy Schools Award (WHSA) scheme, which was developed in the 1990s in England, and has shown positive award-related changes in children's health behaviours. Schools that won awards were found to have a more health-promoting culture than that of the non-awarded health-promoting schools (Lee et al., 2006, 2008; Moon et al., 1999). The HKHSA and WHSA mimic the Social Development Model of Catalano et al. (2004), which suggests children learn their prosocial or antisocial patterns of behaviours from the norms and values held by the social environment in which they are bonded. Those schools achieving a gold award of HKHSA have been shown to sustain positive changes and address the intertwined social, educational, psychological and health needs of school children (Lee et al., 2018).

Taiwan has adapted from HKHSA to develop the Health-Promoting School Accreditation System (HPSAS), which is an objective instrument used to evaluate the HPS programme's process and outcomes (Chen & Lee, 2016). Research on those schools with a gold level of award has shown the significance of school leadership. When the school leadership has established close relationships with their counterparts at local departments of education and health, school administration teams received more resources, technical assistance and support in promoting school health effectively. Therefore, a healthy school policy should be a priority for school management and the government, both of which can be responsible for providing sufficient support to promote the health and wellness of students and staff. The rapid development of a nationwide HPS movement and HPSAS in Taiwan, with its close working relationship with Hong Kong, has illustrated how a robust system of monitoring and evaluation like HKHSA can facilitate development of the HPS to a larger scale with a very rich and diverse data set capturing a large number of implementation processes and outcomes.

The evolutionary development of HPS from identification of needs, professional development of educators in school health promotion and the establishment of HKHSA as system of accreditation of HPS, has influenced recent developments such as GoSmart.net (online Health Education Hub) and New Frontiers (Student Health Leadership training), and it also has supported educational changes. This enables successes to stimulate progress in establishing a professional and community culture that in turn creates a healthy teaching and learning environment (Lee & Cheung, 2017). Lee and Cheung (2017) also claim that the Assessment Program for Affective and Social Outcomes (APASO), used as a tool by schools in Hong Kong, reflected the affective and social developments of the students in the school as a whole, as well as how they relate to the school. HPS has evolved in Hong Kong as a key component of effective schooling, and is more an educational innovation rather than the previous practices in health education where the content and priorities were shaped by the health sector.

6.5   Conclusion

Lawrence St. Leger

The school is a complex setting. Internationally, its prime function is to build the educational outcomes of children and adolescents. Another essential function is to nurture young people as they grow and interact with their peers, families, communities and societies at large. As a setting, the school is influenced by the teachers, families, school administration, local community and various government policies and resource allocations. The students and their contributions to school life also shape it.

The evidence tells us that that schools that have undertaken a wholistic approach to health using evidence-based guidelines, accompanied by adequate financial resources and professional development of staff, have been able to have some small success in improving the health and educational outcomes of students. But the HPS initiatives have largely been driven by the health sector.

There is a slow change emerging. Now schools and the education sector are taking more ownership and initiative in addressing a very important health area, that is, Social and Emotional Well-Being (SEWB). Why? Because schools now know that improving SEWB will significantly improve educational outcomes. In Europe it is seen through the lens of 'citizenship'.

The settings approach to HPS has been mainly driven by the health sector and has seen health promotion actions focused on the setting of the school. Now it emerges that the education sector is rethinking its role as a leader in health, albeit only in SEWB. There is early evidence that health promotion may be moving from health promotion in the school setting to a health promotion setting. For this trend to continue the health sector needs to allow and facilitate more ownership of health by schools to reduce or eliminate short issue-based interventions and programmes and to always provide schools with evidence about how improving certain health behaviours will improve educational outcomes and to ensure teachers are provided ongoing professional development.

References

Adamowitsch, M., Gugglberger, L., & Dür, W. (2017). Implementation practices in school health promotion: Findings from an Austrian multiple-case study. *Health Promotion International, 32*, 218–230.

Baric, L. (1994). *Health promotion and health education in practice module 2. The organization model.* Barns Publications.

Barnekow, V., & Rivett, D. (2000). The European Network of Health Promoting Schools – The alliance of education and health. *Health Education, 100*(2), 61–67.

Bloch, P., Toft, U., Reinbach, H. C., Clausen, L. T., Mikkelsen, B. E., Poulsen, K., & Jensen, B. B. (2014). Revitalizing the setting approach – supersettings for sustainable impact in community health promotion. *International Journal of Behavioral Nutrition and Physical Activity, 11*(1), 118.

Catalano, R. F., Haggerty, K. P., Oesterle, S., Fleming, C. B., & Hawkins, J. D. (2004). The importance of bonding to school for healthy development: Findings from the Social Development Research Group. *Journal of School Health, 74*(7), 252–261.

Chen, F. L., & Lee, A. (2016). Health-promoting educational settings in Taiwan: Development and evaluation of the Health-Promoting School Accreditation System. *Global Health Promotion, 23*(Supp. 1), 18–25.

Clarke, A. M., Morreale, S., Field, C. A., Hussein, Y., & Barry, M. M. (2015). *What works in enhancing social and emotional skills development during childhood and adolescence? A review of the evidence on the effectiveness of school-based and out-of-school programmes in the UK*. A report produced by the World Health Organization Collaborating Centre for Health Promotion Research. National University of Ireland.

Curriculum Development Council. (2001). *Learning to learn: Life-long learning and whole-person development*. Hong Kong SAR Government.

Fathi, B., Allahverdipour, H., Shaghaghi, A., Kousha, A., & Jannati, A. (2014). Challenges in developing health promoting schools' project: application of global traits in local realm. *Health Promotion Perspectives, 4*(1), 9–17. Retrieved April 29, 2021, from https://www.euro.who.int/data/assets/pdf_file/0019/325180/Paris_Declaration_ENG.pdf

Inchley, J., Muldoon, J., & Currie, C. (2006). Becoming a health promoting school: Evaluating the process of effective implementation in Scotland. *Health Promotion International, 22*(1), 65–71.

IUHPE. (2009). *Achieving health promoting schools: Guidelines for promoting health in schools*. IUHPE.

Johnson, A., & Baum, F. (2001). Health promoting hospitals: A typology of different organizational approaches to health promotion. *Health Promotion International, 16*(3), 281–287.

Joyce, A., Dabrowski, A., Aston, R., & Carey, G. (2017). Evaluating for impact: What type of data can assist a health promoting school approach? *Health Promotion International, 32*, 403–410.

Keshavarz Mohammadi, N., Rowling, L., & Nutbeam, D. (2010). Acknowledging educational perspectives on health promoting schools. *Health Education, 110*(4), 240251.

Keshavarz, N., Nutbeam, D., Rowling, L., & Khavarpour, F. (2010). Schools as social complex adaptive systems: A new way to understand the challenges of introducing the health promoting schools concept. *Social Science & Medicine, 70*(10), 1467–1474.

Kochaki, G.-M., Kochaki, A.-M., Charkazi, A.-R., Bayani, A.-A., Esmaeili, A.-L., & Shahnazi, H. (2011). Investigating the effect of implementing the school based health promotion program on students'. *Mental Health Knowledge & Health, 5*(4), 14–19.

Lee, A., Cheng, F., Fung, Y., & St.Leger, L. (2006). Can health promoting schools contribute to the better health and well-being of young people: Hong Kong experience? *Journal of Epidemiology and Community Health, 60*, 530–536.

Lee, A., & Cheung, M. B. (2017). School as setting to create a healthy learning environment for teaching and learning using the model of health promoting school to foster school-health partnership. *Journal of Professional Capacity and Community, 2*(4), 200–214. https://doi.org/10.1108/JPCC-05-2017-0013

Lee, A., Keung, M. K., Lo, S. Y., Kwong, A., & Armstrong, E. (2014). Framework for evaluating efficacy in Health Promoting Schools. *Health Education, 114*(3), 225–242. http://www.emeraldinsight.com/10.1108/HE-07-2013-0035

Lee, A., Lee, S. H., Tsang, K. K., & To, C. Y. (2003). A comprehensive "Healthy Schools Programme" to promote school health: The Hong Kong experience in joining the efforts of health and education sectors. *Journal of Epidemiology and Community Health, 57*, 174–177.

Lee, A., St.Leger, L. H., Ling, K. W. K., Keung, V. M. W., Lo, A. S. C., Kwong, A. C. M., Ma, H. P. S., & Armstrong, E. S. (2018). The *Hong Kong healthy schools award scheme*, school health and student health: an exploratory Study. *Health Education Journal, 77*(8), 857–871.

Lee, A., Wong, M. C. S., Cheng, F., Yuen, H. S. K., Keung, V. M. W., & Mok, J. S. Y. (2008). Can the concept of health promoting schools help to improve students' health knowledge and practices to combat the challenge of communicable diseases: Case study in Hong Kong? *BMC Public Health, 8,* 42.

Moon, A. M., Mullee, M. A., Rogers, L., Thompson, R. L., Speller, V., & Roderick, P. (1999). Helping schools to become health-promoting environments – an evaluation of the Wessex Healthy Schools Award. *Health Promotion International, 14,* 111–122.

Motalebi, G. M., Keshavarz Mohammadi, N., Kuhn, K., Ramezankhani, A., & Azari, M. R. (2017). How far are we from full implementation of health promoting workplace concepts? A review of implementation tools and frameworks in workplace interventions. *Health Promotion International, daw098.*

Nouri, S. M. (2006). *School health.* Vaghefi Publishing Company.

Seel, R. (2000). Culture and complexity: New insights on organisational change. *Organisations & People, 2,* 2–9.

St.Leger, L. H. (2015). Investing in youth health assets. In K. TeRiele & R. Gorur (Eds.), *Interrogating conceptions of 'Vulnerable Youth' in theory, policy and practice.* Sense Publishers.

Vaughan, T., Harris, J., & Caldwell, B. (2017). *Bridging the gap in school achievement through the arts.* Melbourne.

Weare, K. (2015). *What works in promoting social and emotional wellbeing and responding to mental health problems in schools.* National Children's Bureau.

WHO Regional Office for Europe. (2016). *Declaration: Partnerships for the health and well-being for our young and future generations.*

WHO Regional Office for the Western Pacific. (1996). *Health-Promoting Schools Series 5: Regional guidelines. Development of health-promoting schools-A framework for action.* WHO/WPRO.

WHO/EMRO. (2007). *Eastern Mediterranean Network of Health Promoting Schools.* http://www.emro.who.int/school-health/school-news/

World Health Organization. (2006). *Report on the consultation on health- promoting schools in the Eastern Mediterranean Region, Sana'a, Republic of Yemen, 12–14 December 2005*(No. WHO-EM/HSG/310/E). World Health Organization. Regional Office for the Eastern Mediterranean. http://www.who.int/iris/handle/10665/254051

World Health Organization. (2009). *Guidelines and indicators for health promoting schools.* WHO-WPRO.

Yazdi-Feyzabadi, V., Rashidian, A., Keshavarz Mohammadi, N., Omidvar, N., Nedjat, S., & Karimi-Shahanjarini, A. (2018). *Policy formation and implementation analysis of Iran' health promoting schools and the association between school food environment and pupil's dietary behaviors.* PhD thesis. *Tehran University of Medical Sciences, 33*(6), 1010–1021.

Zarei, F., Ghahremani, L., Khazaee-Pool, M., & Keshavarz Mohammadi, N. (2017). Exploring the strengths, challenges and improvement strategy for health-promoting schools from school health experts: A qualitative study. *Journal of Health Education and Health Promotion, 5,* 240–250.

Zimmerman, B., Lindberg, C., & Plsek, P. (1998). *Edgeware: Lessons from complexity science for health care leaders.* VHA Inc.

Chapter 7
Health-Promoting Hospitals

Jürgen M. Pelikan, Birgit Metzler, and Peter Nowak

7.1 Introduction

In relation to health, hospitals are unique organizations and by that pose a specific challenge for health promotion and also for the settings approach. By being a health care organization, the objective and mission of hospitals is oriented at health already. Thus, health promotion is also a specific challenge for hospitals and other health care organizations. Therefore, when offering health promotion to hospitals, two kinds of reactions are common: Either "we are already doing it as we ever have" or "it is not our business, we have no mandate and financing for public health." Hence, health promotion has to argue carefully and demonstrate what added value it can offer to health care services, especially what the difference between caring for health and promoting it is. Or, which meaning does *health* have in health *care* and which in health *promotion*? For this, the Ottawa Charter gives some good arguments. First, by its definition: "Health promotion is the process of enabling people to increase control over, and to improve, their health" (WHO, 1986). Consequently, it is not enough to offer cure and care to patients, but they also have to be enabled and empowered to better control and improve their health themselves.

Second, the Ottawa Charter offers a specific action or strategy just for health care—"Reorient health services"—or more detailed: "The role of the health sector must move increasingly in a health promotion direction, beyond its responsibility

J. M. Pelikan · P. Nowak
WHO Collaborating Centre for Health Promotion in Hospitals and Health Care, Competence
Centre Health Promotion and Health System (Austrian National Public Health Institute),
Gesundheit Österreich GmbH, Vienna, Austria
e-mail: juergen.pelikan@goeg.at; peter.nowak@goeg.at

B. Metzler (✉)
Competence Centre Health Promotion and Health System (Austrian National Public Health
Institute), Gesundheit Österreich GmbH, Vienna, Austria
e-mail: birgit.metzler@goeg.at

© Springer Nature Switzerland AG 2022
S. Kokko, M. Baybutt (eds.), *Handbook of Settings-Based Health Promotion*,
https://doi.org/10.1007/978-3-030-95856-5_7

for providing clinical and curative services. Health services need to embrace an expanded mandate which is sensitive and respects cultural needs. This mandate should support the needs of individuals and communities for a healthier life, and open channels between the health sector and broader social, political, economic and physical environmental components" (WHO, 1986). By that, the Ottawa Charter implicitly diagnosed that health services had a too-narrow mandate and mission, and therefore are in need to be reoriented, at least from the perspective of a new public health, since the title of an earlier version of the Ottawa Charter included "towards a new public health." But, since hospitals cannot define their mandate and mission just by themselves, this reorientation is not only a challenge for hospital organizations, but also for the whole health sector, for health policy, and for the political system of a society.

Third, as far as the setting approach is concerned, the Ottawa Charter offers: "Health is created and lived by people within the settings of their everyday life; where they learn, work, play and love" (WHO, 1986). Interestingly enough, the list does not include, where people "are cured and cared for!" Nevertheless, "work" also holds true for the staff of the hospital as a workplace and "learn" for the training function of the hospital for part of its staff. If we understand health care as coproduction or co-creation and patients as coworkers of health professionals, it holds true also for patients. Thus, health promotion philosophy has to offer a specific widening of the understanding of health care for hospitals' main focus of cure and care of health in the direction of disease prevention, health protection, and health promotion. And that not just for patients' health, but also for staff's health and the health of the residents in the community a hospital serves. Yet, a concrete and comprehensive concept for hospitals as a health-promoting setting and for strategies to implement this concept into already existing hospitals had to be developed, before a Network of Health-Promoting Hospitals (HPH) could be established.

In the following three parts of this chapter, we first we reconstruct and describe the historical development of HPH; second, looking back from the current situation, we reflect how successful HPH has been up to now concerning its reproduction and production; and third, we offer few thoughts on the future of HPH and next steps.

7.2   Historical Background of Health-Promoting Hospitals

There already exist a number of earlier publications (Dietscher, 2012; Dietscher et al., 2014; Pelikan, 2006; Pelikan, 2007a; Pelikan et al., 2001; Pelikan et al., 2010; Pelikan et al., 2014; Pelikan, Dietscher, et al., 2011a; Pelikan, Gröne, & Svane, 2011; Pelikan & Wieczorek, 2019) and some presentations, where the development of HPH has been described and reconstructed in a systematic way. We use an updated table from these publications to give an overview on the HPH history. Different phases of this development have been identified with events and milestones relevant for the career of the HPH movement (see Table 7.1).

Table 7.1 Phases and milestones of development of the international Health-Promoting Hospitals' network (Based on Pelikan, 2007a; Dietscher, 2012, revised and extended for this publication)

Phase 0: Preparations for initiating Health-Promoting Hospitals by WHO/EURO (1986–1989)	
1986	Ottawa Charter for Health Promotion with the demand to reorient health services
1986–	WHO Healthy Cities Project (city of Vienna, Austria was a member from its start)
1988	WHO consultation on the Role of Health-Promoting Hospitals (Milz & Vang, 1989)

Phase 1: Development of concept & initiation of international network structures (1989–1992)	
1989	Feasibility study for a HPH model project
1989–1996	WHO model project "Health and Hospital" at Rudolfstiftung Hospital, Vienna, Austria
1990–	Official start of International HPH Network as a multi-city action plan of the WHO Healthy Cities Project
1990–2001	Coordination and secretariat of International HPH Network by Ludwig Boltzmann Institute for the Sociology of Health and Medicine (LBISHM), Vienna, Austria
1991	Launch of the Budapest Declaration on Health Promoting Hospitals (first HPH policy paper)
1991–1992	Preparations for a European Pilot Hospital Project (EPHP)
1992–	Establishment of WHO Collaborating Centre for Health Promotion in Hospitals and Healthcare at LBISHM, Vienna, Austria

Phase 2: Testing the concept, developing network structures, start of national/regional networks (1993–1998)	
1993–1997	European Pilot Hospital Project (EPHP)
1993–	Annual international HPH conferences, international HPH newsletter
1993	First national/regional HPH networks (Poland, Wales)
1995–	National and regional HPH networks as a strategy by WHO with annual HPH networks coordinators' workshop
1996	Workshop: The Health Promoting Hospital in the European Union, Vienna, Austria
1997	The Vienna Recommendations on Health-Promoting Hospitals
1998–	Launch of website(s) for HPH
1998–2015	HPH task force: Health Promotion in Psychiatric Health Services
1998-	First international project data base of HPH

Phase 3: Standardizing the concept & linking it to quality and evidence methodology (1999–2005)	
1999–2008	HPH task force: HPH and EFQM
2001–2005	Coordination & secretariat of International HPH Network moved to WHO European Office for Integrated Health Care Services in Barcelona, Spain
2001–2006	HPH working group: Putting HPH Policy into Action
2001–2006	HPH working group: Standards for Health-Promoting Hospitals
2002–2011	WHO pilot project: Implementing the HPH Strategy and Standards through a combined application of the EFQM Excellence Model and the Balanced Scorecard (HPH-EFQM-BSC)

(continued)

Table 7.1 (continued)

Phase 0: Preparations for initiating Health-Promoting Hospitals by WHO/EURO (1986–1989)	
2002–2005	EU project: Migrant Friendly and Culturally Competent Hospitals
2004–	Designation of WHO-CC for Evidence-Based Health Promotion in Hospitals and Health Services in Copenhagen, Denmark
2004–	HPH task force: Children and Adolescents in Hospitals
2005–2016	HPH task force: Migrant Friendly and Culturally Competent Health Care
Phase 4: Autonomy, globalizing & extending the scope of the international network (2005–2010)	
2005–	First non-European national/regional network Quebec/Canada joined the International HPH Network
2005–	Coordination & secretariat by WHO-CC for Evidence-Based Health Promotion in Hospitals and Health Services in Copenhagen, Denmark
2006–	Introduction of a general assembly & an elected governance board for the International HPH Network
2006–	Second non-European national/regional network in Taiwan
2008–	"International Network of Health Promoting Hospitals & Health Services (HPH)" founded as an independent association under Swiss law with a constitution
2008–	By the constitution extension of scope of HPH to other health care services and officially also to other WHO regions than WHO/Europe
2008–2012	Project on a Retrospective, Internationally Comparative Evaluation Study on HPH (PRICES-HPH)
2008–2013	HPH task force: Tobacco-Free United
2009–2013	HPH task force: Alcohol and Alcohol Interventions
2009	First time release of a HPH Strategy 2009–2010
2009–2012	HPH DATA Project—Evaluation of a Health Promotion Patient Documentation Model
2010–	HPH task force: HPH and Environment
2010	First Memorandum of Understanding of International HPH Network with WHO/EURO
Phase 5: Further globalizing, evaluation, and strategic communication (2011–2018)	
2011–	Journal: *Clinical Health Promotion*. Research and best practice for patients, staff & community as official journal of the HPH network
2012	First international HPH conference outside Europe—Taipei, Taiwan
2012–2016	WHO-HPH recognition project on fast-track implementation of clinical health promotion
2012–2016	HPH task force: Health-enhancing Physical Activity
2013–	HPH task force: Age-friendly Health Care
2016	Second HPH conference outside Europe—New Haven, USA "New Haven Recommendations on partnering with patients, families and citizens to enhance performance and quality in health promoting hospitals and health"
2016–	HPH working group: HPH and Patient and Family Engaged Health Care
2016–	HPH working group: HPH and Health Literate Health Care Organizations
2016–	HPH task force: Implementation and Monitoring of Standards

(continued)

Table 7.1   (continued)

Phase 0: Preparations for initiating Health-Promoting Hospitals by WHO/EURO (1986–1989)	
2016–2018	HPH task force: Mental Health
2017–	HPH task force: Migration, Equity & Diversity
Phase 6: Starting a transition of HPH and using new means of communication (2019–)	
2019–	Transfer of international HPH Secretariat to OptiMedis AG, Hamburg, Germany
	Relaunch of the HPH website
2020–	Changes of & amendments to the constitution
	New global strategy for HPH 2020–2025
	New umbrella standards of HPH
	Establishing a webinar series on HPH
	Establishment of an online learning and implementation community
	Plan to apply for the Framework of Engagement with Non-State Actors (FENSA) with WHO

Health-Promoting Hospitals (HPH) as a concept, project, network, and movement is a child of the World Health Organization (WHO) and its Ottawa Charter (WHO, 1986). HPH as an international WHO network started already in 1990, initiated by the WHO Regional Office for Europe (WHO/Europe), next to and in relation to the Healthy Cities Project and network, and thus before a number of other settings initiatives. For that, WHO/Europe took three important decisions confining the grand claims of the Ottawa Charter. Instead of focusing on health services more generally or even on the health sector, it chose hospital organizations. Instead of "reorienting" hospitals, it aimed at "health-promoting" hospitals. For implementation, it selected the settings approach, not the other strategies of the Ottawa Charter.

Concerning terminology, alternatives were either "healthy" hospitals or "health-promoting" hospitals. It was decided for "Health-Promoting Hospitals," by that not following the earlier example of "Healthy Cities!" This was a good and realistic decision, not only by directly relating to "health promotion" and not just "health" as the aim of the project. Furthermore, a "healthy" setting or organization is one which is fit for long and good-quality survival in the future, in contrast a "health-promoting" setting or organization aims to increase the health or health gain of all people in different stakeholder roles whose health is impacted or can be affected by the respective setting or organization. Of course, being health promoting, very much depending on the incentives of the health care system in general, can improve the chances of an organization to survive longer and better. But as the development of the health care sector and especially of hospitals in direction of a competitive health care industry shows, being health promoting is only one and a rather minor factor to being a fit survivor in this competition. Therefore, in following the spirit of the Ottawa Charter, we generally favor health-promoting settings over healthy settings.

In a preliminary, preparatory phase 0 (1986–1989), the regional office of the WHO/Europe for starting HPH organized a "Consultation on the role of health promotion in hospitals" in Copenhagen in 1988, which resulted in a first conceptual vision and recommendations for developing HPH (Milz & Vang, 1989).[1] The consultation already used the term "health-promoting hospital," provided a comprehensive vision, and, by proposing to start with model projects, it accepted the complexity of the task to implement health promotion into hospitals' everyday practice. For further procedure, it made practical recommendations (encouraging hospitals to become a force in health promotion, allying with hospital organizations for that purpose, preparing a policy statement on health promotion in hospitals; using the Healthy Cities Network and model projects that demonstrate health promotion in hospitals). Since a later WHO workshop "The health promoting hospital" in London brought no results concerning a host for a model, the WHO, represented by Ilona Kickbusch, found two actors who were willing to take the task in the City Councilman for Health of the "Healthy City" of Vienna and the Ludwig Boltzmann Institute for the Sociology of Health and Medicine (LBI) as a scientific institute.

The developmental phase 1 (1989–1992) started with a feasibility study, where a more detailed concept was developed and a Viennese hospital, the Rudolfstiftung general training hospital, was recruited to host the WHO model project "Health and Hospital," which lasted from 1989 to 1996.

Unique for the approach chosen to develop a health-promoting hospital setting by the team of the LBI were a number of strategic principals concerning implementation of the health-promoting settings concept, which were as follows:

(1) To offer health promotion not as a new and further aim to the hospital, but rather as a new strategy to solve old problems of hospital functioning. A solution of these problems was seen as an entry point for convincing to aim towards and invest into the development of a more health-promoting organization and setting.
(2) To use health promotion strategies to solve existing problems and to become a more health-promoting organization was seen as a complex enterprise of a comprehensive and systemic organizational development process, which needed professional project management and the support of external organizational consultants for implementation, at least at the start and in a model project.
(3) To develop a convincing business case for outreach of the model project, scientific research and evaluation of health-promoting measures and interventions had to be used to create convincing evidence for the added value of health promotion in and by hospitals.
(4) Furthermore, for successful outreach of the model, policy documents and manuals had to be developed and consented and national and regional network infrastructure with administrative hubs secured.

The model project tried to implement these principles by establishing a general project structure and by executing nine different subprojects in the model hospital

---

[1] In the same year, a book *Hospitals Health Promotion* (Sol & Wilson, 1989) was also published in the US, but without much impact on US hospitals. A Canadian health promoter and public health researcher also published an article on 'Creating healthy and health promoting hospitals' (Hancock, 1999).

with resulting manuals for implementation (Pelikan & Halbmayer, 1999a; Pelikan & Halbmayer, 1999b; Nowak & Pelikan, 1999; Nowak, Lobnig, Krajic, & Pelikan, 1999; Nowak, Lobnig, & Pelikan, 1999). An international HPH network was initiated already in 1990 with regular business meetings of interested hospitals and other international partners, coordinated by the LBI, which was designated as the WHO-Collaborating Centre for Health Promotion in Hospitals and Health Care (WHO-CC-HPH) in 1992. In 1991, the Budapest Declaration of Health Promoting Hospitals was adopted, defining 17 specific aims and tasks for a HPH as well as criteria for participation of hospitals as pilot hospitals in a planned European Project of HPH with 13 specific recommendations. In the following business meetings of the HPH network, the concept was further developed and hospitals were recruited for the planned European project.

A second phase of model testing and developing first international network structures and national/regional networks (1993–1998) was determined by the European Pilot Hospital Project on Health Promoting Hospitals (EPHP) which was carried out from 1993 to 1997 (Pelikan et al., 1998; Pelikan et al., 2001; Pelikan & Wolff, 1999). Overall, 20 hospitals from 11 European countries (Austria, Czech Republic, Germany (5), Greece, France, Hungary, Republic of Ireland, Italy (2), Poland (2), Sweden, UK (4: England, Northern Ireland, Scotland, Wales)) followed the methodology to implement a HPH, which had worked well in the Austrian model hospital. The aim was to find out if it was also applicable to other countries with different health care systems and to other types of hospitals. The project was executed by regular business meetings of its participants. In 1993, the fifth business meeting of the International HPH Network was also organized—this time as the first general assembly of the network.

In parallel to the project, also annual international HPH conferences (later with satellite events like annual international summer schools, pre- and post-conference workshops for newcomers and since 2009, a web portal for the conferences), and a HPH newsletter were started. The annual international conferences were important for the HPH network to bring everyone interested in HPH together in a person-to-person meeting, to meet, discuss, and decide network matters in a general assembly of the network and to host business meetings of the EPHP. Later, also meetings of task forces and working groups of the network were organized as satellites. Last, but not least, international conferences were also important to promote upcoming topics relevant for HPH. At the first international conference in Warsaw, Tobacco-Free Hospitals were the additional theme. In 1998, following a conference on this topic, a first HPH task force for Health Promotion in Psychiatric Health Services was started, which lasted until 2015 and produced specific materials and publications (Berger, 2003; Paul et al., 1996; Berger et al., 1999; Berger & Paul, 1998, 1999; Kilian et al., 1999; Berger et al., 2005). Also starting in 1998, websites for HPH were launched and a first international project database on HPH was established.

Already in 1993, two regional or national HPH networks existed, one in Wales and one in Poland. One of the conditions to be accepted as a pilot hospital in EPHP had been to be prepared to establish a regional or national network, if possible jointly with others from the same region or country. To make this happen, WHO promoted regional/national networks as an official strategy of the HPH network in 1995 and initiated a first workshop for network coordinators. To support recruiting countries outside the EPHP, a workshop "The Health Promoting Hospitals in the European Union" was administered in cooperation with the European Commission (Ludwig Boltzman Institute for the Sociology of Health and Medicine, 1996), which led to initiating further regional and national networks in the following years. In 1997, at the fifth international HPH conference in Vienna (Pelikan et al., 1997), the EPHP ended with presenting the Vienna Recommendations on Health Promoting Hospitals.

A third phase (1998–2005) was characterized by standardizing the concept and linking it more explicitly to quality philosophy and tools and the principle of evidence-based health care. Coordination and secretariat of the International HPH Network moved from Vienna to the WHO European Office for Integrated Healthcare Services in Barcelona, Spain. A HPH task force for HPH and EFQM was established and the WHO provided leadership by initiating two international working groups, one on "Standards for Health Promoting Hospitals" (led by the WHO Barcelona office and researchers in Copenhagen) and one on "Putting HPH Policy into Action" (led by the Vienna WHO-CC-HPH). Both working groups delivered documents and publications starting in 2005, the Standards group (Groene, 2006; Groene et al., 2010; Groene & Garcia-Barbero, 2005; Groene & Jorgensen, 2005) as well as the Putting HPH Policy into Action or Strategies group (Pelikan et al., 2005; Pelikan et al., 2006).

Also in 2002, a new project was started within the International HPH Network taking up the important topic of migration for health care by a European Commission supported project "Migrant Friendly and Culturally Competent Hospitals" (http://www.mfheu.net/public/home.htm), which lasted until 2005 and resulted in The Amsterdam Declaration toward Migrant-Friendly Hospitals in an ethno-culturally diverse Europe (MFH Project Group, 2004), presented at a conference "Hospitals in a Culturally Diverse Europe," Amsterdam, The Netherlands, December 9–11, 2004 (Bischoff, 2006; Bischoff et al., 2009; Karl-Trummer & Krajic, 2007; Karl-Trummer, Krajic, et al., 2006; Karl-Trummer, Schulze, et al., 2006; Krajic et al., 2005a, b; Krajic et al., 2006; Novak-Zezula et al., 2006; Pelikan & Krajic, 2007). Within HPH, this led to the formation of a very productive, specific task force on this topic (Chiarenza, 2014) in 2005. Already in 2004, a still ongoing task force on Children and Adolescents in Hospitals had been started (Guerreiro, 2012; Task Force HPH-CA, 2009).

A fourth phase (2005–2010), characterized by becoming independent of the HPH network and widening of its scope, was initiated by the WHO retreating as the coordinating institution of the international network, because of a general change in its setting-oriented policy. Also in 2005, a first regional/national network outside of Europe was established in Quebec, Canada, and in 2006 a second one in Taiwan.

The international secretariat was moved from Barcelona to Copenhagen in 2005 and hosted there by the WHO-CC for Evidence-Based Health Promotion in Hospitals, which was founded in 2004. The retreat of WHO was accompanied by establishing a more formal general assembly and an elected governance board of the

International HPH Network in 2006. By that, a more participatory and democratic structure of the international network was started. The process of emancipating HPH from WHO finally led to legalizing the now named "International Network of Health Promoting Hospitals and Health Services" as an independent association under Swiss law with a specific constitution in 2008. By this constitution, HPH, which was founded as a European project, officially became a global network and included other health services next to still dominating hospitals. HPH was defined as follows: "A Health Promoting Hospital and Health Service (HPH) is understood as an organisation that aims to improve health gain for its stakeholders by developing structures, cultures, decisions and processes. HPH is focused primarily on patients and their relatives, with a specific focus on the needs of vulnerable groups, hospital staff, the community population and—last but not least—the environment" (WHO, 2007). For the first time in 2009, a HPH strategy was released and a Memorandum of Understanding with WHO/Europe was signed in 2010.

Three new task forces were initiated: Tobacco-Free United (2008–2013, later cooperation with the European Network of Smoke-free Hospitals (ENSH) was conducted), on Alcohol and Alcohol Interventions (2009–2013), on HPH and Environment (2010–) (Task Force website: http://www.hph-greenhospital.org/node/7; Global Green and Healthier Hospitals Initiative Agenda (2011) http://green-hospitals.net/wp-content/uploads/2011/10/Global-Green-and-Healthy-Hospitals-Agenda.pdf; *HPH and Environment Manual* (also translated in Chinese) http://www.hphgreenhospital.org/sites/default/files/folder2/hph_and_environment_manual.pdf). Furthermore, related to the Austrian HPH network, a project on the sustainable hospital has been conducted from 2006 to 2009 (Weisz et al., 2011).

Furthermore, two important evaluation projects on HPH were started, a Project on a Retrospective, Internationally Comparative Evaluation Study on HPH (PRICES-HPH) from 2008–2012 (Dietscher, 2012; Dietscher et al., 2011; Pelikan, Dietscher, et al., 2011b; Röthlin, 2013) and the HPH DATA Project—Evaluation of a Health Promotion Patient Documentation Model from 2009 to 2012 (Tønnesen et al., 2012).

A fifth phase (2011–2018) was characterized by further globalization, evaluation, and strategic communication with milestones opening up new activities. The journal *Clinical Health Promotion: Research and Best Practice for Patients, Staff and Community* (2011–) was launched and a Bibliography on Health Promoting Hospitals was included within the Oxford Bibliographies on Public Health for the first time (Dietscher et al., 2014; an update is in progress).

Also based on earlier work (Pelikan et al., 2014, 2013) and newer work, salutogenesis and HPH found inclusion into the *Handbook of Salutogenesis* (Dietscher et al., 2016; Mittelmark et al., 2016; Pelikan, 2016).

A further project "WHO-HPH Recognition Project on Fast-Track Implementation of Clinical Health Promotion" (2012–2016) was initiated (Svane, Chiou, et al., 2018; Svane, Egerod, & Tønnesen, 2018; Tønnesen et al., 2016).

For the first time and also celebrating the twentieth international HPH conference, a HPH conference took place outside of Europe in Taipei, Taiwan (2012), where a strong national network had developed since 2006. A second international conference outside Europe was organized in New Haven, USA (2016), where a regional network in cooperation with Planetree (a nonprofit organization that partners with health care organizations around the world to facilitate person-centered care) was initiated. As a result of this conference, the "New Haven Recommendations on partnering with patients, families and citizens to enhance performance and quality in health promoting hospitals and health" were released (Frampton et al., 2016; Wieczorek et al., 2018). By that, the importance of patient participation in (health-promoting) hospitals was acknowledged and measures to optimally implement this on a micro, meso, and macro level were offered.

New task forces on Health-Enhancing Physical Activity (2012–2016) (HPH Task Force on Health Enhancing Physical Activity in Hospitals and Health Services, 2016), on Age-Friendly Health Care (2013–) (Chiou & Chen, 2009), and on Implementation and Monitoring of Standards (2016–) were established, while two earlier task forces were restarted with a somewhat changed focus, on Mental Health (2016–2018) (Bergerlind, 2018), and on Migration, Equity & Diversity (2017–).

In 2016, the HPH Governance Board approved a new international working group on HPH and Health Literate Organizations, which based on the International Organization for Migration (IOM) concept of "Ten Attributes of a Health Literate Health Care Organization" (Brach et al., 2012) and an extended model and tool by a team at the WHO-CC-HPH in Vienna (Dietscher & Pelikan, 2015, 2017) and further publications (Kickbusch et al., 2013; Pelikan, 2019) provided an international self-assessment tool for organizational health literacy (responsiveness) for hospitals (Working Group HPH & HLO, 2019). This generic English language tool will be translated into further languages and piloted and tested in different countries. Some indicators of this tool were already chosen for a Taiwanese tool for an integrative model of health promotion in hospitals (Wang et al., 2019) and it will also be taken up by the Action Network on Measuring Population and Organizational Health Literacy (M-POHL) under the umbrella of the European Health Information Initiative (EHII) of the WHO/Europe (Dietscher et al., 2019).

The sixth and ongoing phase of HPH (2019–) is starting a kind of transition and relaunch of HPH and introducing the systematic use of new media of communication. Due to changes of the WHO's regulation for the WHO Collaborating Centers, by a call for bids a new host was found for the international secretariat. OptiMedis AG based in Hamburg, Germany, is a renowned health management company for the development of multi-professional regional health networks, whose senior partners, Helmut Hildebrandt and Oliver Groene, have a long tradition of dealing with and supporting of health promotion and HPH specifically. The relaunch is conducted by changes and amendments of the HPH constitution, by a new global strategy of HPH for 2020–2025, a new website, developing new umbrella standards for HPH, establishing a webinar series on HPH and an online learning and implementation community, and planning for the WHO Framework of Engagement with Non-State Actors (FENSA) status with WHO.

How well this transformative relaunch to position HPH for new challenges works will only be seen in the next future.

7.3   Current Situation: How Successful Has HPH Been up to Now?

Evaluating the success of any social system, be it a hospital organization, a social network, or a social movement, and HPH relates to all three of these formats of social systems, has to take two aspects of development into account—its reproduction as a system over time; and its production of a specific vision, mission, aim, goal, objective or added value. To produce or fulfill its mission, a social system has to survive in time, nowadays usually in a complex and dynamic environment, and for that has to be adaptive—reactive and proactive—by adequate internal development to continuously gain necessary resources (money, working time, attention, prestige) from its relevant environments and stakeholders. Therefore, successful reproduction is a prerequisite for successful production, but successful production in most cases also is a precondition for getting the necessary resources for further successful reproduction. Thus, reproduction and production are the main dimensions of evaluating HPH.

Evaluating the success of HPH can be done on three levels: on the level of the international network, on the level of its national/regional networks, and on the level of single member hospitals or other health care services. To do this is difficult in different ways for the three levels and results will differ as well for each of these levels. Since there is more limited data and research for the level of national/regional HPH networks or for single health service organizations as members of these (for the participants of the Pilot Hospital Project, see Pelikan et al., 1998; Pelikan & Wolff, 1999), we will focus our reflection on the level of the International HPH Network.

Concerning reproduction, the International HPH Network has not only survived, but principally has grown in regional representation and involved quite a number of national/regional networks (maximum around 40, at the moment around 25) and also of member institutions (maximum around 900, at the moment rather about 600) over time. The majority of its national/regional networks which were initiated also survived and grew, some after solving critical situations. There are still new networks starting, but some also ceased and shrank. Failure in national/regional networks in Europe mostly was due to changes in general (e.g., economic crisis) or specific (e.g., change in relevance of health promotion in politics) economic and political preconditions or by retreat of important network leaders. Concerning national or regional networks, most countries chose to start immediately with a national network, few with one or more regional networks. For example, Italy was following its regionalized health care system from the beginning, by that some of its regional networks were able to survive in the economic crisis while some were not. A few very big countries like China or the USA just started in one smaller region, other countries with internal cultural–ethnic differences (like Belgium, Canada, Spain) started also with just one specific region. At the beginning, most networks were initiated in Europe either by pilot hospitals of the EPHP or by the initiative of the European Commission. Later, also networks outside Europe have been founded, mainly in Asia and Australia, very few and not very sustainable ones in the Americas, and none in Africa. In some countries, there are only a few individual members of the international network and no regional/national networks at all (e.g., in India, Israel, Slovenia). Thus, while following the new constitution, at least globalization was successful in some continents, but the other widening by the constitution to other health services than hospitals was less successful.

There was no specific strategy for developing other health-promoting health services within HPH, but a European Commission project "Health Promotion in General Practice and Community Pharmacy" (1998–2001) was conducted by the Vienna WHO-CC-HPH, probably too early. The project's results were presented at a European conference on Health Promotion in General Practice and Community Pharmacy—Experiences and Perspectives, Brussels, Belgium, November 10–11, 2000 (Plunger, 2001). The development of health promotion in primary care was lately initiated by a pilot project in Austria (Rojatz et al., 2018) again and got some international support by the new WHO policy on primary care and public health (Astana Declaration). Later, also in relation with the Vienna WHO-CC-HPH, for health-promoting long-term care some interesting research and piloting was conducted in Austria (Cichocki et al., 2015; Krajic et al., 2015; Marent et al., 2018; Quehenberger et al., 2014; Quehenberger & Krajic, 2017).

Regional/national networks considerably differ in size and strength generally, in institutionalization of infrastructure, and in diversity and amount of activities. There is only one internationally comparative study on regional/national networks (Dietscher, 2012) and very few on single networks, for example, Austria (Metzler, 2016), Canada (Graham et al., 2014), Iran (Afshari et al., 2018; Hamidi et al., 2019; Mahmoodi et al., 2019; Yaghoubi & Javadi, 2013), Italy (Gruber, 2016), Taiwan (Huang et al., 2016; Lee et al., 2012, 2014; Lee, Chen, Chien, et al., 2015; Lee, Chen, Powell, & Chu, 2015; Lin & Lin, 2011). Furthermore, there are some studies on the level of single member hospitals in different countries, for example, Croatia (Brkić et al., 2018), Indonesia (Tatang & Mawartinah, 2019), South Africa (Delobelle et al., 2011).

Surviving and growing by establishing and keeping national/regional networks, which recruited organizational network members, was possible, since the international network always had a strong organizational hub and managed the necessary changes in the respective host of the hub or international secretariat well, from a WHO-CC to WHO/Europe, to another WHO-CC and to a renowned health management company. Lastly, it sustainably developed into an autonomous, primarily self-financed, legal organization in the format of an NGO association and established continuous good links to WHO and other important partners. It was successful in getting external institutional and financial support and in recruiting enthusiastic professionals within health services, health politics, and in academia dedicated to serve its mission. Due to being a network of networks, different stronger national/regional networks provided innovation and leadership, took over organizational responsibilities, and offered resources within the different phases of HPH.

Internally, by capacity building, it successfully established diverse infrastructures for managing specific tasks like research projects, task forces, and working groups, got continuous support from several related WHO-CCs and recruited hosts willing to invest in the annual international conferences or in summer schools. By that, it was able to take up and develop newly evolving relevant topics in health care and health promotion for an innovative, widened, and differentiated scope of HPH's content and to provide networks and member organizations with supportive strategic and policy documents and tools, like standards for self-assessment, and to offer training opportunities. By its projects, task forces, and working groups, it was not only able to take up different relevant lifestyle issues (like smoking, nutrition, or physical activity), but also specific needs of vulnerable or disadvantaged groups (like children and adolescents as well as aged people in health care; psychiatric patients and patients in general in the health care system) and lastly of the environment. Furthermore, it established different media, like newsletters, websites, conferences, and workshops for communicating with its members and disseminating and sharing its "products" with possible implementing actors in its relevant environments.

Special importance have the annual—up to now in-person—conferences and their side events for the functioning of the HPH network, going on now for nearly three decades. HPH is the only one of all the WHO setting networks with such regular annual international conferences. International HPH conferences started with about 150 delegates in 1993, had a peak of about 1000, and now most commonly of about 500 participants and around 900 accepted abstracts. These conferences are useful for the different stakeholders of HPH, long-standing members, and newcomers; to present, get feedback, discuss, and learn about relevant themes and developments in health promotion, health care, and public health globally, in different countries and locally; and to network and make new contacts and strengthen already existing ones. By participation in the conference, a common spirit and joint support for being engaged in HPH is updated annually. For the local national/regional network or member health care organization, hosting the international conference is an excellent means to become more visible regionally, strengthen links with important stakeholders, and give attention to local members and staff. Therefore, the COVID-19 pandemic and its social consequences making an in-person conference impossible at the moment is a real challenge for HPH. By the international conferences, projects, task forces, and working groups, themes mainly related to developments in the three overarching topics health care, health promotion, and relevant burning societal issues have been promoted.

Health care: **Reorienting health services** (governance & leadership, HPH as a health policy issue); **Quality philosophy & management** (strategies & standards, EFQM, monitoring, evaluation, reporting); **Cost containment** (effectivity, cost-effectiveness, evidence-based healthcare); **Patient-centered healthcare** (pain-free & palliative care) & coproduction of health (patient empowerment, self-help-friendly hospitals, patient-reported outcomes); **Change management & culture change** (organizational development, sustainable health systems); **Other services of health care than hospitals** (primary health care, medical doctors, health promotion in continuous & integrated care).

Health promotion: **Issue related** (tobacco, alcohol/drugs, nutrition, physical exercise; violence; social determinants, noncommunicable diseases); **Vulnerable population related** (baby-friendly hospitals, children and adolescents, aged citizens/healthy aging, gender issues, migrants, mental health, and psychiatric care; somato-psycho-social health needs); **Setting related** (workplace health promotion, community health promotion, salutogenic hospitals, organizational capacity building, cooperation with other settings, partnerships in healthy alliances); **Communication & health literacy** (health education, health literate hospitals); **Methods & techniques** (evidence-based health promotion, risk prediction models, information and communications technology, long-term effects of interventions).

Relevant burning societal issues: **Environmental & ecological issues** (environment-friendly & sustainable health care); **Migrants & cultural diversity** (refugees and asylum seekers, multiethnic society); **Global health inequalities** (cooperation with developing countries, solidarity and equity in health, secondary prevention and inequalities); Aging populations; Digitalization in health care and beyond.

Unfortunately, due to a lack of available documentation and research, we cannot give a systematic description of capacity building on the level of regional/national networks or hospital and health service organizations beyond the first model project and the following pilot hospital project. But at least we could demonstrate that the reproduction of HPH as an international network has been quite successful over three decades since it was established by WHO in 1990.

It is more difficult to evaluate the success of HPH concerning its "production." What actually is the intended "product" of HPH, or more generally, what is principally offered to actors and systems by health promotion in its relevant environment? To be realistic, health promotion can only offer symbolic or intellectual products, like arguments (on the "what," "why," and "how" of health promotion), supporting evidence by facts and figures (based on research) and descriptions of evidence-based health promotion good practices (based on experience and research) to better protect and promote the health of people, and communicate these "products"— more or less effectively—to the relevant actors and systems, who are in a position to use and implement these. In the case of HPH, this will be the stakeholders of hospitals and other health services, like owners, financers, managers, health professionals, and patients, who can impact and change the everyday functioning of these organizations and by that finally the health gain for the people affected by it in different roles. The actors and systems who are supposed to implement health promotion have to be informed and motivated by social marketing and lobbying to "buy" the health promotion mission and be enabled by documents and tools (e.g., for needs assessment, implementation, capacity building, health impact assessment) as well as by consultation and training to effectively use health promotion for their own ends. For that, a precondition was to define a vision, mission, model, or concept outlining the scope and objectives of HPH and furthermore developing policy documents, strategies, action plans, standards, etc. on how to implement and execute these in everyday life of the respective health service organization or setting.

The first step was to develop a more detailed concept or model to define what the vision and mission of HPH is all about. Background was of course the Ottawa Charter generally and its action area Reorienting Health Services especially, but already more focused and limited by the results of the WHO consultation (Milz & Vang, 1989) just to Health-Promoting Hospitals. Therefore, some later critique of the results of HPH being that HPH did not have succeeded in fully Reorienting Health Services (de Leeuw, 2009; Wise & Nutbeam, 2007), which of course was a correct diagnosis, nevertheless was partly misled, because that was not the mandate of HPH. The description in the Ottawa Charter of the action area Reorienting Health Services was more realistic in this respect by highlighting: "The responsibility for health promotion in health services is shared among individuals, community groups, health professionals, health service institutions and governments. They must work together towards a health care system which contributes to the pursuit of health. [...] Health services need to embrace an expanded mandate [...] Reorienting health services also requires stronger attention to health research as well as changes in professional education and training" (WHO, 1986). This definitely and realistically cannot be achieved alone, and partly not even initiated, just by health promotion–oriented hospital organizations or settings themselves, it needs reorientation and support by a wider society. However, Wise and Nutbeam (2007) correctly have argued that, while HPH has concentrated on the hospital sector, broader health system reform toward health promotion needs yet to be achieved. By its constitution, HPH officially widened its scope at least to other health services and even changed its name to International Network of Health Promoting Hospitals and Health Services in 2008, but not many efforts have been invested to prepare the necessary products to support this to happen. De Leeuw's editorial reflects the discourse on HPH in the wider community of health promotion research.

Although the early conception of Milz and Vang (1989) did not try to operationalize Reorienting Health Services, it nevertheless had a wide and comprehensive whole systems conception of Health-Promoting Hospitals and not just single health promotion projects within the hospital setting. It already was focusing on health and wellness for and participation of patients, staff, and the community; understanding hospitals also as a workplace, an educational institution, an important partner in communities; relating health promotion to quality assurance, monitoring, and evaluation; and hinting at the importance of architecture and ecological aspects of hospitals. Based on that, the Viennese feasibility study (1989) for the model project Health and Hospital produced a more detailed concept on the possible content of a health-promoting hospital. The next official document on HPH, the Budapest Declaration on Health Promoting Hospitals (1991), defining the vision for the EPHP, entailed 17 comprehensive characteristics for content and aims for hospitals participating in HPH beyond the assurance of good quality medical services and health care.

At the end of the Pilot Hospital Project, the Vienna Recommendations on Health Promoting Hospitals (1997) reiterated the concept by six fundamental principles and four strategies for implementation of HPH and gave three criteria for participation in the WHO Health Promoting Hospitals Network.

The official definition of HPH in WHO's Health Promotion Glossary (Nutbeam, 1998a, p. 357) was adapted from the Budapest Declaration and defined HPH as follows:

> A health promoting hospital does not only provide high quality comprehensive medical and nursing services, but also develops a corporate identity that embraces the aims of health promotion, develops a health promoting organizational structure and culture, including active, participatory roles for patients and all members of staff, develops itself into a health promoting physical environment and actively cooperates with its community. Health promoting hospitals take action to promote the health of their patients, their staff, and the population in the community they are located in. Health promoting hospitals are actively attempting to become 'healthy organizations'. The Health Promoting Hospital is a concept in development since 1988. An international network has developed to promote the wider adoption of this concept in hospitals and other health care settings.

The qualifications of the Budapest Declaration, the fundamental principles and implementation strategies of the Vienna Recommendations, and the definition of the Health Promotion Glossary definitely fulfill the criteria for Type 4 "Being a health promotion setting and improving the health of the community" (as opposed to Type 1 "Do a health promotion project," Type 2 "Delegate health promotion to a specific division, department or staff," and Type 3 "Being a health-promotion setting"), as defined in the typology of different organizational approaches to health promotion by Johnson and Baum (2001), who knew about and related to the Vienna Model Project. The WHO's concept and model from its beginning and the following documents of the HPH network integrated the four types or better strategies of a HPH for the settings approach.

A peer-reviewed article in the same year on HPH (Pelikan et al., 2001) outlined what reorientation of health care services may mean for the main hospital functions: "These include: the health promoting hospital setting; health promoting workplaces, the provision of health (related) services, training, education and research; the hospital as an advocate and 'change agent' for health promotion in its community/environment; the 'healthy' (metaphorically speaking) hospital organisation." Furthermore, it stated: "It is argued that the further development of the HPH Network will have to take into account some major changes that have occurred in the hospital landscape since the start of the network: the quality movement and, as a subset of this, the increasing importance of Evidence Based Medicine."

Already in 1999, a HPH task force HPH and EFQM had been started by an initiative of the German national network on HPH which published a handbook relating implementation of HPH first to the European Forum on Quality Management (EFQM) methodology (Brandt, 2001) and somewhat later also to the Balanced Score Card methodology by a WHO pilot project from 2002 to 2011: Implementing the HPH Strategy and Standards through a combined application of the EFQM Excellence Model and the Balanced Scorecard (HPH-EFQM-BSC) (Brandt et al., 2005; Groene et al., 2009). Also in 2001, HPH started to take quality and evidence-based methodology even more seriously by starting two international HPH working groups on "Putting HPH Policy into Action" and "Standards for Health Promoting Hospitals," which both produced documents and publications on HPH strategies and standards (Groene & Garcia-Barbero, 2005) (Strategies: Pelikan et al., 2005; Pelikan et al., 2006; Standards: Groene, 2006).

The Putting HPH Policy into action working group provided a matrix of 18 strategies (cf. Table 7.2) to define the comprehensive systems approach of HPH and linked implementation to quality methodology by further seven strategies. Columns in the matrix refer to the three stakeholder groups whose health and health gain is focused by HPH: patients (and their families), staff (and their families), and residents in the community which the hospital serves. The six rows of the matrix relate to the specific functions a hospital has to fulfill for these stakeholders to be health promoting for them.

Strategy one, empowerment for health promoting self-reproduction, takes into account that all stakeholders coming into contact with the hospital do that as representatives of a specific role, for example, as patients, staff or visitors with specific role-related challenges, but also as biopsychosocial human beings that have to self-reproduce their organism, psyche and social status independently of their specific roles within the setting. For that they need enablement and empowerment by a supporting material–cultural–social process of the setting as their temporary environment (cf. Pelikan, 2007b, 2009).

Strategy two, empowerment for health-promoting coproduction, relates directly to the specific role fulfillment, be it of a co-productive patient or staff or visitor. For that role, incumbents need to be enabled and empowered for healthy participation in coproduction by the setting as a supportive workplace for all roles involved. Concerning coproduction with services outside the hospital within its community, this is about enabling effective cooperation processes of the hospital with these.

Strategy three, developing a safe and health-promoting setting, relates to health-promoting structures and infrastructures of a hospital as a material, cultural, and social setting and as a necessary framework for enabling the processes of strategies one and two. All three strategies together can be seen as defining specific qualities for the core cure and care functions of hospitals, that is, diagnosis, treatment, and rehabilitation. Therefore, these strategies can be expected from every hospital, since they mainly guarantee good clinical outcome and well-being for patients and protection of the health and well-being of staff and also taking into account the hospital's possible impact on the health of the residents of the community the hospital serves.

In contrast, the next three strategies can be done by health services outside the hospital as well and—if expected from a hospital—widen the mandate and the functions of hospitals. Therefore, to become a realistic and attractive opportunity for hospitals, these functions need to be officially added to and integrated into the mandate and financing schemes of hospitals, which has to be specifically regulated by health policy.

Strategy four, empowerment for illness management, expects more responsibility for the recuperation process of the patients after discharge from the hospital, by empowering them for self-management and prevention in relation to their specific disease. The same holds true for occupational diseases of staff or empowerment for prevention and self-management of specific diseases for residents in the community.

Table 7.2 Eighteen core strategies as a comprehensive framework for health promotion activities for a HPH (Pelikan et al., 2005, p. 59)

HP for/by	Patients	Staff	Community
HP quality development of treatment & care, by empowerment of stakeholders for health-promoting **self-reproduction**	Empowerment of patients for health-promoting self-care/self-maintenance/self-reproduction in the hospital (PAT-1)	Empowerment of staff for health-promoting self-care/self-maintenance/self-reproduction in the hospital (STA-1)	Empowerment of community health-promoting self-care/self-reproduction by adequate access to hospital (COM-1)
HP quality development of treatment & care, by empowerment of stakeholders for health-promoting **coproduction**	Empowerment of patients for health-promoting participation/coproduction in treatment and care (PAT-2)	Empowerment of staff for health-promoting participation/coproduction in treatment and care (STA-2)	Empowerment of health professionals in the community for health-promoting coproduction in treatment and aftercare of patients (COM-2)
HP quality development for health-promoting & empowering **hospital setting** for stakeholders	Development of hospital into a supportive, health-promoting & empowering setting for patients (PAT-3)	Development of hospital into a supportive, health-promoting & empowering setting for staff (STA-3)	Development of hospital into a health-promoting & empowering setting for the community (COM-3)
Provision of specific HP services—empowering **illness management** (patient education) for stakeholders	Empowerment of patients for health-promoting management of chronic illness (after discharge) (PAT-4)	Empowerment of staff for health-promoting management of occupational illness (STA-4)	Empowerment of community population for health-promoting management of chronic illness (COM-4)
Provision of specific HP services—empowering **lifestyle development** (health education) for stakeholders	Empowerment of patients for health-promoting lifestyle development (after discharge) (PAT-5)	Empowerment of staff for health-promoting lifestyle development (STA-5)	Empowerment of community population for health-promoting lifestyle development (COM-5)
Provision of specific HP activities—participation in health-promoting & empowering **community development** for stakeholders	Participation in health-promoting & empowering development of community infrastructures for specific patient needs (PAT-6)	Participation in health-promoting & empowering development of community infrastructures for specific needs of staff (STA-6)	Participation in health-promoting & empowering community development for general population (COM-6)

Reprinted from *Health Promotion in Hospitals: Evidence and Quality Management* (Oliver Groene and Mila Garcia-Barbero, Editors). Jürgen M. Pelikan, Christina Dietscher, Karl Krajic, & Peter Nowak. Eighteen core strategies for Health Promoting Hospitals, pp. 59–60, Copyright 2005. https://www.euro.who.int/__data/assets/pdf_file/0008/99827/E86220.pdf. Accessed on October 19, 2021

Strategy five, empowerment for lifestyle development, is somewhat more far reaching and relates to empowering for healthy lifestyle changes of all three stakeholder groups.

And strategy six, (co-)developing health-promoting living conditions in the community, is even more far reaching, since it expects hospitals not only to care also for people who are not their patients, but furthermore to engage (with other agents) in improving the living conditions in the community to better the health of people who are affected by these.

Thus, these strategies define a really comprehensive concept of a HPH, but at the same time they also demonstrate that it is not taken for granted at all that hospitals are in a situation to realistically be able and willing to take up all these strategies as a package for implementation, if the preconditions for that will not be changed adequately before. Hospitals definitely need a widened mandate, new financial regulations, and specific incentives to take up the full package of the comprehensive whole systems model of HPH.

Since at least the first three strategies can be definitely seen just as quality improvement aspects of hospital services and the other three also as quality issues, but with a widened mandate of hospitals, HPH chose to recommend and offer quality philosophy and methodology for implementation of HPH. Quality reform strategies have become more and more prominent for hospital and health services development in the last decades, which seems to be rather specific for the health care setting. Using a shortened quality circle (cf. Table 7.3), health promotion

Table 7.3 Seven implementation strategies for health promotion in health care organizations following quality circle and aspects (Pelikan, 2007a)

Quality of... Quality Functions	Structures of services (& settings)	Processes of services (& settings)	Outcomes/impacts of services (& settings)
1. Definition	S1 Define HP criteria & standards for structures	P1 Define HP guidelines & standards for processes	O1 Define targets for HP outcomes & impacts
2. Assessment, monitoring, evaluation	S2 Assess for HP of structures	P2 Assess for HP of processes	O2 Assess for HP of outcomes & impacts
3. Assurance, development, improvement	S3 Improve HP of structures by organizational, personal and technical development	X	X

criteria and standards have first to be defined for hospital structures, processes, and outcomes and impacts; for second to be assessed, monitored, and evaluated; and third, based on results of assessment, structures can be developed and improved by specific measures and interventions. These, hopefully, will result in more health-promoting processes and lastly in better outcomes and impacts, since one has to accept that processes, outcomes, and impacts cannot directly be improved. (That only could be done by cooking of statistics and accounts!)

In line with the importance of standards and criteria for measurement, benchmarking and improvement of quality aspects, the Standards Working Group developed 5 standards with 24 substandards and 40 measureable elements following criteria and methodology of the International Society for Quality in Health Care (ISQua). These standards (cf. Table 7.4) are not taking up the full content of the 18 strategies of a HPH, for what they partly have been criticized, but they include important aspects mainly of the three quality strategies. These standards have been translated into different languages and been used for monitoring and implementation studies by national/regional networks (e.g., Hamidi et al., 2019) and further single hospitals (Amiri et al., 2016; Tatang & Mawartinah, 2019). A systematic review (Mahmoodi & Shaghaghi, 2019) found by analyzing 24 studies that "availability of resources, leadership and management support, intra health system collaboration/partnership and organizational capacity building for the HPH implementation" (2019, p. 235) are the most commonly reported facilitators. Whereas "scarcity of resources, insufficiency of leadership and/or management support, paucity of skilled and in-formed/committed personnel, deficiency of evaluation programmes, not having health promoting approach amongst personnel, low priority of health promotion activities in hospitals and overall policy resistance to change" (2019, p. 235) are among the most frequently reported barriers.

Table 7.4 Five Standards for implementing health promotion in hospitals (Source: Groene, 2006)

Standard 1: **Management policy**
The organization has a written policy for health promotion. The policy is implemented as part of the overall organization quality improvement system, aiming at improving health outcomes. This policy is aimed at patients, relatives and staff
Standard 2: **Patient assessment**
The organization ensures that health professionals, in partnership with patients, systematically assess needs for health promotion activities
Standard 3: **Patient information and intervention**
The organization provides patients with information on significant factors concerning their disease or health condition, and health promotion interventions are established in all patient pathways
Standard 4: **Promoting a healthy workplace**
The management establishes conditions for the development of the hospital as a healthy workplace
Standard 5: **Continuity and cooperation**
The organization has a planned approach to collaboration with other health service providers and other institutions and sectors on an ongoing basis

Another review, just on health-promoting hospitals in Iran (Hamidi et al., 2019), found 10 studies which showed that the HPH standards in the hospitals studied were generally very poor and that the standard of management policy had the lowest mean value. Results of the reviewed interventional studies showed that the implementation of HPH standards and educational interventions increase the standard of HPH. The review furthermore indicated that the main challenge in achieving the HPH standards is the more treatment-oriented hospital policy of Iran.

Furthermore, some of the taskforces and working groups have developed, marketed, and partly implemented specific standards and self-assessment tools for children and adolescents (Guerreiro, 2012), migrants (Chiarenza, 2014), age-friendly health care (Chiou & Chen, 2009), HPH and environment (HPH and Environment Task Force, 2010), for health-literate hospitals (Working Group HPH & HLO, 2019), for sustainable and health-promoting hospitals, (partly) based on the original five standards. Also the concept of self-help friendly hospitals (Forster et al., 2013; Trojan et al., 2016) has been researched mostly outside HPH, but partly taken up by HPH.

If being health promoting is understood as a specific aspect of the quality of health promotion, it makes sense to also integrate developing health promotion in a hospital into its quality management system. For that it is important that quality management gets a specific mandate and specific resources for monitoring and developing health promotion within the hospital setting. Of course, also a specific health promotion unit can be established in parallel to quality management, or, if there is no quality management system, as a standalone. But for giving the comprehensive whole systems HPH settings approach a chance, there is definitely a need for a specific technical unit for health promotion development, the closer to top management, the better.

The European HPH Network has been criticized for being under-researched and there were calls for more evaluation on the effectiveness of the approach (Whitehead, 2004). In his response, Groene (2005) rejected some of the critical arguments raised and provided evidence for progress in HPH.

While from the start, the development of HPH had been linked with research and evaluation mainly by the Model Project and the EPHP, later developments have not been researched as systematically or at all. But systematic evaluation was started again by the Project on a Retrospective, Internationally Comparative Evaluation Study of HPH (PRICES-HPH), which was conducted from 2008 to 2012 (Dietscher, 2012, 2017; Dietscher et al., 2011; Pelikan, Dietscher, et al., 2011b; Röthlin et al., 2015).

The project aimed at a systematic documentation and evaluation of structures, processes, and outcomes regarding the health promotion qualities of national/regional HPH networks and the member organizations in these networks. A specific evaluation model—the PRICES-HPH evaluation model—was developed to guide evaluation of health promotion implementation on the level of national/regional HPH networks and on the level of their member organizations to find out which role networks play in supporting the implementation of health promotion capacities and strategies at the hospital level (see Fig. 7.1). Coordinators of all 35 networks that

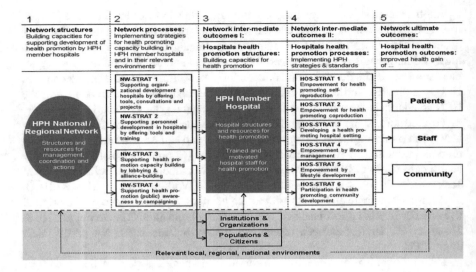

Fig. 7.1 The comprehensive framework of the PRICES-HPH Evaluation Model for national/regional networks and member hospitals (Pelikan, Dietscher, et al., 2011b) (HOS: Hospital, NW: Networks, STRAT: Strategy). ©WHO Collaboration Centre for Evidence-based Health Promotion in Hospitals & Health Services, Bispebjerg University Hospital, Copenhagen 2011

existed at the time of data collection were invited to participate. Of these, 28 completed questionnaires were received, which equals a return rate of 80% of all networks. Also, 529 coordinators of member hospitals were invited to participate in an online survey; 180 returned a completed questionnaire, which equals a response rate of 34%.

The PRICES-HPH evaluation model (see Fig. 7.1) was developed to guide evaluations of health promotion implementation in member hospitals within national/regional HPH networks and to find out which role networks play in supporting this implementation. The model applies and integrates concepts from various discourses: quality in health care, evaluation, and capacity building in health promotion and specific HPH documents. The model distinguishes between two kinds of actors and systems: firstly the member hospitals of national/regional HPH networks, and secondly, the national/regional networks themselves. It allows observation and evaluation of hospitals' and networks' health promotion qualities of their structures, processes, and outcomes (following Donabedian's (1966) quality paradigm and Nutbeam's (1998b) hierarchy of outcomes). The model relates to the capacity-building debate in health promotion by acknowledging that settings for effective health promotion interventions need adequate infrastructure and resources to be successful. Outcomes were the self-reported degree of implementation of the 18 core strategies for putting health promotion policy into action and the perceived strengthening by participation in HPH. In line with the main goal of HPH, the ultimate outcome of the model is defined as improved health gain of patients and their relatives or carers, staff, and their relatives as well as members of the community whose health interests are served by hospitals. However, health gain could not be measured by the design of the PRICES study, because this would need a more complex long-time-study design, and there are special studies demonstrating the principal effects of certain health promotion interventions on people's or patient's health.

Main results were, firstly, HPH capacities enable implementation of HP activities for patients, staff, and community by the following infrastructures and resources: HPH hospital coordinator, HP personnel and structures, HP policies and standards, HP financial resources, HP quality assessment, HP outcome monitoring, cooperation with partners for HP. Secondly, HPH network strategies have relevant effects on implemented HP capacities in member hospitals. A number of capacities are effective in supporting organizational development of hospitals by offering initiatives and tools, HP implementation tools (e.g., guidelines), specific task forces, respective membership criteria, a written HP policy, HP assessment (e.g., five standards, national indicators), or supporting personnel development of hospital staff by regular network conferences. Thirdly, national/regional regulations for HP have effects on implemented HP capacities, if legal regulations for HP exist specifically in health care and funding options for HP in health care (e.g., DRGs) or if HP is part of vocational training of health professionals.

In summary, the national/regional HPH networks and their member hospitals have implemented the HPH strategies to a substantial degree. They consider their involvement in HPH networks as a relevant influence for this purpose. The extent of implementation however varied by type of HPH strategy and by affiliation to the networks. Later studies and reviews partly found similar results and discussed furthering and hindering factors for successful implementation of HPH in more detail (Lee et al., 2014, Lee, Chen, Powell, & Chu, 2015; Pelikan et al., 2014; Wieczorek et al., 2015; Svane, Chiou, et al., 2018; Yaghoubi et al., 2018).

7.4   The Future of HPH and Next Steps

Since health promotion and even health-promoting settings cannot be implemented in a special health promotion world, but in a world where health promotion is just a minor factor determining developments, the success of health promotion as a vision, mission, and movement in this outer world mainly depends on other factors, even more so, as far as the future is concerned. But, of course, to a certain degree, health promotion's success is also dependent on the quality of the products it offers for making health promotion attractive in its outside world and for supporting effective and efficient implementation.

For health promotion in health care settings generally and in hospitals specifically, all that holds true in a unique way. Health care is already about health and thus has its own understanding of "health," which only partly overlaps with that of health promotion. Health care is a rather dynamic setting, driven mainly by progress in clinical technology, especially now by digitalization, which in turn is driven by big industry, and furthermore by the demographic change toward aging societies. These trends have the effect to expand the demand for health care and by that also its cost, and, therefore, in most countries the relative share of the Gross National Product spent on health care is rising. Since the state, more directly or indirectly, is responsible for and involved in health care financing, with economic crises of the state, cost containment is another strong driver for the development of the health care sector.

Thus, already in the past and up to the present, the success of HPH has been influenced by general societal trends and by specific ones within the health care sector to a high degree. The early growth of HPH and its later shrinking by the numbers of networks and member hospitals, very much is a consequence of economic situations, health policies, and availability of leading people. It is difficult to foresee these factors in the future, and COVID-19 and its social consequences, which definitely will affect health care, are increasing the insecurity of any prognosis.

Yet, these are not reasons to give up the vision of a comprehensive, whole-systems HPH settings approach. Seen from a perspective of optimizing health gain, this is a very sensible approach. But successful implementation and real reorientation of health services requires more than integrating health promotion into the core business of hospitals and good capacity building at the level of hospital settings and national/regional networks as well as strengthening connections with relevant parallel agendas. That has already been mostly achieved by HPH. It is also important that the international HPH network is repositioning itself and starting transformation. However, to guarantee a stronger movement for HPH and better reorientation of health services in the near and long-term future, a shift in (health) policy is needed to change the mandate of health services and hospitals, adapt financing systems, innovate the training of health professionals, and invest more in health promotion research.

References

Afshari, A., Mostafavi, F., Latifi, A., Ghahnaviyeh, L.A., Pirouzi, M., & Eslami, A.A. (2018). Hospitals reorientation towards health promotion: A qualitative study of barriers to and strategies for implementation of health promotion in hospitals of Isfahan. Journal of Education and Health Promotion, 7 (1) [online]. Available at: https://doi.org/10.4103/jehp.jehp_135_17

Amiri, M., Khosravi, A., Riyahi, L., & Naderi, S. (2016). The impact of setting the standards of health promoting hospitals on hospital indicators in Iran. PloS One, 11(12) [online]. Available at: https://doi.org/10.1371/journal.pone.0167459

Berger, H. (2003). Health promotion-a new approach in psychiatry. *Psychiatrische Praxis* [online]. Available at: https://doi.org/10.1055/s-2003-38547

Berger, H., Krajic, K., & Paul, R. (1999). Health promoting hospitals in practice: Developing projects and networks. In *Proceedings of the 6th International Conference on Health Promoting Hospitals, Darmstadt, April 29th-May 2nd*. Health Promotion Publications.

Berger, H., & Paul, R. (1998). The health promoting psychiatric hospital – What is the difference? Experiences from the Philipps hospital Pilot Hospital Project in Riedstadt. In J. M. Pelikan, M. Garcia-Barbero, H. Lobnig, & K. Krajic (Eds.), *Pathways to a health promoting hospital. Experiences from the European Pilot Hospital Project* (pp. 71–94). Conrad.

Berger, H., & Paul, R. (1999). From establishing a HPH-taskforce on health promoting mental health services to HPMHS network activities'. In H. Berger, K. Krajic, & R. Paul (Eds.), *Health promoting hospitals in practice: Developing projects and networks* (pp. 73–76). Conrad.

Berger, H., Paul, R., & Heimsath, E. (2005). *Task Force on Health Promoting Psychiatric Services* [online]. Available at: http://hph.mhil.at/archive/palanga06/htm/proceedings/II-1.1_Berger.pdf

Bergerlind, L-l.R. (2018). *Examples and contributions of HPH to mental health promotion and mental illness prevention* [online]. Available at: https://www.hphconferences.org/fileadmin/user_upload/P3_Bergerlind.pdf

Bischoff, A. (2006). *Caring for migrant and minority patients in European hospitals. A review of effective interventions*. SFM-Report 43.

Bischoff, A., Chiarenza, A., & Loutan, L. (2009). "Migrant-friendly hospitals": A European initiative in an age of increasing mobility. *World Hospitals and Health Services: The Official Journal of the International Hospital Federation, 45*(3), 7–9.

Brach, C., Keller, D., Hernandez, L. M., Baur, C., Parker, R., Dreyer, B., Schyve, P., Lemerise, A. J., & Schillinger, D. (2012). *Ten attributes of health literate health care organizations*. Institute of Medicine.

Brandt, E. (2001). *Qualitätsmanagement und Gesundheitsförderung im Krankenhaus: Handbuch zur EFQM-Einführung [Quality management and health promotion in hospitals: Manual for the introduction of EFQM]*. Luchterhand.

Brandt, E., Schmidt, W., Dziewas, R., & Groene, O. (2005). Implementing the health promoting hospitals strategy through a combined application of the EFQM excellence model and the balanced scorecard. In O. Groene & M. Garcia-Barbero (Eds.), *Health promotion in hospitals: Evidence and quality management* (pp. 80–99). WHO-Regional Office for Europe.

Brkić, M. Z., Šogorić, S., Lovrić, S., Sertić, V., Galinec, A., Tomas, M., Mikulan, M., Gašparić-Sikavica, M., & Markovčić, D. (2018). Health promoting hospitals-self-assessment of health promotion activities at department of psychiatry, Dr. Tomislav Bardek general hospital, Koprivnica. *Acta Medica Croatica, 72*(2), 233–239.

Chiarenza, A. (2014). *Standards for equity in health care for migrants and other vulnerable groups self-assessment tool for pilot implementation*. HPH Task Force on Migrant-Friendly and Culturally Competent Health Care.

Chiou, S. T., & Chen, L. K. (2009). Towards age-friendly hospitals and health services. *Archives of Gerontology and Geriatrics, 49*(2) [online]. Available at: https://doi.org/10.1016/S0167-4943(09)70004-4

Cichocki, M., Quehenberger, V., Zeiler, M., Adamcik, T., Manousek, M., Stamm, T., & Krajic, K. (2015) Effectiveness of a low-threshold physical activity intervention in residential aged care–results of a randomized controlled trial. *Clinical Interventions in Aging* [online]. Available at: https://doi.org/10.2147/CIA.S79360

de Leeuw, E. (2009) Have the health services reoriented at all?. *Health Promotion International, 24*(2) [online]. Available at: https://doi.org/10.1093/heapro/dap015

Delobelle, P., Onya, H., Langa, C., Mashamba, J., & Depoorter, A. M. (2011). Pilot health promoting hospital in rural South Africa: Evidence-based approach to systematic hospital transformation. Global Health Promotion, 18(1) [online]. Available at https://doi.org/10.1177/1757975910393171

Dietscher, C. (2012). *Interorganizational networks in the settings approach of health promotion - The case of the International Network of Health Promoting Hospitals and Health Services (HPH)*. PhD Thesis. Faculty of Social Sciences. University of Vienna [online]. Available at: https://doi.org/10.25365/thesis.24185

Dietscher, C. (2017). How can the functioning and effectiveness of networks in the settings approach of health promotion be understood, achieved and researched? *Health Promotion International, 32*(1) [online]. Available at: https://doi.org/10.1093/heapro/dat067

Dietscher, C., & Pelikan, J. M. (2015). Gesundheitskompetente Krankenbehandlungs-organisationen. *Prävention und Gesundheitsförderung* [online]. Available at: https://doi.org/10.1007/s11553-015-0523-0

Dietscher, C., & Pelikan, J. M. (2017). Health-literate hospitals and healthcare organizations. Results from an Austrian feasibility study on the self-assessment of organizational health literacy in hospitals. In D. Schaeffer & J. M. Pelikan (Eds.), *Health Literacy, Forschungsstand und Perspektiven* (pp. 303–313). Hogrefe.

Dietscher, C., Pelikan, J. M., Bobek, J., Nowak, P., & World Health Organization. Regional Office for Europe. (2019). The action network on measuring population and organizational health literacy (M-POHL): a network under the umbrella of the WHO European health information initiative (EHII). *Public Health Panorama, 5*(1), 65–71.

Dietscher, C, Pelikan J. M., & Schmied, H. (2014). Health promoting hospitals. *Oxford Bibliographies in Public Health* [online]. Available at: https://doi.org/10.1093/OBO/9780199756797-0131

Dietscher, C., Schmied, H., Röthlin, F., & Pelikan, J. M. (2011). *Project on a Retrospective, Internationally Comparative Evaluation Study of HPH (PRICES – HPH): Characteristics of national / regional networks of the International Network of Health Promoting Hospitals (HPH). The PRICES – HPH Network Survey. Report 1* (Working Paper 11). Ludwig Boltzmann Institute Health Promotion Research.

Dietscher, C., Winter, U., & Pelikan, J. M. (2016). The application of Salutogenesis in hospitals. In M. B. Mittelmark, S. Sagy, M. Eriksson, G. F. Bauer, J. M. Pelikan, B. Lindström, & G. A. Espnes (Eds.), *The handbook of Salutogenesis* (pp. 277–298). Springer International.

Donabedian, A. (1966). Evaluating the quality of medical care. *The Milbank Memorial Fund Quarterly, 83*(4) [online]. Available at: https://doi.org/10.1111/j.1468-0009.2005.00397.x

Forster, R., Rojatz, D., Schmied, H., & Pelikan, J. M. (2013). Self-help groups and health promoting hospitals - a promising alliance for health [Selbsthilfegruppen und Gesundheitsförderung im Krankenhaus - eine entwicklungsfähige Allianz für Gesundheit]. *Prävention und Gesundheitsforderung, 8*(1), 9–14.

Frampton, S. B., Pelikan, J. M., & Wieczorek, C. C. (2016). *The New Haven Recommendations on partnering with patients, families and citizens to enhance performance and quality in health promoting hospitals and health services.* International Network of Health Promoting Hospitals and Health Services. Available at: http://hph.mhil.at/fileadmin/user_upload/HPH_Declarations/New-Haven-Recommendations.pdf

Graham, R., Boyko, J. A., & Sibbald, S. L. (2014). Health promoting hospitals in Canada: A Proud past, an uncertain future. *Clinical Health Promotion, 4*(2), 70–75.

Groene, O. (2005). Evaluating the progress of the health promoting hospitals initiative? A WHO perspective. Commentary On: Whitehead, D. (2004). The European health promoting hospitals (HPH) Project: How far on?. *Health Promotion International, 20*(2) [online]. Available at: https://doi.org/10.1093/heapro/dah613

Groene, O. (2006). *Implementing health promotion in hospitals: Manual and self-assessment forms.* WHO Regional Office for Europe. [online]. Available at: Retrieved October 19, 2021, from http://www.euro.who.int/__data/assets/pdf_file/0009/99819/E88584.pdf

Groene, O., Alonso, J., & Klazinga, N. (2010). Development and validation of the WHO self-assessment tool for health promotion in hospitals: Results of a study in 38 hospitals in eight countries. *Health Promotion International, 25*(2), 221–229.

Groene, O., Brandt, E., Schmidt, W., & Moeller, J. (2009). The balanced scorecard of acute settings: Development process, definition of 20 strategic objectives and implementation. *International Journal for Quality in Health Care, 21*(4), 259–271.

Groene, O., & Garcia-Barbero, M. (2005). *Health promotion in hospitals: Evidence and quality management.* World Health Organization.

Groene, O., & Jorgensen, S. J. (2005). Health promotion in hospitals-a strategy to improve quality in health care. *The European Journal of Public Health, 15*(1), 6–8.

Gruber, G. (2016). *Das italienische Health Promoting Hospitals (HPH) Netzwerk als Mitglied des internationalen HPH- Netzwerkes – Entwicklungen, Strukturen und Besonderheiten [The Italian HPH network as a member of the international HPH network – developments, structures and characteristics].* Master Thesis, Faculty of Social Sciences, University of Vienna [online]. Available at: https://doi.org/10.25365/thesis.44122

Guerreiro, A. I. F. (2012). *Children's rights in Hospital and Health Services: Manual and tools for assessment and improvement.* Task Force HPH-CA.

Hamidi, Y., Hazavehei, S. M. M., Karimi-Shahanjarini, A., Rabiei, M. A. S., Farhadian, M., Alimohamadi, S., & Moghadam, S. M. K. (2019). Health promoting hospitals in Iran: A review of the current status, challenges, and future prospects. *Medical Journal of the Islamic Republic of Iran, 33.*

Hancock, T. (1999). Creating healthy and health promoting hospitals: A worthy challenge for the twenty-first century. *International Journal of Health Care Quality Assurance Incorporating Leadership in Health Services, 12*(2–3) [online]. Available at: https://doi.org/10.1108/13660759910266784

HPH Environment Task Force. (2010). *HPH and environment manual.* Copenhagen: International Network of Health Promoting Hospitals [online]. Available at: https://www.hphnet.org/knowledge-innovation/#content-task-forces

HPH Task Force on Health Enhancing Physical Activity in Hospitals and Health Services: "Implementation of physical activity in health care - facilitators and barriers", Supplementto. *Clinical Health Promotion*; Vol. 6, Supplementum 2, Dec 2016 [online]. Available at: https://www.clinicalhealthpromotion.org/2016-supplementum-2

Huang, N., Chien, L. Y., & Chiou, S. T. (2016). Advances in health promotion in Asia-Pacific: Promoting health through hospitals. *Global Health Promotion, 23*(1) [online]. Available at:. https://doi.org/10.1177/1757975916635504

International Network of Health Promoting Hospitals. (1997). *The Vienna Recommendations on Health Promoting Hospitals.* Vienna [online]. Available at: https://www.hphnet.org/wp-content/uploads/2020/03/Vienna-Recommendations.pdf

International Working Group Health Promoting Hospitals and Health Literate Healthcare Organizations (Working Group HPH & HLO). (2019). *International Self-Assessment Tool for Organizational Health Literacy (Responsiveness) of Hospitals (OHL-Hos) SAT-OHL-Hos-v1.0-EN-international.* WHO Collaborating Centre for Health Promotion in Hospitals and Healthcare (CC-HPH).

Johnson, A., & Baum, F. (2001). Health promoting hospitals: A typology of different organizational approaches to health promotion. *Health Promotion International, 16*(3) [online]. Available at: https://doi.org/10.1093/heapro/16.3.281

Karl-Trummer, U., & Krajic, K. (2007). Migrant friendly hospitals: Organisations learn sensitivity for differences. In C. B. Cuadra & S. Cattacin (Eds.), *Migration and health: Difference sensitivity from an organisational perspective* (pp. 40–61). Malmö University.

Karl-Trummer, U., Krajic, K., Novak-Zezula, S., & Pelikan, J. M. (2006). Prenatal courses as health promotion intervention for migrant/ethnic minority women: High efforts and good results, but low attendance. *Diversity in Health and Social Care, 3*(1), 55–58.

Karl-Trummer, U., Schulze, B., Krajic, K., Novak-Zezula, S., Nowak, P., & Pelikan, J. M. (2006). *SF_MFQQ: Short form – Migrant friendly quality questionnaire.* Ludwig Boltzmann Institut für Medizinsozologie.

Kickbusch, I., Pelikan, J. M., Apfel, F., & Tsouros, A. D. (2013). *Health literacy. The solid facts.* WHO Regional Office for Europe.

Kilian, R., Paul, R., Berger, H., & Angermeyer, M. C. (1999). *The psychiatric hospital as a health promoting hospital. Health promoting hospitals in practice: Developing projects and networks* (pp. 54–60). Conrad.

Krajic, K., Cichocki, M., & Quehenberger, V. (2015). Health-promoting residential aged care: A pilot project in Austria. *Health Promotion International, 30*(3) [online]. Available at: https://doi.org/10.1093/heapro/dau012

Krajic, K., Karl-Trummer, U., Novak-Zezula, S., Wirtenberger, M., & Pelikan, J. M. (2005a). *Migrant-friendly hospitals in an ethno-culturally diverse Europe. Experiences from a European Pilot Hospital Project.* Final Report. Summary and CD-Rom. LBIMGS. http://www.mfh-eu.net

Krajic, K., Straßmayr, C., Karl-Trummer, U., Novak-Zezula, S., & Pelikan, J. M. (2005b). Improving ethnocultural competence of hospital staff by training: Experiences from the European 'Migrant-friendly Hospitals' project. *Diversity in Health and Social Care, 2*(4), 280–290.

Lee, C. B., Chen, M. S., Chien, S. H., Pelikan, J. M., Wang, Y. W., & Chu, C. M. Y. (2015) Strengthening health promotion in hospitals with capacity building: A Taiwanese case study. *Health Promotion International, 30*(3) [online]. Available at: https://doi.org/10.1093/heapro/dat089

Lee, C. B., Chen, M. S., Powell, M., & Chu, C. M. Y. (2012). Achieving organizational change: Findings from a case study of health promoting hospitals in Taiwan. *Health Promotion International, 29*(2) [online]. Available at: https://doi.org/10.1093/heapro/das056

Lee, C. B., Chen, M. S., Powell, M. J., & Chu, C. M. Y. (2015). Self-Reported changes in the implementation of hospital-based health promotion in Taiwan. *American Journal of Health Promotion, 29*(3) [online]. Available at: https://doi.org/10.4278/ajhp.120816-ARB-397

Lee, C. B., Chen, M. S., & Wang, Y. W. (2014). Barriers to and facilitators of the implementation of health promoting hospitals in Taiwan: A top-down movement in need of ground support. *The International Journal of Health Planning and Management, 29*(2) [online]. Available at:. https://doi.org/10.1002/hpm.2156

Lin, Y. W., & Lin, Y. Y. (2011). Health-promoting organization and organizational effectiveness of health promotion in hospitals: A national cross-sectional survey in Taiwan. *Health Promotion International, 26*(3) [online]. Available at: https://doi.org/10.1093/heapro/daq068

Ludwig Boltzmann Institute for the Sociology of Health and Medicine. (1996). *The Health Promoting Hospital in the European Union.* Workshop. Vienna, 17–18 May.

Mahmoodi, H., Sarbakhsh, P., & Shaghaghi, A. (2019). Barriers to adopt the Health Promoting Hospitals (HPH) initiative in Iran: The Q method derived perspectives of front line practitioners. *Patient Education and Counseling, 102*(4) [online]. Available at: https://doi.org/10.1016/j.pec.2018.10.030

Mahmoodi, H., Shaghaghi, A. (2019). Barriers and gateways to adapt standards of the Health Promoting Hospitals: A rigorous consolidation of the global research evidence. *International Journal of Health Promotion and Education, 57*(5) [online]. Available at: https://doi.org/1 0.1080/14635240.2019.1610025

Marent, B., Wieczorek, C. C., & Krajic, K. (2018). Professionals' perspectives towards health promotion in residential aged care: An explorative study in Austria. *Health Promotion International, 33*(2) [online]. Available at: https://doi.org/10.1093/heapro/daw075

Metzler, B. (2016). *Effektivität interorganisationaler Netzwerke im Setting-Ansatz der Gesundheitsförderung [Effectiveness of interorganizational networks in the settings approach of health promotion. A sociological case study using the example of the Austrian HPH Network].* MA Thesis. Faculty of Social Sciences. University of Vienna.

MFH Project Group. (2004). *The Amsterdam Declaration. Towards Migrant-Friendly Hospitals in an ethno-culturally diverse Europe* [online]. Available at: https://ec.europa.eu/health/ph_projects/2002/promotion/fp_promotion_2002_annex7_14_en.pdf

Milz, H., & Vang, J. (1989). Consultation on the role of health promotion in hospitals. *Health Promotion International, 3*, 425–427.

Mittelmark, M. B., Sagy, S., Erikson, M., Bauer, G. F., Pelikan, J. M., Lindström, B., & Espnes, G. A. (2016). *The handbook of Salutogenesis.* Springer International Publishing AG.

Novak-Zezula, S., Schulze, B., Karl-Trummer, U., Krajic, K., & Pelikan, J. M. (2006). Improving interpreting in clinical communication: Models of feasible practice from the European project "Migrant-friendly hospitals". *Diversity in Health and Social Care, 3*(1), 55–58.

Nowak, P., Lobnig, H., Krajic, K., & Pelikan, J. M. (1999). Case Study Rudolfstiftung Hospital, Vienna, Austria – WHO-Model Project "Health and Hospital". In J. M. Pelikan, M. Garcia-Barbero, H. Lobnig, & K. Krajic (Eds.), *Pathways to a health promoting hospital. Experiences from the European Pilot Hospital Project 1993-1997* (2nd ed., pp. 47–66). Conrad Health Promotion Publications.

Nowak, P., Lobnig, H., & Pelikan, J. M. (1999). Projektorganisation am Beispiel des Wiener WHO-Modellprojektes "Gesundheit und Krankenhaus". In J. M. Pelikan & S. Wolff (Eds.), *Das gesundheitsfördernde Krankenhaus. Konzepte und Beispiele zur Entwicklung einer lernenden Organisation* (pp. 13–36). Juventa.

Nowak, P., & Pelikan, J. M. (1999). The WHO Model Project "Health and Hospital" at the Viennese Hospital Rudolfstiftung. In D. N. G. Krankenhäuser (Ed.), *Pathways towards Health Promoting Hospitals. Practical examples from England, France, Ireland, Italy, Austria and Sweden* (pp. 187–212). Health Promotion Publications.

Nutbeam, D. (1998a). Health promotion glossary. *Health Promotion International, 13*(4), 349–364.

Nutbeam, D. (1998b). Evaluating health promotion - Progress, problems and solutions. *Health Promotion International, 13*, 27–44.

Paul, R., Berger, H., & Kilian, R. (1996). Health promotion in a psychiatric healthcare institution. *Newsletter Health Promotion Hospitals, 8*, 4–5.

Pelikan, J. M. (2006). Linking health promotion and health care in the interest of a new public health. In H. R. Noack & D. Kahr-Gottlieb (Eds.), *Promoting the public's health. Conference Report EUPHA 2005*. Health Promotion Publications.

Pelikan, J. M. (2007a). Health promoting hospitals-assessing developments in the network. *Italian Journal of Public Health, 4*(4), 261–270.

Pelikan, J. M. (2007b). Understanding differentiation of health in late modernity - By use of sociological system theory. In D. V. McQueen, I. S. Kickbusch, L. Potvin, J. M. Pelikan, L. Balbo, & T. Abel (Eds.), *Health and modernity: The role of theory in health promotion* (pp. 74–102). Springer.

Pelikan, J. M. (2009). Ausdifferenzierung von spezifischen Funktionssystemen für Krankenbehandlung und Gesundheitsförderung oder: Leben wir in der "Gesundheitsgesellschaft"? *Österreichische Zeitschrift für Soziologie, 34*(2), 28–47.

Pelikan, J. M. (2016). The application of salutogenesis in healthcare settings. In M. B. Mittelmark, S. Sagy, M. Eriksson, G. F. Bauer, J. M. Pelikan, B. Lindström, & G. A. Espnes (Eds.), *The handbook of salutogenesis* (pp. 261–266). Springer International.

Pelikan, J. M. (2019). Health-literate healthcare organizations. In O. Okan, U. Bauer, D. Levin-Zamir, & K. Sorensen (Eds.), *International handbook of health literacy – research, practice and policy across the Life-Span* (pp. 539–554). Policy Press.

Pelikan, J. M., Dietscher, C., Krajic, K., & Nowak, P. (2005). Eighteen core strategies for health promoting hospitals. In O. Groene & M. Garcia-Barbero (Eds.), *Health promotion in hospitals: Evidence and quality management* (pp. 46–63). WHO Regional Office for Europe. Available at: Retrieved October 19, 2021, from https://www.euro.who.int/__data/assets/pdf_file/0008/99827/E86220.pdf

Pelikan, J. M., Dietscher, C., Röthlin, F., & Schmied, H. (2011a). *Hospitals as organizational settings for health and health promotion.* (Working Paper LBIHPR 5). LBIHPR.

Pelikan, J. M., Dietscher, C., Röthlin, F., & Schmied, H. (2011b). A model and selected results from an evaluation study on the International HPH Network (PRICES-HPH). *Clinical Health Promotion, 1*(1), 9–15.

Pelikan, J. M., Dietscher, C., & Schmied, H. (2013). How far is the health promoting hospital a salutogenic hospital, and how can it be developed? In G. F. Bauer & G. J. Jenny (Eds.), *Salutogenic organizations and change: The concepts behind organizational health intervention research* (pp. 149–165). Springer.

Pelikan, J. M., Garcia-Barbero, M., Lobnig, H., & Krajic, K. (Eds.). (1998). *Pathways to a health promoting hospitals. Experiences from the European Pilot Hospital Project 1993-1997*. Health Promotion Publications.

Pelikan, J. M., Gröne, O., & Svane, J. K. (2011). The international HPH network - A short history of two decades of development. *Clinical Health Promotion, 1*(1), 32–36.

Pelikan, J. M., & Halbmayer, E. (1999a). Gesundheitswissenschaftliche Grundlagen zur Strategie des Gesundheitsfördernden Krankenhauses. In J. M. Pelikan & S. Wolff (Eds.), *Das gesundheitsfördernde Krankenhaus. Konzepte und Beispiele zur Entwicklung einer lernenden Organisation* (pp. 13–36). Juventa.

Pelikan, J. M., & Halbmayer, E. (1999b). A basis from health sciences for health promoting hospital strategies. In J. M. Pelikan & S. Wolff (Eds.), *Das gesundheitsfördernde Krankenhaus. Konzepte und Beispiele zur Entwicklung einer lernenden Organisation* (pp. 13–36). Juventa.

Pelikan, J. M., & Krajic, K. (2007). The European migrant friendly hospitals program and its link to the health promoting hospital. In L. Epstein (Ed.), *Proceedings of the Workshop: Culturally appropriate health care by culturally competent health professionals* (pp. 33–39).

Pelikan, J. M., Krajic, K., & Dietscher, C. (2001). The health promoting hospital (HPH): Concept and development. *Patient Education and Counselling, 45*(4), 239–243.

Pelikan, J. M., Krajic, K., Dietscher, C., & Nowak, P. (2006). *Putting HPH policy into action. Working paper of the WHO collaborating centre on health promotion in hospitals and health care.* WHO Collaborating Centre for Health Promotion in Hospitals and Health Services at Ludwig Boltzmann Institute for the Sociology of Health and Medicine.

Pelikan, J. M., Krajic, K., & Lobnig, H. (1997). Feasibility, effectiveness, quality and sustainability of health promoting hospital projects. In *Proceedings of the 5th international conference on health promoting hospitals. Vienna, Austria, April 16–19.* Health Promotion Publications.

Pelikan, J. M., Schmied, H., & Dietscher, C. (2010). Prävention und Gesundheitsförderung im Krankenhaus. In K. Hurrelmann, T. Klotz, & J. Haisch (Eds.), *Lehrbuch Prävention und Gesundheitsförderung* (3rd ed., pp. 290–301). Huber.

Pelikan, J. M., Schmied, H., & Dietscher, C. (2014). Improving organizational health: The case of health promoting hospitals. In G. F. Bauer & O. Hämmig (Eds.), *Bridging occupational, organizational and public health* (pp. 133–153). Springer.

Pelikan, J. M., & Wieczorek, C. C. (2019). Gesundheitsförderung in der Krankenversorgung, mit Schwerpunkt Krankenhaus. In M. Staats (Ed.), *Die Perspektive(n) der Gesundheitsförderung* (pp. 99–116). Beltz Juventa.

Pelikan, J. M., & Wolff, S. (1999). *Das gesundheitsfördernde Krankenhaus. Konzepte und Beispiele zur Entwicklung einer lernenden Organisation.* Juventa.

Plunger, P. (2001). *Health promotion in general practice and community pharmacy - A European project.* Ludwig Boltzmann-Institut for Sociology of Health and Medicine.

Quehenberger, V., Cichocki, M., & Krajic, K. (2014). Sustainable effects of a low-threshold physical activity intervention on health-related quality of life in residential aged care. *Clinical Interventions in Aging, 9,* 1853–1864.

Quehenberger, V., & Krajic, K. (2017). Applications of salutogenesis to aged and highly-aged persons: Residential care and community settings. In M. B. Mittelmark, S. Sagy, M. Eriksson, G. Bauer, J. M. Pelikan, B. Lindström, & G. A. Espnes (Eds.), *The handbook of salutogenesis* (pp. 325–335). Springer.

Rojatz, D., Nowak, P., Christ, R., & World Health Organization. Regional Office for Europe. (2018). The Austrian health care reform: An opportunity to implement health promotion into primary health care units. *Public Health Panorama, 04*(04), 627–631.

Röthlin, F. (2013). Managerial strategies to reorient hospitals towards health promotion: Lessons from organisational theory. *Journal of Health Organization and Management, 27*(6) [online]. Available at: https://doi.org/10.1108/JHOM-07-2011-0070

Röthlin, F., Schmied, H., & Dietscher, C. (2015). Organizational capacities for health promotion implementation: Results from an international hospital study. *Health Promotion International, 30*(2) [online]. Available at: https://doi.org/10.1093/heapro/dat048

Sol, N., & Wilson, P. K. (1989). *Hospital health promotion.* Human Kinetics Books.

Svane, J. K., Chiou, S. T., Groene, O., Kalvachova, M., Brkić, M. Z., Fukuba, I., Härm, T., Farkas, J., Ang, Y., Andersen, M. Ø., & Tønnesen, H. (2018). A WHO-HPH operational program versus usual routines for implementing clinical health promotion: An RCT in health promoting hospitals (HPH). *Implementation Science, 13*(1) [online]. Available at. https://doi.org/10.1186/s13012-018-0848-0

Svane, J. K., Egerod, I., & Tønnesen, H. (2018). Staff experiences with strategic implementation of clinical health promotion: A nested qualitative study in the WHO-HPH recognition process RCT. *Sage Open Medicine*, 6 [online]. Available at: https://doi.org/10.1177/2050312118792394

Task Force HPH-CA. (2009). *Self-evaluation Model and Tool (SEMT) on the Respect of Children's Rights in Hospital.*

Tatang, E., & Mawartinah, T. (2019). Evaluation study of health promotion hospital (HPH) in Muhammadiyah hospital in DKI Jakarta, Indonesia. *KEMAS: Journal Kesehatan Masyarakat of Public Health, 14*(3), 410–418.

Tønnesen, H., Svane, J. K., Groene, O., & Chiou, S. T. (2016). The WHO-HPH recognition project: Fast-track implementation of clinical health promotion - A protocol for a multi-center RCT. *Clinical Health Promotion, 6*(1), 13–20.

Tønnesen, H., Svane, J. K., Lenzi, L., Kopecky, J., Surrorg, L., Rashida Khan Bukholm, I., & Masiello, M. G. (2012). Handling clinical health promotion in the HPH DATA model: Basic documentation of health determinants in medical records of tobacco, malnutrition, overweight, physical inactivity & alcohol. *Clinical Health Promotion, 2*(1), 5–11.

Trojan, A., Nickel, S., & Kofahl, C. (2016). Implementing 'self-help friendliness' in German hospitals: A longitudinal study. *Health Promotion International, 31*(2), 303–313.

Wang, Y.-W., Chia, S.-L., Chou, C.-M., Chen, M. S., Pelikan, J. M., Chu, C., Wang, M.-H., & Lee, C. B. (2019). Development and validation of a self-assessment tool for an integrative model of health promotion in hospitals: Taiwan's experience. *International Journal of Environmental Research and Public Health, 16*(11) [online]. Available at. https://doi.org/10.3390/ijerph16111953

Weisz, U., Haas, W., Pelikan, J. M., & Schmied, H. (2011). Sustainable hospitals: A socio-ecological approach. *GAIA – Ecological Perspectives for Science and Society, 20*(3), 191–198.

Whitehead, D. (2004). The European health promoting hospitals (HPH) project: How far on?. *Health Promotion International, 9*(2) [online]. Available at: https://doi.org/10.1093/heapro/dah213

WHO. (2007). *The international network of health promoting hospitals and health services: Integrating health promotion into hospitals and health services.* WHO.

Wieczorek, C. C., Nowak, P., Frampton, S. B., & Pelikan, J. M. (2018). Strengthening patient and family engagement in healthcare – The New Haven Recommendations. *Patient Education and Counselling, 101*(8) [online]. Available at. https://doi.org/10.1016/j.pec.2018.04.003

Wise, M., & Nutbeam, D. (2007). Enabling health systems transformation: What progress has been made in re-orienting health services? *Promotion & Education, 14*(25) [online]. Available at: https://doi.org/10.1177/10253823070140020801x

World Health Organization. (1986). *Ottawa Charter for health promotion.* WHO.

World Health Organization. (1991). *Budapest Declaration on Health Promoting Hospitals* [online]. Available at: http://www.ongkg.at/downloads-links/downloads.html?no_cache=1&download=02_Budapest-Declaration.pdf&did=88

Yaghoubi, M., & Javadi, M. (2013). Health promoting hospitals in Iran: How it is. *Journal of Education and Health Promotion, 2,* [online]. Available at: https://doi.org/10.4103/2277-9531.115840

Yaghoubi, M., Karamali, M., Bahadori, M. (2018). Effective factors in implementation and development of health promoting hospitals: A systematic review. *Health Promotion International, 34*(4) [online]. Available at: https://doi.org/10.1093/heapro/day024.

Wieczorek, C.C., Marent, B., Osrecki, F., Dorner, T.E., & Dür, W. (2015). Hospitals as professional organizations: challenges for reorientation towards health promotion. *Health Sociology Review, 24*(2), [online]. Available at: https://doi.org/10.1080/14461242.2015.1041541

Chapter 8
Health-Promoting Higher Education

Mark Dooris

8.1 Introduction

It has been widely argued that significant improvements in public health will occur only through a "Health in All Policies" approach, embedding health into programs and policies in nonhealth sectors. Higher education is an important and fast-growing sector, while universities have over many years been characterized as élitist and privileged settings—a reality that prevails in many parts of the world—governments have also championed policies to widen access and participation, resulting in a more diverse student body (UNESCO, 2017; Universities UK, 2017). Universities thus have enormous potential to support and promote health through maximizing opportunities to:

- impact positively on the health of students and staff—through core activities and specific interventions
- benefit the local community—through citizen engagement, community service, and campus design and planning
- contribute to the long-term health improvement of the population—through education, research, and knowledge exchange
- and, generate health, justice, and sustainability in families, neighborhoods, and society—through focusing on their corporate social and environmental responsibility and their potential to "future-shape" students (and, indeed, staff) as local and global citizens.

In turn, it is increasingly acknowledged that a commitment to health and well-being can enhance a university's core mandate through impacting positively on key

M. Dooris (✉)
Institute of Citizenship, Society and Change/Healthy and Sustainable Settings Unit, University of Central Lancashire, Preston, Lancashire, UK
e-mail: mtdooris@uclan.ac.uk

© Springer Nature Switzerland AG 2022   151
S. Kokko, M. Baybutt (eds.), *Handbook of Settings-Based Health Promotion*,
https://doi.org/10.1007/978-3-030-95856-5_8

enablers such as achievement, performance, productivity, and reputation (Universities UK, 2020). As one study observed, "there was awareness that the health and wellbeing of staff and students are strongly influenced by the organisational context, that the health of the organisation strongly influences performance, and that both the health of staff and students and the performance of the organisation are continuously co-produced by the ongoing interaction between them, suggesting a reciprocal relationship" (Newton et al., 2016, p. 62).

Universities have a long history of delivering specific health-related interventions and activities on topical issues, resulting in student-focused guidance on themes such as mental health, drugs, and alcohol, alongside a growing focus on staff well-being (Dooris & Doherty, 2010a). It is only relatively recently, however, that there has been a shift from delivering "health promotion in the university setting" to develop more holistic and strategic health-promoting university initiatives (Doherty & Dooris, 2006; Dooris, 2001; Dooris & Doherty, 2010b).

8.2   History and Development

The first few health-promoting university initiatives were established at Lancaster University and the University of Central Lancashire (UCLan) in the UK in the mid-1990s, following an international conference on setting-based health promotion (Theaker & Thompson, 1995). As Beattie (1995) commented at this time, health-promoting universities had been slow to get going compared to health-promoting schools and hospitals, due to the absence of visible leadership or infrastructures at national or international levels. These UK developments catalyzed the involvement of the WHO Regional Office for Europe, with an international conference, a round table meeting and the publication of *Health Promoting Universities: Concept, Experience and Framework for Action* (Tsouros et al., 1998), which proposed a strategic framework for future development within the context of WHO's European Healthy Cities Project. While the book raised the profile of health-promoting universities, WHO's engagement dissipated along with the expectation that a European program and network would be developed.

However, as the timeline illustrates (see Table 8.1), momentum had been established and interest in the concept and practice of health-promoting universities steadily grew. In parallel to UK developments, Germany established a Health Promoting Universities Network in 1995, and in 2003, the First International Health Promoting Universities Congress was held in Chile. This was followed by a Second International Congress in 2005 in Canada, which resulted in the Edmonton Charter for Health Promoting Universities (2005), a series of largely Spanish-speaking congresses, and the establishment of a growing number of national and regional networks.

Fast forward to 2015, when the University of British Columbia hosted the International Health Promoting Universities and Colleges Conference

Table 8.1 History and Development of Health-Promoting Universities—Timeline

1986	Ottawa Charter for Health Promotion
1994/5	First HPU Initiatives established: Lancaster and University of Central Lancashire, UK
1995	German Network established
1996	International HPU Conference, Lancaster, UK
1998	WHO Book "HPUs: Concept, Experience & Framework for Action"
2003	I International HPU Congress
2005	II International HPU Congress and Edmonton Charter
2006	UK and Spanish Networks established
2007	Ibero-American Network established
2009	Austrian and Swiss Networks established
2014	ASEAN Network established
2015	Okanagan International HPU and Colleges Conference and Charter
	TWANZ [New Zealand] Network established
2016	International HPU and Colleges Network/Steering Group established
	Canadian Network established
2019	International Symposium, Rotorua, NZ
2020	USA Network established

(incorporating the seventh International Congress), the expanded reach and significance of the movement were evident. Although research relating to the effectiveness
of health-promoting universities *per se* remained scant (Newton, 2014), it was by
this point in time possible to draw on studies and reviews from the wider education
sector to suggest that complex comprehensive multicomponent "whole-system"
approaches are more likely to result in positive outcomes for students, staff, and
institutions (St Leger et al., 2009; Stewart-Brown, 2006; Warwick et al., 2008).
Alongside this growing evidence base, in the UK at least, policy-makers were
increasingly using the language of "the whole university approach" and referencing
health-promoting universities in formulating guidance on key topics such as student
mental health and violence and relationships (Universities UK, 2015, 2016, 2017).
The conference was attended by 375 researchers, practitioners, administrators, students, and policy-makers from over 30 countries and resulted in the co-production
of the influential international Okanagan Charter (2015). A pledge to implement the
Charter was signed not only by individuals and networks, but also by representatives of the World Health Organization, Pan American Health Organization, and
UNESCO. This in turn led to the formation of an International Steering Group for
Health Promoting Universities and Colleges, which currently comprises representatives from 12 networks around the world and oversees international network developments (https://www.healthpromotingcampuses.org/).

8.3   Context, Concepts, and Theory

In considering how the setting-based approach can be applied to universities, it is necessary to take account of the particularities of the higher education context, appreciating that universities have their own distinctive culture and ethos and have multiple roles in society (Abercrombie et al., 1998; Dooris et al., 2012), as:

- centers of learning and development, with roles in education, research, capacity-building, and knowledge exchange
- foci for creativity and innovation, developing knowledge and understanding within and across disciplines, and applying them to the benefit of society
- places within which students undergo life transition—exploring and experimenting, developing independence and life skills, and facing particular health challenges
- workplaces and businesses, concerned with performance and productivity within a competitive marketplace
- contexts that "future-shape" students and staff as they clarify values, grow intellectually, and develop capabilities that can enhance current and future citizenship within families, communities, workplaces, and society as a whole
- resources for and influential partners and corporate citizens within local, regional, national, and global communities.

This contextual focus has been developed further by Suárez-Reyes and Van den Broucke (2016), who report on a systematic review exploring how the health-promoting university approach has been implemented in culturally different contexts.

In a scoping review of literature pertaining to health-promoting universities, Dooris et al. (2014) identified a number of theoretical influences that are also found within wider literature on health-promoting settings—specifically salutogenesis, socioecology, and sociological perspectives relating to structure and agency, systems thinking, and organization development. They explored how engagement with these theories could elucidate inter-related questions: What does it mean to consider the university as a setting? What is health and how is it created in the university? Why is the setting approach an important and useful means of promoting health in universities? How can health promotion be introduced into and embedded within the university setting? Drawing from these theoretical perspectives, Dooris (2006) proposed a conceptual framework, which he has subsequently expanded and applied to higher education (Dooris, 2015, 2018)—contending that the settings approach has five key characteristics:

- First, it represents a shift of focus toward a salutogenic view concerned not only with preventing and addressing illness, but with well-being and what makes people thrive and flourish (Antonovsky, 1996)—fostering health potentials inherent in the university setting and strengthening the resources that can empower people to increase control over the determinants of health (Kickbusch, 1996).

- Second, it adopts an ecological model. It appreciates that health is multilayered and determined by a complex interaction of personal, social, behavioral, and environmental factors, and it addresses human health within the framework of ecosystem health (Hancock, 2015). Recognizing the interplay between structure and agency, it appreciates that different "stakeholders" have different degrees of access to and control over the determinants of their health and well-being.
- Third, it views the university as a dynamic complex system, acknowledging interconnectedness and synergy between its component parts and recognizing that it is connected to the world around it (Dooris, 2001; Naaldenberg et al., 2009).
- Fourth, it adopts a comprehensive holistic change focus, drawing on learning from organization and community development and using multiple, interconnected interventions to embed health within the university's culture, ethos, structures, processes, and routine life (Dooris, 2009).
- And fifth, it appreciates that universities, like many other settings, do not have health as their main mission or raîson d'etre and that it is therefore essential to advocate for health in terms of impact on or outflow from core business (Dooris, et al., 2012).

The Okanagan Charter (2015, p. 2) sets out a bold and inspiring vision, looking to Health Promoting Universities and Colleges to: "Transform the health and sustainability of our current and future societies, strengthen communities and contribute to the wellbeing of people, places and the planet...[and] infuse health into everyday operations, business practices and academic mandates. By doing so [they] enhance the success of our institutions; create campus cultures of compassion, well-being, equity and social justice; improve the health of the people who live, learn, work, play and love on our campuses; and strengthen the ecological, social and economic sustainability of our communities and wider society." The Charter goes on to issue two calls to action (p. 3):

1. **Embed health into all aspects of campus culture, across the administration, operations, and academic mandates:** This sets out a whole university approach, using the five focus areas of the Ottawa Charter (WHO, 1986) as a framework (healthy policies, supportive environments, community action, personal development, and re-orientation of services).
2. **Lead health promotion action and collaboration locally and globally:** This looks outwards to propose a whole-system approach, concerned to enhance research for health promotion; position the university as a leader and advocate for local and global action; and embed health, well-being, and sustainability in and across multiple disciplines, so that students—whether studying nursing, engineering, architecture, or urban planning—gain a critical understanding and become fired up as change agents in families, communities, workplaces, and society as a whole.

Laying out an aspiration that accords with the Okanagan Charter, the UK Healthy Universities Network suggests that a Health Promoting University: "adopts an holistic understanding of health; takes a whole university approach; and aspires to create a learning environment and organisational culture that enhances the health,

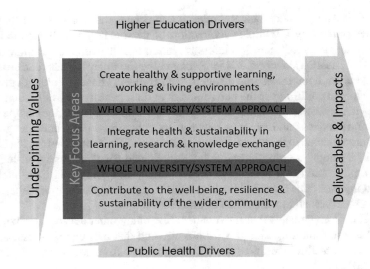

Fig. 8.1 Healthy universities—a model for conceptualizing and applying the healthy setting approach to higher education (source: adapted from Dooris et al. (2010))

wellbeing and sustainability of its community and enables people to achieve their full potential" (UK Healthy Universities Network, n.d.). Informed by this vision and drawing on the early work of Barić (1993, 1994), its membership helped to produce a model for applying healthy settings thinking within higher education (see Fig. 8.1).

The model is structured to show how underpinning values (e.g., equity, participation, empowerment, partnership) come together with public health and higher education policy drivers to inform whole university and whole-system action and deliver impacts, across three focus areas:

- create learning, working, and living environments that support and sustain the health and well-being of the university population and help people to flourish
- integrate health and sustainable development within the university's core business of learning, research, and knowledge exchange
- connect with and contribute to the well-being, resilience, and sustainability of local, regional, national, and global communities.

As noted by Dooris et al. (2012), a whole university and whole-system approach not only requires anticipating and balancing higher education and public health priorities, but also involves securing high-level commitment and leadership, engaging a wide range of stakeholders, and combining high visibility health-related projects with system-level organization development and change. Subsequent research has further reinforced this thinking: A study conducted into the use of the UK Healthy Universities Network's Self-Review Tool highlighted how its use within institutions had been a catalyst to senior-level stakeholders coming together across boundaries to review progress and plan ahead (Dooris et al., 2018a); and a project examining leadership for health, well-being, and sustainability highlighted characteristics of a successful whole-system approach (Dooris et al., 2018b).

Newton et al. (2016) reported on a doctoral study exploring how the concept of a healthy university is operationalized in two case study universities. Although it was not possible to evidence a causal relationship between the adoption of a healthy university approach and a salutogenic organizational culture, the contrasting case studies suggested that such benefits may well be catalyzed or reinforced by an intentional and explicit commitment to health and well-being. Other literature has largely reported on experience drawn from practice or reported on detailed studies framed within the conceptual context of healthy universities—in Germany and Lithuania (Meier et al., 2007; Stock et al., 2001, 2003); Hong Kong and China (Lee, 2002; Xiangyang et al., 2003); the Americas (Stanton et al., 2013; Kosarchyn, 2014; Suárez-Reyes & Van den Broucke, 2016); the UK (Dooris et al., 2016; Dooris & Doherty, 2010a, 2010b; Holt et al., 2015; Holt & Powell, 2016); and Australia and New Zealand (Taylor et al., 2018; Waterworth & Thorpe, 2017).

8.4   Current Situation

As noted above, health-promoting universities have gathered momentum and become established as a worldwide movement, as evidenced by the involvement of multiple national and regional networks within the International Health Promoting Universities and Colleges Steering Group and emerging Network. While there is broad consensus about the need for a whole university and whole-system approach (Dooris et al., 2019), different countries and different institutions have inevitably been informed by different priorities and used different entry points to develop their work. While student enrolment to higher education is now growing fastest in middle-income countries, with low-income countries picking up speed (UNESCO, 2017), it is noticeable that the majority of the established networks are in high-income countries.

The examples in Boxes 8.1–8.3 provide insights into how three universities in different parts of the world have developed and implemented their vision of the health-promoting university.

> **Box 8.1 University of British Columbia (UBC), Canada**
> Building on longstanding commitments to sustainability and to human and ecological well-being, UBC Well-being was established in 2014 as a university-wide priority—a collaborative effort to make the university a better place to live, work, and learn through a system-wide and setting-based approach across its two campuses.
>
> (continued)

Box 8.1 (continued)

UBC Well-being is overseen by a High-Level Steering Committee of academic leaders, senior administrators, and student executives. At each campus, advisory committees provide guidance, partnership, and expertise to align strategic initiatives with well-being priorities, and a Strategic Support Team works with faculties, units, and departments to integrate well-being into their practices, policies, and cultures. Additionally, multistakeholder working groups support each UBC Well-being priority area (Built and Natural Environments; Inclusion and Connection; Food and Nutrition; Mental Health and Resilience; and Physical Activity and Sedentary Behaviour). Each working group develops a framework for action to help guide goal-setting and facilitate cross-cutting initiatives in alignment with health promotion principles.

UBC Well-being has a clear commitment to a whole university approach. It has combined senior-level commitment with bottom-up engagement and prioritized a distributed approach to leadership and implementation by embedding "health promotion" and "well-being" into multiple people's roles, gradually building well-being into and creating a cultural shift across the entire university. The Okanagan Charter has proved enormously helpful in moving things forward through UBC formally adopting it and integrating its principles and calls to action in strategic and operational plans. Active participation in the Canadian Network for Health Promoting Universities and Colleges has also proved enormously beneficial in facilitating peer-to-peer support and building momentum.

Source: This example draws from a case study provided by Dr. Matt Dolf profiled in Dooris et al., (2018b). This case study has been developed with the use of the publication "Healthy Universities: Whole University Leadership for Health, Wellbeing and Sustainability," which is owned by Advance HE. © 2018 Advance HE. All rights reserved.

Box 8.2 University of Central Lancashire (UCLan), UK

Building on academic interest in setting-based health promotion, UCLan established its health-promoting university (now called "Healthy University") initiative in 1995. Coordinated from the Healthy and Sustainable Settings Unit, it aspires to create a learning environment and organizational culture that enhances the health, well-being, and sustainability of its community and enables people to achieve their full potential. This aspiration is supported at a strategic level through the University Strategy 2015–2020 expressing commitment to "the health, safety, and well-being of all" and the Campus Masterplan Framework pledging to create "a healthy, safe, active, and sustainable campus."

(continued)

Box 8.2 (continued)

The Healthy University Coordinator reports to a high-level cross-institution Steering Group, which oversees the implementation of a Healthy University Plan by a number of multi-service, multidisciplinary (and, where appropriate, multiagency) activities, and working groups. The plan's purpose is to foster a whole university and whole-system approach; to take proactive and co-productive approaches to planning and prioritizing for health and well-being; to guide and facilitate the implementation of evidence-informed interventions and best practice; and to support "habits for life" for individuals and communities to create and maintain healthy lifestyles. It is structured to ensure that the Healthy University supports the University's and Students' Union's core business and contributes to the delivery of other key strategies. To coincide with the development and launch of a new university strategy, UCLan is planning to reconfigure and strengthen its decision-making and implementation structures, to ensure a strong university-wide commitment to health, well-being, and sustainability supported by groupings focused on student health, staff health, and infrastructure/environment/climate change.

The Okanagan Charter has been used within the university and has been helpful in demonstrating that UCLan is part of a large global movement. The vice-chancellor is strongly committed to the Healthy University initiative and has signed the executive membership form for the UK Network, affirming that the university "recognises that promoting health and sustainability within the context of higher education is essential to achieving our full potential in learning and teaching, research, innovation and engagement, and to ensuring human and ecological wellbeing and flourishing."

The university has coordinated and co-chaired the UK Healthy Universities Network over many years and currently co-chairs the International Health Promoting Universities and Colleges Steering Group.

Source: This example draws from a case study provided by Sharon Doherty profiled in Dooris et al., (2018b). This case study has been developed with the use of the publication "Healthy Universities: Whole University Leadership for Health, Well-being and Sustainability," which is owned by Advance HE. © 2018 Advance HE. All rights reserved.

Box 8.3 University of Puerto Rico (UPR), Puerto Rico
Founded in 1903, the University of Puerto Rico (UPR) is the country's public university, comprising eleven campuses with 55,000 students and 3200 professors. It is strongly committed to the values of health, well-being, and quality of life for the university community and has, over several decades, developed various initiatives relating to and supporting the movement for health-promoting universities. For example:

(continued)

Box 8.3 (continued)

- In 1989, the Puerto Rican Consortium of University Resources for Drugs, Alcohol and Violence (CRUSADA) was instituted as an inter-university organization, committed to fostering university environments free from the use and abuse of alcohol, other drugs, and violence, as well as promoting positive and healthy lifestyles in university communities.
- In 1997, UPR established its Quality of Life Program with the purpose of promoting healthy lifestyles among university students.
- In 2007, UPR assumed a leadership role in the development of the movement for health-promoting universities at national and international levels. Since then, it has led the Ibero-American Network of Health Promoting Universities (RIUPS).

UPR-own Health Promoting University initiative is led from the University's WHO/PAHO Collaborating Center and has a Systemic Coordinating Committee, located structurally at the highest level of the University's Central Administration. The initiative is governed by a philosophical–conceptual document, an institutional policy endorsed by the university administration and a work plan that is reviewed and evaluated annually. The conceptual framework of the initiative is dominated by the principles of health promotion, the healthy setting approach, the academic and professional networking approach, and the foundations of university social responsibility. Health promotion actions are operationalized in a decentralized manner in and across the eleven university campuses: Each campus has a steering committee that develops health promotion, health education, prevention, and sustainable development activities.

Source: This example draws from a case study provided by Dr. Hiram V. Arroyo, Director, Collaborating Center of the World Health Organization (WHO/PAHO) for Training and Research in Health Promotion & Health Education, University of Puerto Rico. Used with permission.

8.5 Looking to the Future

The challenges and opportunities involved in developing and implementing health-promoting universities have been discussed elsewhere (Dooris et al., 2012). Looking ahead in the context of the Okanagan Charter and underpinning theory, there are a number of pertinent observations.

First, even while struggling with the real-world challenges involved in translating rhetoric to action, health-promoting universities need to hold onto a vision characterized by whole university and whole-system perspectives. If we are to move beyond delivering health promotion interventions in the higher education context to implement a setting-based approach, then we need to break down silos and connect different parts of the system. This means valuing and celebrating the work people do in their own particular service or role, but appreciating that this is part of a greater whole and that we can achieve more by knitting together disparate areas of activity and forging connections between people, issues, components, policies, and agendas (Dooris, 2006). More broadly, we know that a transdisciplinary approach to research is most likely to lead to innovation by focusing on synergy generated at the interface of different subject disciplines and that interprofessional approaches to learning and working are most likely to address societal needs and challenges.

Second, while continuing to prioritize student and staff experience, health-promoting universities need also to look outwards and appreciate their wider roles in generating health and well-being in society at large. Locally, the ongoing debate about the purpose and value of universities has led to a renewed focus on the idea of the "civic university," of the university being actively engaged with its local communities and able to communicate a compelling and integrated narrative about its societal value, within the context of "place" (Campbell, 2018). Globally, our work takes place within the context of huge challenges, in a world in which converging crises such as environmental degradation, climate change, resource depletion, and social, economic, and ecological injustice are intensifying (Poland et al., 2011). To be truly health-promoting, universities need to recognize that many determinants of health are situated outside their immediate locus of control and reassert their roles in society as leaders, agenda-setters, and generators of knowledge and maximize their public value through practicing meaningful corporate social and environmental responsibility. As a sector, higher education has a potentially powerful role in advocating for and being a prominent voice for transformative social, political, cultural, economic, and environmental change that will promote health, well-being, and justice. Our institutions also need to clarify their values and ensure that these infuse their organizational cultures and learning, working, and living environments—thereby "future-shaping" students and staff as local and global citizens and as influencers within families, neighborhoods, workplaces, and government.

Third, health-promoting universities need to find ways of operating within an increasingly competitive marketplace, while countering and re-orienting the dominant sectoral culture that prioritizes instrumental relations—where people are viewed and used as commodities, where success being talked about in terms such as "student numbers," "recruitment and retention statistic," and "income generation" and where league tables are glorified (Waddington, 2016). In such a culture, it will be important to prioritize and assert values such as compassion that run counter to prevailing trends and can truly support well-being, through shifting the organizational culture to one characterized by relationships built on mutual respect, care, kindness, and trust.

Fourth, health-promoting universities need to prioritize a joined-up commitment to salutogenesis (Antonovsky, 1996) and regenerative/restorative sustainability (Brown, 2016; Robinson & Cole, 2015). Sustainability and health promotion both look beyond lifestyle influences, highlighting the intersection of environmental, social, and economic determinants. In their operations, universities have for many years implemented environmental sustainability management systems and preventive health interventions. However, sustainability and health promotion have largely been viewed as separate domains, despite the growing convergence of agendas and emphasis on co-benefits (Orme & Dooris, 2010), and have generally focused on "reducing the negatives" rather than achieving "net positive" impacts. By bringing together the common perspectives that flow from a commitment to salutogenesis and regenerative/restorative sustainability, we can raise our aspirations so that our campus design, operational management, research focus, and curricular orientation and promote the well-being and flourishing of people, place, and planet.

8.6 Summary

This chapter began by providing a background to and brief historical overview of health-promoting universities, which first took root in the mid-1990s. It then explored the context for developing health-promoting universities and examined some key theoretical and conceptual underpinnings, before offering three contrasting examples of current practice in Europe, North America, and Latin America. It concluded by reflecting on future directions, highlighting the importance of developing a truly joined-up and whole-system approach; a willingness to look outwards and be future-oriented, thereby engaging with local and global concerns and challenges and using leverage to bring about change; courage to prioritize values such as compassion that may not readily "fit" with dominant sectoral cultures; and a commitment to salutogenesis and regenerative sustainability.

References

Abercrombie, N., Gatrell, T., & Thomas, C. (1998). Universities and health in the 21st century. In A. Tsouros, G. Dowding, J. Thompson, & M. Dooris (Eds.), *Health promoting universities: Concept, experience and framework for action*. WHO Regional Office for Europe. http://www.euro.who.int/document/e60163.pdf

Antonovsky, A. (1996). The salutogenic model as a theory to guide health promotion. *Health Promotion International, 11*(1), 11–18.

Barić, L. (1993). The settings approach – implications for policy and strategy. *Journal of the Institute of Health Education, 31*(1), 17–24.

Barić, L. (1994). *Health promotion and health education in practice. Module 2: The organisational model*. Barns Publications.

Beattie, A. (1995). Editorial: new agendas for student health. *Health for All 2000 News, 31*, 2–3.

Brown, M. (2016). *FutuREstorative: Working towards a new sustainability*. RIBA Publishing.

Campbell, C. (2018). *Integrated thinking and reporting: Telling a different story of HE*. WONKHE. https://wonkhe.com/blogs/integrated-thinking-and-reporting-telling-a-different-story-of-he/

Doherty, S., & Dooris, M. (2006). The healthy settings approach: The growing interest within colleges and universities. *Education and Health, 24*, 42–42.

Dooris, M. (2001). The 'health promoting university': A critical exploration of theory and practice. *Health Education, 101*, 51–60.

Dooris, M. (2006). Healthy settings: Challenges to generating evidence of effectiveness. *Health Promotion International, 21*, 55–65.

Dooris, M. (2009). Holistic & sustainable health improvement: The contribution of the settings-based approach to health promotion. *Perspectives in Public Health, 129*, 29–36.

Dooris, M. (2015). *Promising paths: Health promoting higher education: Reflections, challenges & future frontiers* (Presentation at International Conference on Health Promoting Universities & Colleges). University of British Columbia. 22-25 June. https://open.library.ubc.ca/cIRcle/collections/53926/items/1.0224787

Dooris, M. (2018). *Healthy and sustainable universities and colleges.* Presentation at Welsh HE/FE Networking Event, Cardiff, 23 January. http://www.wales.nhs.uk/sitesplus/888/page/82249#higher

Dooris, M., Cawood, J., Doherty, S., & Powell, S. (2010). *Healthy universities: Concept, model and framework for applying the healthy settings approach within higher education in England.* Final Project Report – March 2010. UCLan/RSPH.

Dooris, M., & Doherty, S. (2010a). Healthy Universities: current activity and future directions – findings and reflections from a national-level qualitative research study. *Global Health Promotion, 17*, 6–16.

Dooris, M., & Doherty, S. (2010b). Healthy Universities: Current activity and future directions – findings and reflections from a national-level qualitative research study. *Health Promotion International, 25*, 94–106.

Dooris, M., Doherty, S., Cawood, J., & Powell, S. (2012). The healthy universities approach: Adding value to the higher education sector. Chapter. In A. Scriven & M. Hodgins (Eds.), *Health promotion settings: Principles and practice.* Sage.

Dooris, M., Doherty, S., & Orme, J. (2016). The application of Salutogenesis in universities. In M. B. Mittelmark, S. Sagy, M. Eriksson, et al. (Eds.), *The handbook of Salutogenesis [Internet].* Springer. 2017. Chapter 23. Available from: https://link.springer.com/chapter/10.1007/978-3-319-04600-6_23

Dooris, M., Farrier, A., Doherty, S., Holt, M., Monk, R., & Powell, S. (2018a). The UK healthy universities self-review tool: Whole system impact. *Health Promotion International, 32*(3), 448–457.

Dooris, M., Farrier, A., & Powell, S. (2018b). *Healthy universities: Whole university leadership for health, wellbeing & sustainability.* Leadership Foundation for Higher Education/Advance HE. https://www.advance-he.ac.uk/knowledge-hub/healthy-universities-whole-university-leadership-health-wellbeing-and-sustainability

Dooris, M., Powell, S., & Farrier, A. (2019). Conceptualising the 'whole university' approach: An international qualitative study. *Health Promotion International.* https://doi.org/10.1093/heapro/daz072

Dooris, M., Wills, J., & Newton, J. (2014). Theorising healthy settings: A critical discussion with reference to healthy universities. *Scandinavian Journal of Public Health, 42*(Suppl 15), 7–16.

Edmonton Charter for Health Promoting Universities and Institutions of Higher Education. 2nd Pan-American International Conference on Health Promoting Universities. (2005). http://www.gesundheitsfoerdernde-hochschulen.de/Inhalte/E_Gefoe_HS_internat/2005_Edmonton_Charter_HPU.pdf

Hancock, T. (2015). Population health promotion 2.0: An eco-social approach to public health in the Anthropocene. *Canadian Journal of Public Health, 106*(4), e252–e255.

Holt, M., Monk, R., Powell, S., & Dooris, M. (2015). Student perceptions of a healthy university. *Public Health, 129*, 674–683.

Holt, M., & Powell, S. (2016). Healthy Universities: A guiding framework for universities to examine the distinctive health needs of its own student population. *Perspectives in Public Health, 137*(1), 53–58.

Kickbusch, I. (1996). Tribute to Aaron Antonovsky: What creates health? *Health Promotion International, 11*(1), 5–6.

Kosarchyn, C. (2014) Creating a framework for a health promoting university. *Virginia Journal, 35*(2):7–11. http://c.ymcdn.com/sites/vahperd.site-ym.com/resource/resmgr/Communicator-Journal/Vahperd_Fall14_PROOF.PDF

Lee, S. (2002). Health promoting university initiative in Hong Kong. *Promotion & Education, 9*(S1), 15.

Meier, S., Stock, C., & Krämer, A. (2007). The contribution of health discussion groups with students to campus health promotion. *Health Promotion International, 22*, 28–36.

Naaldenberg, J., Vaandrager, L., Koelen, M., Wagemakers, A., Saan, H., & de Hoog, K. (2009). Elaborating on systems thinking in health promotion practice. *Global Health Promotion, 16*, 39–47.

Newton, J., Dooris, M., & Wills, J. (2016). Healthy universities: An example of a whole-system health-promoting setting. *Global Health Promotion, 23*(Suppl. 1), 57–65.

Okanagan Charter: An International Charter for Health Promoting Universities and Colleges. (2015). https://open.library.ubc.ca/cIRcle/collections/53926/items/1.0132754

Orme, J., & Dooris, M. (2010). Integrating health and sustainability: The higher education sector as a timely catalyst. *Health Education Research, 25*, 425–437.

Poland, B., Dooris, M., & Haluza-Delay, R. (2011). Securing 'supportive environments' for health in the face of ecosystem collapse: Meeting the triple threat with a sociology of creative transformation. *Health Promotion International, 26*(Supplement 2), ii202–ii215.

Robinson, J., & Cole, R. (2015). Theoretical underpinnings of regenerative sustainability. *Building Research & Information, 43*(2), 133–143.

St Leger, L., Young, I., Blanchard, C., & Perry, M. (2009). *Promoting health in schools: from evidence to action*. International Union for Health Promotion and Education. Retrieved November 18, 2010, from www.iuhpe.org/?page=516 & lang=en.

Stanton, A., Chernenko, V., Dhaliwal, R., Gilbert, M., Goldner, E., Harris, C., Jones, W., & Mroz, M. (2013). Building healthy campus communities: The adaptation of a workplace tool to understand better student wellbeing within higher education settings. *Education & Health, 31*(3), 84–90.

Stewart-Brown, S. (2006). *What is the evidence on school health promotion in improving health or preventing disease and, specifically, what is the effectiveness of the health promoting schools approach?* WHO Regional Office for Europe. [Health Evidence Network Report. Retrieved March 5, 2010, from www.euro.who.int/document/e88185.pdf]

Stock, C., Kücük, N., Miseviciene, I., Habil, D., Guillen-Grima, F., Petkeviciene, J., Aguinaga-Ontoso, I., & Krämer, A. (2003). Differences in health complaints among university students from three European countries. *Preventive Medicine, 37*, 535–543.

Stock, C., Wille, L., & Krämer, A. (2001). Gender-specific health behaviors of German university students predict the interest in campus health promotion. *Health Promotion International, 16*, 145–154.

Suárez-Reyes, M., & Van den Broucke, S. (2016). Implementing the health promoting university approach in culturally different contexts: a systematic review. *Global Health Promotion, 23*(Suppl. 1), 46–56.

Taylor, P., Saheb, R., & Howse, E. (2018). Creating healthier graduates, campuses and communities: Why Australia needs to invest in health promoting universities. *Health Promotion Journal of Australia*. https://doi.org/10.1002/hpja.175

Theaker, T., & Thompson, J. (1995). *The settings-based approach to health promotion: Conference Report*. Hertfordshire Health Promotion.

Tsouros, A., Dowding, G., Thomson, J., & Dooris, M. (Eds.). (1998). *Health promoting univer-sities: Concept, experience and framework for action*. WHO Regional Office for Europe. Retrieved November 18, 2010, from [www.euro.who.int/document/e60163.pdf]

UK Healthy Universities Network. (n.d.). What is a Healthy University? Available from: https://healthyuniversities.ac.uk/healthy-universities/what-is-a-healthy-university/

UNESCO (2017) *Six ways to ensure higher education leaves no one behind* (Policy Paper 30). UNESCO. http://unesdoc.unesco.org/images/0024/002478/247862E.pdf

Universities UK. (2015). *Guidelines on student mental health policies and procedures for higher education*. Universities UK. https://www.universitiesuk.ac.uk/policy-and-analysis/reports/Pages/student-mental-wellbeing-in-higher-education.aspx

Universities UK. (2016). *Changing the culture: Report of Universities UK Taskforce examining violence against women, harassment and hate crime affecting university students*. Universities UK. http://www.universitiesuk.ac.uk/policy-and-analysis/reports/Pages/changing-the-culture-final-report.aspx

Universities UK. (2017). *Higher Education in Numbers*. Universities UK. https://www.universitiesuk.ac.uk/facts-and-stats/Pages/higher-education-data.aspx

Universities UK. (2020). *Stepchange: Mentally healthy universities*. Universities UK. https://www.universitiesuk.ac.uk/policy-and-analysis/reports/Documents/2020/uuk-stepchange-mhu.pdf

Waddington, K. (2016). The compassion gap in UK universities. *International Practice Development Journal, 6*(1), 1–9.

Warwick, I., Statham, J., & Aggleton, P. (2008). *Healthy and health promoting colleges – Identifying an evidence base*. Thomas Coram Research Unit, University of London.

Waterworth, C., & Thorpe, A. (2017). Applying the Okanagan Charter in Aotearoa New Zealand. *Journal of the Australian and New Zealand Student Services Association, 25*(1), 49–61.

World Health Organization (WHO). (1986). *Ottawa Charter for health promotion*. WHO.

Xiangyang, T., Lan, Z., Xueping, M., Tao, Z., Yuzhen, S., & Jagusztyn, M. (2003). Beijing health promoting universities: Practice and evaluation. *Health Promotion International, 18*, 107–113.

Chapter 9
Health-Promoting Workplaces

Karl Kuhn and Cordia Chu

The workplace influences workers' health and the potential spread of disease in various ways. While work can be financially and socially rewarding, and a resource for personal development and the enhancement of personal skills), it can also cause ill-health if workplaces create hazardous, stressful, and health-damaging work conditions. For example, work may provide a nonsupportive workplace culture, poor work organization and workloads, and inadequate skills to deal with changing work tasks. There is mounting evidence from around the world that there has been a significant rise in healthcare costs from work-related stress, occupational injuries, and chronic illnesses, which bring associated socioeconomic costs, including productivity losses (ILO, 2010, 2014; Pronk, 2013). Thus, it is important for work organizations to develop appropriate workplace health programs to protect and promote worker health.

To effectively promote workplace health, the multi-casual nature of health and illnesses, health determinants, and the relationship between the workplace and health must be considered. The term "workplace health promotion" (WHP) should be viewed in its societal context, while emphasizing the significant role that both employers and employees have in promoting health at work.

A broadly accepted definition of "workplace health promotion" in Europe is the *Luxembourg Declaration* (1997). Adopted by the European Network for WHP (ENWHP, 1997), workplace health promotion is defined as follows:

> the combined efforts of employers, employees and society to improve the health and well-being of people at work. This can be achieved through a combination of:

K. Kuhn (✉)
European Network for Workplace Health Promotion (ENWHP),
Fröndenberg, North Rhine-Westphalia, Germany

C. Chu
Centre for Environment and Population Health, Griffith University, Nathan, QLD, Australia
e-mail: c.chu@griffith.edu.au

© Springer Nature Switzerland AG 2022
S. Kokko, M. Baybutt (eds.), *Handbook of Settings-Based Health Promotion*,
https://doi.org/10.1007/978-3-030-95856-5_9

- improving the work organization and the working environment
- promoting active participation
- encouraging personal development.

The concept of WHP has evolved, influenced by the ILO's international standards and WHO's health promotion principles, and in response to the rapid transformation of the world of work, the globalized world economy, and the development of management principles (Chu & Dwyer, 2002). It has shifted away from a narrow focus on health education and individual responsibility to a broader, more comprehensive, integrative approach to health and health determinants (Chu, 2004; Pham et al., 2019).

9.1 International Standards

To advance workplace health promotion, many international organizations, such as the International Labour Organization (ILO) and World Health Organization (WHO), have attempted to create international workplace health standards that include prerequisite legal requirements.

The **ILO's** mandate for work in the field of occupational health and safety is found in the Preamble of its Constitution, which provides the protection of workers against sickness, disease, and injury arising from their employment. It is also found in the 1944 Declaration of Philadelphia, which recognizes the ILO's obligation to promote programs that protect the life and health of workers in all occupations. The ILO has adopted more than 40 standards dealing specifically with occupational safety and health, as well as over 40 Codes of Practice. Nearly half of the ILO's instruments deal directly or indirectly with occupational health and safety issues (ILO, 2003).

The Occupational Safety and Health Convention (No. 155), adopted in 1981, provides the formulation and implementation of national policies on occupational safety, health, and the working environment. To achieve this goal, both the government and enterprises must take action. Convention No. 155 is complemented by the 1981 *Occupational Safety and Health (OHS) Recommendation* (No. 164), which further elaborates on the actions that may be undertaken to address these issues.

In 1985, the ILO adopted the *Occupational Health Services Convention* (No. 161), which provides the establishment of enterprise-level occupational health services that are entrusted with preventive functions and are responsible for advising all interested parties on maintaining a safe and healthy working environment. More recently, in 2006 the *Promotional Framework for Occupational Safety and Health Convention* (No. 187) was adopted to promote a preventive safety and health culture, and to progressively achieve a safe and healthy working environment. In addition, the ILO adopts Codes of Practice, which set out practical guidelines on safety and health at work for public authorities, employers, workers, enterprises, and other bodies.

In sum, the right to health and safety at work has been enshrined in international instruments, mostly adopted by the ILO and WHO, which create sound legal standards in this field.

In 1995, at the Twelfth Session of a joint committee of the ILO and the WHO, ILO and WHO sought to revise the 1950 definition of "occupational health" and reorient toward three objectives:

- The maintenance and promotion of workers' health and working capacity;
- Improving working environments and work to make them conducive to safety and health; and
- To develop work organization and working cultures that support health and safety at work, and thereby promote a positive social climate and smooth operations and may enhance productivity of the undertaking.

The **WHO** has also been active in protecting workers' occupational health since its creation in 1948. The WHO Constitution empowers the organization to work toward improving working conditions. In 2007, the World Health Assembly endorsed the *WHO Global Plan of Action on Workers' Health* (2008–2018) (WHO, 2007), which follows the *WHO Global Strategy on Occupational Health for All*, adopted by the World Health Assembly in 1996. In 1993, the WHO Western Pacific Regional Office offered training workshops and sponsored pilot projects to guide the regional development of healthy workplaces in the Asia-Pacific (WHO-WPRO, 1999). Furthermore, WHO also provides a number of workplace health technical guidelines, such as the 2010 World Health Organization Guidelines for Healthy Workplaces.

As formulated in the WHO's *Ottawa Charter* (1986), the aim of health promotion is to promote health by initiating processes that enable everyone a greater degree of self-determination on their health. Health promotion thus becomes a social responsibility and not just a matter of individual lifestyle. This development led to the formulation of important principles for developing workplace health promotion:

- All people are addressed in their daily lives rather than exclusively targeting specific risk groups;
- Health promotion aims to influence the conditions for good health and eliminate the causes of poor health;
- Health promotion combines different but complementary actions and approaches;
- Health promotion aims especially at achieving the general public's active and effective participation.

These objectives, formulated at the Ottawa Conference, led to several key programs that, true to the fundamental idea, were implemented in various life settings. The original target group, the family, was followed by the "health-promoting school," and then, the focal point was "healthy cities." Finally, the world of work was selected as an area for health promotion activities.

9.2   Conceptualization and Implementation of Workplace Health Promotion

Workplace health promotion (WHP) has existed since the 1970s when the primary concept focused on changing a single lifestyle habit or individual behavior. The 1980s were dominated by more comprehensive wellness programs at work, but still focused on the individual. By the 1990s, a more interdisciplinary approach to promoting health developed from an increased understanding of the multi-causal nature of, and the importance of organizational measures to, employee health. Thus, for the first time, an approach was developed that involved workers and management collectively trying to create a health-promoting workplace. WHP continues to widen, and its scope now covers environmental, social, ergonomic, and organizational work issues, as well as individual, family, and community health issues. The trend is to view the worker in a holistic rather than purely medical manner, as is the case in most occupational health services today (Chu, Allen, et al., 2000; Chu, Breucker, et al., 2000; Motalebi et al., 2018; Pham et al., 2019).

Summarizing: The health-promoting workplace (HPW) approach has been translated into many different conceptual frameworks with several domains and characteristics; however, there is no unified version of a HPW. For example, WHO's healthy workplace framework attributes several domains to HPW, but does not provide it with specific characteristics. In addition, there are regional-, national-, and local-level frameworks with different and similar domains, and numerous tools have been developed to help evaluate the characteristics of an HPW. Workplace health promotion programs also vary in goals, objectives, and implementing procedures, depending on needs identified by employees and other parties involved.

However, while WHP concepts vary, all WHP models set up a variety of central principles to guide employers, employees, and health professionals to develop quality and effective HPW programs. The WHO Guidelines suggest developing healthy workplaces must occur around the principles of comprehensiveness, participation and empowerment, multi-sectoral and multidisciplinary cooperation, social justice, and sustainability. The central formulation of WHP concepts is the WHO healthy workplace model (Burton & WHO, 2010). It creates a "healthy workplace model": an abstract representation of the structure, content, processes, and system of the healthy workplace concept. The model includes both the content of the issues that should be addressed in a healthy workplace and also the process that will ensure the success and sustainability of healthy workplace initiatives.

While WHP strategies are often based on the principles set out in the Ottawa Charter (WHO-WPRO, 1999), in order to be applicable, they must be placed in the specific context of working life and culture in which they are operating. Thus, in the Ottawa Charter WHP is based on:

- The building of a healthy corporate policy.
- The creation of a supportive working environment.
- The development of employee skills conducive to health—supporting personal and social development is a central concept of health promotion. The opportunities for workplaces to provide information and enhance skills are many and varied.
- Strengthening a workforce's actions toward health. Enabling workers to influence, control, and gain ownership of workplace practices and activities that influence their health (both for the better and worse) is of great importance.
- The re-orientation of occupational health services. Occupational health services play a vital part in maintaining employees' ability to work.

9.3   Key Elements and Success Factors of WHP

Workplace health promotion has been shown to have number of beneficial outcomes for workers and companies including improving productivity, decreasing sickness absence, improving working relationships and employee morale, and creating a better public image for organizations that implement WHP programs.

While specific program goals and objectives vary with the identified needs of individual enterprises, key principles of the management of workplace health promotion are to:

- improve work organization and the working environment,
- develop healthy company policy and culture,
- encourage active participation by all involved,
- foster personal development, work styles, and lifestyles conducive to health, and to
- ensure health promotion and disease prevention strategies become an integral part of management practices.

For workplace health promotion to be successful and sustainable, it must be integrated into corporate policy and regular management practice and should be coordinated by members within the work organization rather than by costly external consultants.

As demonstrated by international examples (Motalebi et al., 2018; Pham et al., 2019; WHO-WPRO, 1999; Wynne, 1998), a successful WHP program can ensure a flexible and dynamic balance between fulfilling organizational targets on the one hand and employees' skills and health needs on the other. This is a desirable and essential ingredient for competing successfully in the modern world, not only for companies, but also for nations, whose sustainable social and economic development depends on the development of WHP. Box 9.1 highlights the features of successful WHP good practices in promoting employee health.

Box 9.1

Research based on a large number of models of good practice in enterprises from all over the world shows the common success factors for workplace health promotion. These include:

- Workplace health action should be based on an analysis of an enterprise's health requirements and needs;
- Health actions should take a participatory approach by involving all stakeholders in enterprises, especially the workers, and representatives of intermediary organizations;
- WHP actions should seek to improve the quality of working life and conditions as well as focusing on individual workers' behavior;
- Workplace health action should become an integral part of management practices and daily working life at all levels of an enterprise.
- These general characteristics of successful workplace health practice are independent of enterprise size and economic sector.

These criteria are intended to provide assistance in the planning and implementation of successful, high-quality health promotion measures for all those responsible for health at the workplace.

The terms "health" and "health promotion" are largely defined by concepts created by the WHO, and they form the basis for the term "workplace health promotion." WHP is the process of enabling workplaces to increase control over and to improve the health of all members of the organization. WHP is as follows:
directed toward action on the various determinants of workplace health
any combination of health, education, economic, political, spiritual, or organizational initiatives designed to bring about positive attitudinal, behavioral, social, or environmental changes, conducive to improving the health of members of the workplace.

As a result, the link between the idea of health promotion, granting everyone a greater degree of self-determination over their physical, mental, and social well-being and thus enabling them to improve their health, and the social preconditions found in organizations such as companies lead to "workplace health promotion." It comprises all the action and projects aimed at improving health at work that is implemented in response to statutory provisions or is offered voluntarily and that creates costs for the company.

WHP contributes to a wide range of work factors that improve employees' health (WHO, 2010). These include:

- management principles and methods recognizing that employees are a necessary success factor for the organization instead of a mere cost factor;
- a culture and corresponding leadership principles that encourage employee participation and motivate and place personal responsibility on all employees;

- work organization principles that provide employees with an appropriate balance between job demands, control over their own work, level of skills, and social support;
- a personnel policy that actively incorporates health promotion issues; and
- an integrated occupational health and safety service.

9.4 Transformation of the World of Work and the Future of Workplace Health Promotion

The world of work is undergoing profound changes, not least the transformative effect of new technology, changing demographics, and climate change and the shift toward the green economy. Technologies affect where we work, how we work, how we are compensated, and whether and how we are employed (Berger & Frey, 2016). These changes will bring about new challenges and opportunities for the safety and health of the world's workers (Pham et al., 2019).

The most important drivers and trends shaping tomorrow's world of work include:

- digitalization, which creates new technological foundations and possibilities for collaboration, production, company organization, and the sale of goods and services. Digital technologies have given efficiency, rationalization, value creation, and profit maximization a new dynamic as they open up the perspective of replacing people in tasks, jobs, and professional roles in many sectors while at the same time creating new opportunities and professions (European Agency for Safety and Health at Work, 2018; Pham et al., 2019);
- globalization, boosted by digitalization, has significantly expanded companies' and workers' spheres of action in recent decades and facilitated cross-border trade and communication, but has also led to a marked rise in migration flows. Economic globalization has resulted in increasing flows of capital, labor, goods, and services between national economies. Open trade and investment policies have triggered major changes in the structure and organization of work, with greater opportunities to outsource work to lower-wage economies and to tap into global labor markets.
- demographic change, which determines who, and with what skills, can participate in value creation now and in the future. There are two sides to the impact of demography on the labor market. In most developed economies including Europe, population growth is stagnant or shrinking and life expectancy is increasing, resulting in an older population with growing needs for care, as well as an urgent need for payments into social security systems by younger people. It is crucial that healthy aging is supported by actions to promote health and prevent disease throughout the lifespan by tackling key issues including poor nutrition, insufficient physical activity, alcohol, drug and tobacco consumption, environmental risks, traffic accidents, and accidents in the home. Improving the health of children, adults of working age, and older people will help create a healthy,

productive population and support healthy aging now and in the future (Pham et al., 2019).

- ongoing cultural and societal change, which is transforming consumption patterns and relationships etc., and exerts a significant influence on which innovations are accepted and catch on, and which are not; and finally,
- technological advances, which increase the threats of job insecurity and transform the work environment.

Based on the Intergovernmental Panel on Climate Change's *Fifth Assessment Report on Climate Change* (2014), the future will be characterized by increasing temperatures, changing precipitation patterns, and the increased occurrence and intensity of extreme weather events (such as droughts, storms, and floods). New diseases and health risks will emerge, there will be biodiversity loss, air, water, and soil pollution, and natural resources will decline due to overexploitation. Climate change and environmental degradation will shape safety and health at work and the actions that are needed to protect workers, as they introduce or amplify risks in the future (WHO, 2008).

In summary, the combination of technology, demographics, and globalization will be among the most significant forces that transform the nature and role of work. These mega-trends are affecting ideas of what a job is, what work is, and how the workplace is designed. Work and workplaces are constantly changing with the introduction of new technologies, substances and work processes, changes in the structure of the workforce and the labor market, and new forms of employment and work organization. This may give rise to new risks and challenges to workers' safety and health. These must be anticipated and addressed to ensure safe and healthy workplaces in the future.

The ILO Commission on the Future of Work (ILO, 2019) outlines a vision for a human-centered agenda based on investing in people's capabilities, institutions of work, and decent and sustainable work. Potential harms and new types of stress and strain need to be identified and prevented early, alongside finding new resources to promote employee health.

The term "workplace health promotion" should be viewed in its societal context, while emphasizing the significant role both employers and employees have within the workplace in promoting health at work. The definition makes clear that to achieve its maximum potential workplace health promotion relies upon the active engagement of all key stakeholders, for example, at a societal level, government (ministries of labor, and health), national and local health services, and providers of occupational health, while for employees the role of trade unions in embracing the workplace health agenda cannot be underestimated.

Anticipating risks is a crucial first step to effectively managing them and to building a preventive health culture in an ever-changing world. This requires a consideration of:

- How to integrate psychosocial risks in risk assessments as part of occupational safety and health (OSH) management systems in order to develop targeted prevention and hazard management strategies, interventions, and evaluations;

- How to develop a psychosocial safety climate and better manage mental health at the workplace; and
- The dynamics of antecedents of stress (unhealthy work stressors) and the antecedents of well-being (including demand resource models and issues related to the individual), organization, and the environment.

If work is recognized as a social determinant of health, then there is a need for greater attention to the connections between safety, health, and public health, and on possible new roles for occupational health, for example, in health promotion, and the prevention and management of emerging psychosocial risks, mental health disorders, and noncommunicable diseases.

The link between public health and OSH can be recognized in the need to promote healthy work environments (including work practices) that support health and prevent diseases through organizational improvements. Issues such as nutrition (access to affordable and healthy food during working hours), increased physical activity, good sleep, addressing psychosocial hazards, preventing substance abuse, and other addictions can all be positively influenced by working environments. These precipitate the need for a strong bridge among various mechanisms (occupational health services and public/private health services) to support worker health. This may require that worker protection is expanded through public health approaches and services, and more research to be done on the combination of procedures governing occupational and environmental health, that consider, for example, aspirations for a better quality of life that are closely joined with other activities relating to the protection of the human environment.

References

Berger, T., & Frey, C. (2016). *Structural transformation in the OECD: Digitalization, deindustrialization and the future of work* (OECD Social, Employment and Migration Working Papers, No. 193). OECD Publishing. Retrieved from https://www.oecd-ilibrary.org/docserver/5jlr068802f7-en.pdf?expires=1552228107&id=id&accname=guest&checksum=A2602163D20F58022978 0F9184E61B0E

Burton, J., & WHO. (2010). *Healthy workplace framework and model: Background and supporting literature and practice.* WHO, S. 75. Retrieved from https://apps.who.int/iris/bitstream/handle/10665/113144/9789241500241_eng.pdf

Chu, C. (2004). From Workplace Health Promotion to Integrative Workplace Health Management. In *Global occupational health network newsletter (GOHNET)* (Vol. 6, pp. 1–4). WHO.

Chu, C., Allen, J., Dwyer, S., et al. (2000). Workplace health promotion: The Australian experience. In G. Breucker (Ed.), *Towards better health at work: Successful European strategies* (pp. 337–371). BKK.

Chu, C., Breucker, G., Harris, N., Stitzel, A., Gan, X., Xueqi, G., & Dwyer, S. (2000). Health-promoting workplaces—international settings development. *Health Promotion International, 15*(2), 155–167.

Chu, C., & Dwyer, S. (2002). Employer role in integrative workplace health management. *Disease Management and Health Outcomes, 10*(3), 175–86.12.

ENWHP (The European Network for Workplace Health Promotion). (1997). *Luxemburg declaration on Workplace Health Promotion in the European Union*. https://www.enwhp.org/resources/toolip/doc/2018/05/04/luxembourg_declaration.pdf

European Agency for Safety and Health at Work. (2018). EU-OSHA ISSN: 1831-9343, Foresight on new and emerging occupational safety and health risks associated with digitalization by 2025. *European Risk Observatory*. Retrieved from https://osha.europa.eu/en/tools-and-publications/publications?sort_by=search_api_relevance&direction=desc&page=4

ILO, (2003). ILO standards-related activities in the area of occupational safety and health: An in-depth study for discussion with a view to the elaboration of a plan of action for such activities, 91st Session 2003, International Labour Organization. http://www.ilo.org/global/standards/subjects-covered-by-international-labourstandards/occupational-safety-and-health/lang--en/index.htm.

ILO. (2010). *Emerging risks and new patterns of prevention in a changing world of work*. Programme on Safety and Health at Work and the Environment (SafeWork), International Labour Organization.

ILO. (2014). *Safety and health at work: A vision for sustainable prevention*. XX World Congress on Safety and Health at Work 2014: Global Forum for Prevention; 24–27 August 2014. ILO Publications.

ILO. (2019). *The future of work*. https://www.ilo.org/global/topics/future-of-work/lang%2D%2Den/index.htm

IPCC (2014) *The Fifth Assessment Report on Climate chanage-2022*. https://www.ipcc.ch/report/ar5/syr/

Motalebi, M. G., Mohammadi, N. K., Kuhn, K., Ramezankhani, A., & Azari, M. R. (2018). How far are we from full implementation of health promoting workplace concepts? A review of implementation tools and frameworks in workplace interventions. *Health Promotion International, 33*(3), 488–504.

Pham, C. T., Lee, C. B., Nguyen, T. L. H., Lin, J. D., Ali, S., & Chu, C. (2019). Integrative settings approach to workplace health promotion to address contemporary challenges for worker health in the Asia-Pacific. *Global Health Promotion*, 1757975918816691. https://doi.org/10.1177/175918816691. https://journals.sagepub.com/doi/10.1177/1757975918816691

Pronk, N. P. (2013). Integrated worker health protection and promotion programs: Overview and perspectives on health and economic outcomes. *Journal of Occupational and Environmental Medicine., 55*(12), S30.

The Luxembourg Declaration. (1997). https://www.enwhp.org/?i=portal.en.policies-and-declarations

WHO. (2007). *Workers' health: global plan of action*. https://www.who.int/occupational_health/WHO_health_assembly_en_web.pdf

WHO. (2008). *New and emerging environmental threats to human health. Executive Summary*. First Interministerial Conference on Health and Environment in Africa: Health Security thr;2008.

WHO. (2010). *Healthy workplaces: A model for action: for employers, workers, policy-makers and practitioners*. WHO Press, World Health Organization.

WHO-WPRO. (1999). *Regional guidelines for the development of healthy workplaces*. WHO.

Wynne, R. (1998). *What makes workplace health promotion work? Findings from the European Foundation's Research Programme. lit—Success factors of workplace health promotion* Essen: BKK (Bundesverband) Federal Association of Company Health Insurance Funds.

Chapter 10
Prisons as a Setting for Health

James Woodall and Michelle Baybutt

10.1 Introduction

Globally, prisoners tend to come from marginalised and socially disadvantaged sections of society and exhibit a disproportionately high incidence of ill health, linked to social exclusion and multiple complex needs (Ismail & de Viggiani, 2018; Baybutt et al., 2018). On any given day, more than 11 million people globally are estimated to be in prison. In Western countries, the prison population continues to increase with prison services not keeping pace placing enormous financial burden on governments and threatening social cohesion of societies (Penal Reform International, 2020). Changes to prison demography are posing particular challenges, for example penal systems are struggling to cope with the rising number of older prisoners and this is creating new pressures and particular challenges. In the UK, there are triple the number of people aged 60 and over than there was 15 years ago the fastest growing age group in the prison estate (Prison Reform Trust, 2019).

Overcrowding is a salient and multidimensional issue for the majority of prison systems and has clear implications for health and well-being of prisoners and staff, including the transmission of disease and the propensity to accelerate poor mental health (WHO, 2014). Mental health and well-being in prison can be impacted greatly by a range of additional factors such as violence, enforced solitude, a lack of privacy, a lack of meaningful activity and isolation from social networks

J. Woodall (✉)
School of Health, Leeds Beckett University, Leeds, UK
e-mail: j.woodall@leedsbeckett.ac.uk

M. Baybutt
Healthy and Sustainable Settings Unit, School of Community Health and Midwifery,
University of Central Lancashire, Preston, Lancashire, UK
e-mail: mbaybutt@uclan.ac.uk

© Springer Nature Switzerland AG 2022
S. Kokko, M. Baybutt (eds.), *Handbook of Settings-Based Health Promotion*,
https://doi.org/10.1007/978-3-030-95856-5_10

(de Viggiani, 2007; WHO, 2008). Studies for mental health issues in prisons show that prison mental illness, and suicide is consistently higher than the general population.

The majority of prisoners (>90%) across the world are adult men (Penal Reform International, 2020), with epidemiological data consistently recognising that prisoners in general have poor health when measured against a range of health indicators (Stürup-Toft et al., 2018). The health profile of people in prison is complex with co-occurring physical and mental health problems with the poor health status of this population that is typically set against a backdrop of entrenched and intergenerational social disadvantage (WHO, 2019). Many of those entering the criminal justice system have been subjected to a lifetime of social exclusion, including poor educational backgrounds, low incomes, meagre employment opportunities, lack of engagement with normal societal structures, low self-esteem and impermanence in terms of accommodation (including bouts of homelessness) and poor relationships with family members (Department of Health, 2009; Levy, 2005; Senior & Shaw, 2007). The Social Exclusion Unit (2002), in their highly cited report, claimed that prisoners were thirteen times more likely to have grown up in care and more likely to have run away from home as a child. They revealed that most prisoners had disrupted educational experiences and were less likely to have any qualifications or basic skills.

Accessing people in the places they live their lives and make choices is a key public health approach (Dooris, 2012). Prisons are, therefore, a prime opportunity to address the disproportionate health and social circumstances of prisoners and offer a way of tackling inequalities in health and justice, through promoting health, reducing reoffending and facilitating community integration (Baybutt et al., 2018). While prisons are not necessarily in the primary business of promoting health, they do provide access to marginalised groups who would otherwise be classified as 'hard to reach' in the wider community. Further, the majority of people in prison return to the community, with many moving repeatedly between both settings (Kinner & Young, 2018) and serving to emphasise the importance of prison health as a concern for broader society and public health. Prisons are thus a key setting for health promotion to ensure health and well-being and to achieve the United Nations Sustainable Development Goals (WHO, 2019).

10.2   The Health-Promoting Prison Concept

The notion that prisons should be health-promoting has emerged in recent times as a response to the disease burden in this environment (Woodall & Dixey, 2015). While the health-promoting prison is a relatively new concept, several definitions have been proposed. One states that the health-promoting prison is as follows:

> …a place of compulsory detention in which the risks to health are reduced to a minimum; where essential prison duties such as the maintenance of security are undertaken in a caring

atmosphere that recognizes the inherent dignity of all prisoners and their human rights; where health services are provided to the level and in a professional manner equivalent to what is provided in the country as a whole; and where a whole-prison approach to promoting health and welfare is the norm. (Gatherer et al., 2009, p. 89)

There is relatively little practical guidance, which would enable prisons to shift towards being more 'health-promoting'. Some have advocated the Ottawa Charter as a useful way of conceptualising and realising the health-promoting prison (Woodall et al., 2014). The Charter attempts to address both structural forces that influence health (e.g. prison policy and the prison environment) and also the individual health choices that people make (Rütten & Gelius, 2011). The Charter provides five principal areas for action in prison: building healthy public policy; creating supportive environments; strengthening community action; developing personal skills; and re-orientating health services (WHO, 1986).

Theoretically, the health-promoting prison concept does not only concern prisoners who '(temporarily) live' there, but they also seek to consider staff need and those of visitors into the environment. Yet, the focus to date has been almost exclusively on prisoners (Woodall, 2016). It seems clear though, that for prisoners to be rehabilitated and released into the community as law abiding, healthy citizens, prison staff need to feel valued and in good physical, mental and psychosocial health (Bögemann, 2007). One of the underpinning principles, therefore, includes a focus on all those within the setting and a 'whole-prison approach' to health and well-being (Baybutt & Chemlal, 2016). A whole-system focus in the prison context means using organisational development to introduce and manage change throughout the prison with a concern to:

- Ensure living and working environments promote health and effectively rehabilitate prisoners;
- Integrate health and well-being within the culture and core business of the prison; and.
- Forge connections to the wider community, beyond the prison setting.

By applying the settings approach in the creation of a health-promoting prison, it seeks to establish an environment that is safe, secure and reforming underpinned by a commitment to participation, equity, partnership, human rights, respect and decency.

Drawing together these key elements provides a possible framework for health-promoting prisons:

- Creation of an environment within each prison, through procedural and capacity-building measures, that is supportive of health and ensuring the prison regime supports prisoners well-being (concept of decency; rehabilitative culture);
- Implementation of policies that specifically promote the health and well-being of prisoners and staff; and.
- Delivery of disease prevention, health education and health-promoting initiatives that seek to address health needs in each prison.

10.3   History and Development

The exact origins of the health-promoting prison concept are difficult to accurately pinpoint, although some have suggested that this was in October 1995 when an international meeting with senior prison health representatives from eight selected European countries agreed that the public health importance of prisoner health had been neglected (Gatherer et al., 2005). After this meeting, WHO Europe outlined its view of health promotion in prison, which was underpinned by core values—such as holism, a multidisciplinary approach and empowerment—and operationalised through a 'settings approach' (WHO, 1995). The first international conference on Healthy Prisons the following year proved to be a catalyst to foster discussion, along with opportunity for WHO to reaffirm their commitment (Squires & Strobl, 1996). A presentation at the conference, delivered by a WHO official, stated the following:

> In the World Health Organization (WHO) we have for too long now overlooked the problem of health in prisons…The Healthy Cities Project has now been running for over ten years and there was no way, ten years ago, we could have predicted the potential of that project. Healthy Cities has become a movement, a global movement….And I would like to think at an occasion like this that it is possible to start a similar movement as we did for Health Cities but now for prisons. (Goos, 1996, p. 20)

The WHO Health in Prisons Programme (HIPP) developed from a pilot network to include most of the Member States in the WHO Europe Region. The purpose of the network has been to exchange experience in tackling health issues that face prisoners and people working in prisons and to produce consensual statements of advice (Gatherer et al., 2005). Building on the definition of health as a 'state of complete physical, mental and social well-being, and not merely the absence of disease or infirmity' (WHO, 1948), WHO's principle objectives were to address prisoners health needs and risks, to recognise and mitigate against the harmful impacts of imprisonment and, consistent with these objectives, to safeguard prisoners' human rights and access to healthcare comparable/equivalent to those available to the general population (Ismail & de Viggiani, 2018).

The UK has been one of the leaders in developing health promotion in prison (although other work has been happening in Europe, for example France (Baybutt & Chemlal, 2016)), with the health-promoting prison concept comprehensively outlined in the English and Welsh strategy 'Health Promoting Prisons: A Shared Approach' (Department of Health, 2002). This document used the discourse of a 'whole-prison' approach with a core philosophy of creating environments that were supportive of health, with an emphasis on the wider determinants of prisoner health (Department of Health, 2002).

The strategy was subsequently converted into practical guidance through means of a Prison Service Order on Health Promotion (PSO 3200) in 2003 (HM Prison Service, 2003). Prison Service Orders (PSOs) are instructions that were issued until 31 July 2009. They were long-term, mandatory instructions, which were intended to last indefinitely and as such do not have an expiry date. The PSO was considered a major breakthrough for health promotion within the prison setting because the translation of a Department of Health strategy into an auditable prison document was a crucial step forward as it provided a level of commitment to health promotion within the offender management system. The PSO sets out required actions for prison governors to promote health as part of a whole-prison approach. Such policy drivers showed a great deal of promise within the health-promoting prisons field at the time; however, there has been minimal investment in fully embedding and evaluating the approach and some are unclear as to the impact that these documents have made to prisons and prisoners' health. Indeed, recent analysis has shown real challenges in applying a 'whole-prison' approach in most prisons. The analysis suggests that 44% of prisons in England and Wales demonstrated a whole-prison approach to promoting health and well-being, but the constituent activities comprising this were not clear (Woodall & Freeman, 2020). Where health promotion has been developed in prisons, it tends to follow a medical model, viewing health primarily as the absence of disease and focusing on individual lifestyle choices rather than wider determinants (Woodall et al., 2014). Yet, it is clear that prisoners' health is influenced by a complexity of 'deprivation' and 'importation' factors that relate to imprisonment itself and to circumstances predating incarceration (de Viggiani, 2006b).

10.4   Current Situation

The authors have consistently noted the challenges that have been faced when moving from the concept of the health-promoting prison to practice (Baybutt & Chemlal, 2016). The distance between the rhetoric of health promotion in prison, which adopts a settings approach, and translating this into practical guidance to aid delivery has been a major barrier. The WHO has itself acknowledged that policy formulation at a strategic level may not always be implemented properly in practice (van den Bergh and Gatherer, 2010), but the key question is why? A number of explanations of the current situation are offered:

1. 'Lifestyle drift', or the inclination for policy that recognises the need to act on upstream social determinants only to drift downstream to focus on individual lifestyle factors (Popay et al., 2010), has been evident in prison health promotion for some time. There has undoubtedly been an obsession with addressing prisoners' 'lifestyle' choices without fully acknowledging the need to also tackle their wider social context, which often includes poverty, unemployment and fractured family dynamics (de Viggiani, 2006a).
2. To operationalise the strategic vision of health-promoting prisons, there need to be coherent partnerships with organisations not traditionally seen to have a 'health' focus. In order to do this effectively, Dooris (2013) has suggested that settings should connect 'beyond health' making linkages to alternative agendas to maximise the contribution that settings can make to health and well-being. At

the moment, prisons have struggled to engage fully in broader agendas, although the situation may be changing in relation to the sustainability agenda in prisons in parts of the UK (Baybutt & Chemlal, 2016).

3. It is likely that strategic policy implementation of the health-promoting prison may break down at the stage where it is meant to be implemented by those 'on the ground'. Prison staffing levels have not kept pace with rising prison populations in some parts of the world—this has meant that staff may not always be able to implement policy or directives (see, e.g., staff reluctance to implement smoke-free policy in the UK (Woodall & Tattersfield, 2018)).

4. Whether 'standardised' measures are useful to assess the extent prisons that are achieving the optimum levels of health promotion is debatable. That said that prison inspections, which occur in many countries, should consider key pillars of activity that provide strong foundation for the health-promoting prison and embed this in their audit and monitoring of establishments.

5. Those tasked with translating the rhetoric of health-promoting prisons into reality have had to navigate a delicate and difficult policy path in which wider public and political opinion is an ever present force (Tabreham, 2014). The political and public views on whether prisons are 'deserving' of support have arguably tempered strategic values from being implemented fully.

6. A further challenge to the health-promoting prison has been the global inactivity. While global consensus has been reached on school settings, for example, this has not been replicated in the prison context. One predicted indicator of success for the health-promoting prison movement was the expansion of activity beyond European borders (Gatherer et al., 2005); yet, two decades since the European model was put forward there has been very limited policy or practice. Dixey et al. (2015) discussing the situation in the African continent point to resource challenges and extremity of health need, which has meant that African prisons have been unable to engage in health-promoting actions. Moreover, the United States has failed to engage with agenda for various reasons including the sheer magnitude of the incarcerated population in the United States and the lack of political will or momentum to address the needs of prisoners (Woodall, 2018).

Practice Case Study
Horticulture as a Vehicle for Joined-Up, Whole-System Health Improvement: Greener on the Outside for Prisons [GOOP]

Established in 2008, Greener on the Outside of Prisons (GOOP) is a programme of therapeutic horticulture that continues to operate in all North West England public sector prisons and is unique because it takes a 'whole-prison approach'—particularly, that it embeds education [e.g. key skills and related horticultural qualifications] and health within the programme alongside wider prison and 'through the gate' input, while supporting resettlement, impacting on the drive to reduce reoffending and contributing to the creation of a rehabilitative prison culture. GOOP continues to be delivered in all public sector

(continued)

prisons in the North West and four in the South West and has been piloted in a further five prison sites outside of the region. Engaging with some of the most challenging and complex people in our society, GOOP recognises that those who go to prison generally return to the community, thus taking with them their health and social care issues. It therefore uses the potential of prison as a place to intervene, tackle health inequalities and change the lives of individuals and their families.

The aim of the programme is, through engagement with nature, to:

- Reduce inequalities and achieve sustainable improvements in health, well-being and learning outcomes for prisoners with a particular focus on mental health, physical activity and healthier eating.

Markedly understudied and under-represented in policy and practice, prison-based horticulture is one intervention that can positively impact on entrenched cycles of deprivation and poor health. The consistent message from a diverse body of research is that contact with the natural environment improves psychological health and mental well-being. Increasing evidence suggests nature and the outdoors is a dynamic environment that stimulates creativity and enables learning to happen faster while improving health and well-being and providing an opportunity to impact positively on attitudes and self-esteem. In the context of the current UK prison reform agenda, GOOP offers multiple benefits and makes a significant contribution to the creation of safer, more secure, supportive and health-enhancing prison environments.

GOOP is more than working in the prison Gardens Department. It is most effective when working joined-up and across the whole prison and beyond, for example:

Involving health care in the referral process to the GOOP project by identifying prisoners who would benefit the most—perhaps those with identified mental health problems, experiencing problems with depression, anxiety or more challenging behaviours such as substance misuse and self-harm, issues with violence and aggression or those who are struggling to integrate. Health care in prison is the key department to undertake baseline and follow-up health assessments, monitoring change over time, while prisoners are participating in GOOP.

Involving the education provider to deliver a range of qualifications such as relating directly to horticulture and land-based activities, or relating to more creative and art-based skill development that improve the environment; and concurrently embedding key skills such as literacy and numeracy into GOOP is a resource to the Gardens department and wider prison, supporting prisoners to become better and more appropriately qualified.

Working with the catering department to find ways of utilising produce grown by prisoners is a way of encouraging prisoners to learn about and try new vegetables and salads while complimenting their diet with fresh foods locally produced.

(continued)

Engaging with residential staff so that they are aware of what prisoner participation in the GOOP project can achieve. This awareness can enable residential staff to help direct prisoners into appropriate work and education programmes. It can also help by increasing awareness of how the value of GOOP can extend to more stability on the wing particularly with younger people or those with more challenging behaviour and complex health and social care issues.

Some key ingredients that make GOOP work:

- Top-down support and bottom-up engagement: support and endorsement from the Governing Governor and Senior Management Team and a solid partnership between the garden staff, education provider, and health provider as well as residential staff.
- Wider community involvement: engaging with national partners for environment, biodiversity, ecology and sustainability, and with local community partners, agencies and organisations such as garden centres and suppliers, social cooperatives, farmers' markets and local cafes.

Impact

GOOP has been found to have a positive impact on participants' mental health and well-being. In improving skills and employability, GOOP also encourages physical activity and healthy eating and develops social and interpersonal skills. GOOP can also have a calming effect on participants, including prisoners who may be more vulnerable, challenging or aggressive and has been found to reduce self-harm and aggressive behaviour.

Over 4500 prisoners in the North West prisons participated in the evaluation of the first phase of the GOOP programme up to 2015 (which continues to be evaluated in 2022). The research found that participation in GOOP had a positive impact on prisoners' mental health and well-being including reducing incidents of self-harm. This was assessed using questionnaires of mental health indicators and through interviews with prisoners. In total, 88.2% of participants stated that from participating in GOOP, they felt more confident to manage their everyday lives. Prisoners also felt that their confidence levels and self-efficacy had been boosted by participating. Participants described how GOOP helped them with their own mental health and well-being:

I have suffered with mental health problems for over 25 years but working in the [horticulture] project has helped me to feel more confident. (Male prisoner)

Being involved in the group has helped me with my social anxieties and helped me gain self-belief again. (Female prisoner)

It is clear that prisoners have valued and forged connections to nature and that this experience has helped them to cope with or resolve challenges:

...being out[side] actually helps tremendously, or shall I say...allows you to deal with your problems a lot better. (Male prisoner)

(continued)

In addition to data related to the mental health outcome indicators, the study revealed multiple layers of 'added value' related to mental health arising from engagement with horticultural work in a prison setting. Positive impacts on prisoners' mental health and well-being included increased confidence, social interactions with staff and other prisoners, and gaining skills and qualifications and work experience, and increasing potential for post-release employment. The impact on drug and alcohol users has also been significant—it provides a calming area to work, provides prisoners with responsibility and something different to focus on.

Looking to the future, horticulture in prisons offers an important opportunity to connect policy agendas through enhancing learning and health literacy; building skills and enhancing employability; developing social and interpersonal skills and the competence to maintain family relationships; and promoting models of good citizenship (Baybutt & Chemlal, 2016). Though facing challenges in providing healthy environments, prison offers opportunities to improve health and reduce health inequalities through whole-system place-based public health programmes such as GOOP. Key to the success of GOOP has been the role of horticulture in connecting different parts of the prison system (at local, regional and national levels) with opportunities for health improvement (in its broadest sense) and embedding understanding of the roles and responsibilities for health in the systems and structures of the prison setting.

10.5 Looking to the Future

A major challenge to developing the health-promoting prison is to facilitate connections and links with other settings. Developing partnerships with workplaces, communities, education and training institutions pose several challenges—none more so than marrying together the different cultures and ways of working—and moreover, this needs to be prioritised if prison populations are supported to take more control over their health and wider determinants. Broadly speaking, if a settings approach is to be fully realised, a more radical, upstream and holistic outlook is required in prisons. This would include embracing the idea of salutogenesis in prison and recognising 'what creates health' for those incarcerated (Baybutt & Chemlal, 2016). This would create a greater shift away from the current deficit models of health towards greater consideration of positive health and well-being (Danks & Bradley, 2018). Indeed, the majority of prisons inspected in England and Wales in 2018 were exceptionally proficient at managing and screening for diseases in prison. The analysis suggested that 88% of prisons enabled easy access to health checks, disease prevention and screening programmes. There were few instances where support and healthcare provision were deficient in this domain (Woodall & Freeman, 2020). Finally, while managing modern prison systems is complex, there is a need for enlightened global leadership for the settings approach to truly flourish across the world. At the moment, there is little doubt that policy and practice are, at best, patchy and in some continents nonexistent.

10.6 Key Principles for a Health-Promoting Prison

The health-promoting prison should include all facets of prison life, from address-ing individual health need to organisational factors and the physical environment. The Ottawa Charter (WHO, 1986), alluded to earlier, is a useful framework to envis-age these facets of prison life and has been used by others to map health promotion work in prisons (Ramaswamy & Freudenberg, 2007). Figure 10.1 attempts to dem-onstrate the applicability of the Ottawa Charter to the health-promoting prison.

10.7 Summary

The WHO Health in Prisons Programme has had inherent challenges (Woodall, 2016); however, it has been widely argued that the settings approach that it endorses offers opportunities to realise the potential of prisons to embrace health promotion and meaningfully tackle health inequalities (Baybutt & Chemlal, 2016). Appreciating that health is created and lived within the settings of everyday life (WHO, 1986), the approach embraces a socioecological model of health, a salutogenic orientation concerned with what creates well-being and makes people thrive, a system perspec-tive and a focus on holistic change (Dooris, 2013). Applied in this context, the set-tings approach prioritises a whole-prison perspective and involves revisiting notions of control, choice and empowerment and utilising a determinant-focused framework.

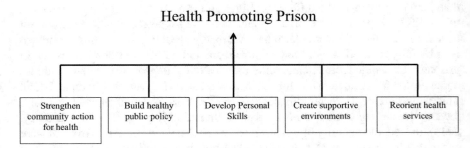

Fig. 10.1 The Ottawa Charter as a framework for action within the health-promoting prison

Ultimately, good prison health is a global concern for the whole of society, with prisoners coming from and returning to the wider community (WHO, 2014). Therefore, accessing people in the environments in which they lead their lives and make life choices is an essential approach to tackling health inequalities and promoting public health (Devine et al., 2019). It is argued therefore that the prison setting offers a unique opportunity to address health and social issues; however, translating the health-promoting prisons' concept into practice is a real challenge (Baybutt & Chemlal, 2016).

References

Baybutt, M., & Chemlal, K. (2016). Health-promoting prisons: Theory to practice. *Global Health Promotion, 23*, 66–74.

Baybutt, M., Dooris, M., & Farrier, A. (2018). Growing health in prison settings. *Health Promotion International.* https://doi.org/10.1093/heapro/day037

Bögemann, H. (2007). Promoting health and managing stress among prison employees. In L. Møller, H. Stöver, R. Jürgens, A. Gatherer, & H. Nikogosian (Eds.), *Health in prisons*. WHO.

Danks, K., & Bradley, A. (2018). Negotiating barriers: Prisoner and staff perspectives on mental wellbeing in the open prison setting. *Journal of Criminal Psychology, 8*, 3–19.

de Viggiani, N. (2006a). A new approach to prison public health? Challenging and advancing the agenda for prison health. *Critical Public Health, 16*, 307–316.

de Viggiani, N. (2006b). Surviving prison: Exploring prison social life as a determinant of health. *International Journal of Prisoner Health, 2*, 71–89.

de Viggiani, N. (2007). Unhealthy prisons: Exploring structural determinants of prison health. *Sociology of Health and Illness, 29*(1), 115–135.

Department of Health. (2002). *Health promoting prisons: A shared approach*. Crown.

Department of Health. (2009). *Improving health, supporting justice: The national delivery plan of the health and criminal justice programme board*. Department of Health.

Devine, H., Baybutt, M., & Meeks, R. (2019). Producing food in English and Welsh prisons. *Appetite.* https://doi.org/10.1016/j.appet.2019.104433

Dixey, R., Nyambe, S., Foster, S., Woodall, J., & Baybutt, M. (2015). Health promoting prisons–an impossibility for women prisoners in Africa? *Agenda*, 1–8.

Dooris, M. (2012). Settings for promoting health. In L. Jones & J. Douglas (Eds.), *Public health: Building innovative practice*. Sage.

Dooris, M. (2013). Expert voices for change: Bridging the silos—Towards healthy and sustainable settings for the 21st century. *Health & Place, 20*, 39–50.

Gatherer, A., Møller, L., & Hayton, P. (2005). The World Health Organization European health in prisons project after 10 years: Persistent barriers and achievements. *American Journal of Public Health, 95*, 1696–1700.

Gatherer, A., Møller, L., & Hayton, P. (2009). Achieving sustainable improvement in the health of women in prisons: The approach of the WHO health in prisons project. In D. C. Hatton & A. Fisher (Eds.), *Women prisoners and health justice*. Radcliffe.

Goos, C. (1996). Perspectives on healthy prisons. In N. Squires & J. Strobl (Eds.), *Healthy prisons a vision for the future, 24–27th March, 1996*. The University of Liverpool, Department of Public Health.

HM Prison Service. (2003). *Prison service order (PSO) 3200 on health promotion*. HM Prison Service.

Ismail, N., & de Viggiani, N.(2018, March 13). *What are the barriers prison governors and staff face in implementing the healthy prisons agenda? South west public health scientific confer-*

ence 2018, Bristol, UK. (pp. 1–14). Centre for the Development and Evaluation of Complex Interventions for Public Health Improvement (DECIPHer). Available from http://eprints.uwe. ac.uk/36233

Kinner, S. A., & Young, J. T. (2018). Understanding and improving the health of people who experience incarceration: An overview and synthesis. *Epidemiologic Reviews, 40*(1), 4–11. https:// doi.org/10.1093/epirev/mxx018

Levy, M. (2005). Prisoner health care provision: Reflections from Australia. *International Journal of Prisoner Health, 1*, 65–73.

Penal Reform International. (2020). *Global prison trends 2020*. Penal Reform International.

Popay, J., Whitehead, M., & Hunter, D. J. (2010). Injustice is killing people on a large scale—But what is to be done about it? *Journal of Public Health, 32*, 148–149.

Prison Reform Trust. (2019). *Bromley briefings. Prison Factfile*. Prison Reform Trust.

Ramaswamy, M., & Freudenberg, N. (2007). Health promotion in jails and prisons: An alternative paradigm for correctional health services. In R. B. Greifinger, J. Bick, & J. Goldenson (Eds.), *Public health behind bars. From prisons to communities*. Springer.

Rütten, A., & Gelius, P. (2011). The interplay of structure and agency in health promotion: Integrating a concept of structural change and the policy dimension into a multi-level model and applying it to health promotion principles and practice. *Social Science & Medicine, 73*, 953–959.

Senior, J., & Shaw, J. (2007). Prison healthcare. In Y. Jewkes (Ed.), *Handbook on prisons*. Willan Publishing.

Social Exclusion Unit. (2002). *Reducing re-offending by ex-prisoners*. Crown.

Squires, N., & Strobl, J. (1996). *Healthy prisons, a vision for the future : Report of the 1st international conference on healthy prisons, Liverpool, 24–27 March 1996*. University of Liverpool.

Stürup-Toft, S., O'Moore, E., & Plugge, E. (2018). Looking behind the bars: Emerging health issues for people in prison. *British Medical Bulletin, 125*, 15–23.

Tabreham, J. D. (2014). *Prisoners' experience of healthcare in England: Post-transfer to National Health Service responsibility: A case study* (PhD). University of Lincoln.

WHO. (1948). *Constitution*. WHO.

WHO. (1986). Ottawa Charter for health promotion. *Health Promotion, 1*, iii–v.

WHO. (1995). *Health in prisons. Health promotion in the prison setting. Summary report on a WHO meeting, London 15–17 October 1995*. WHO.

WHO. (2014). *Prisons and health*. WHO.

WHO. (2019). *Status report on prison health in the WHO European Region*. WHO Regional Office.

Woodall, J. (2016). A critical examination of the health promoting prison two decades on. *Critical Public Health, 26*, 615–621.

Woodall, J. (2018). Why has the health-promoting prison concept failed to translate to the United States? *American Journal of Health Promotion, 32*, 858–860.

Woodall, J., de Viggiani, N., Dixey, R., & South, J. (2014). Moving prison health promotion along: Toward an integrative framework for action to develop health promotion and tackle the social determinants of health. *Criminal Justice Studies, 27*, 114–132.

Woodall, J., & Dixey, R. (2015). Advancing the health promoting prison: A call for global action. *Global Health Promotion, 24*, 58–61.

Woodall, J., & Freeman, C. (2020). Promoting health and Well-being in prisons: An analysis of one year's prison inspection reports. *Critical Public Health, 30*(5), 555–566.

Woodall, J., & Tattersfield, A. (2018). Perspectives on implementing smoke-free prison policies in England and Wales. *Health Promotion International, 33*, 1066–1073.

World Health Organization. (2008). *Trencin statement on prisons and mental health*. World Health Organization.

Chapter 11
Health Promotion in Sports Settings

Aurélie Van Hoye, Susanna Geidne, Jan Seghers, Aoife Lane, Alex Donaldson, Matthew Philpott, and Sami Kokko

11.1 Introduction

The setting-based health promotion approach was introduced and developed in certain official institutional and traditional settings like cities, schools and hospitals as demonstrated in this book. After initial steps in the mid-1990s, more initiatives were established, and in the early 2000s, the potential of sports-related settings was

A. Van Hoye (✉)
EA4360 APEMAC, Université de Lorraine, Nancy, France
e-mail: aurelie.van-hoye@univ-lorraine.fr

S. Geidne
School of Health Sciences, Örebro University, Örebro, Sweden
e-mail: susanna.geidne@oru.se

J. Seghers
Physical Activity, Sport & Health Research Group, Department of Movement Sciences,
University of Leuven (KU Leuven), Leuven, Belgium
e-mail: jan.seghers@kuleuven.be

A. Lane
Department of Sport and Health Sciences, SHE Research Group, Technological
University of the Shannon, Athlone, Ireland
e-mail: alane@tus.ie

A. Donaldson
Centre for Sport and Social Impact, La Trobe University, Melbourne, Australia
e-mail: a.donaldson@latrobe.edu.au

M. Philpott (✉)
European Healthy Stadia Network, Liverpool, UK
e-mail: Matthew.Philpott@healthystadia.eu

S. Kokko (✉)
Research Center for Health Promotion, Faculty of Sport and Health Sciences,
University of Jyväskylä, Länsi-Suomi, Finland
e-mail: sami.p.kokko@jyu.fi

© Springer Nature Switzerland AG 2022
S. Kokko, M. Baybutt (eds.), *Handbook of Settings-Based Health Promotion*,
https://doi.org/10.1007/978-3-030-95856-5_11

noted and initiatives were developed focusing on sports clubs (health-promoting sports club) and sports stadiums (Healthy Stadia). Although these two concepts and settings overlap to a certain degree, they also have unique features and evolution. Therefore, they are presented in separate sections of this chapter.

The health-promoting sports club (HPSC) concept was established in 2004 in Finland, and it has spread to other countries thereafter, mainly in Europe. The aim of HPSC is to integrate health promotion actions into sports activities in order to further support and develop the core business of sports clubs. The HPSC recognizes sports clubs as an entity, meaning that the whole system within a club is acknowledged. In addition, external actors are recognized and collaborations are established. Over the past 20 years, a lot of research has been done on the concept of the HPSC. The framework and fundamentals of the health-promoting sports club and its evolution are presented in Sect. 11.2.

Healthy Stadia was established in 2004 in the UK. The emphasis is on sports stadiums, but sports clubs are also acknowledged. A Healthy Stadium has been defined as '...one which promotes the health of visitors, fans, players, employees and the surrounding community. It is a place where people can go to have a positive healthy experience playing or watching sport' (Skille, 2010). The European Healthy Stadia network was initiated in 2007, and it extends to an increasing number of sports stadiums, clubs and governing bodies that are developing health-promoting sports settings. The concept and principles of the Healthy Stadia are presented in Sect. 11.3.

11.2 Health-Promoting Sports Club

Aurélie Van Hoye, Susanna Geidne, Jan Seghers, Aoife Lane, Alex Donaldson, and Sami Kokko

11.2.1 Introduction

The potential of sports clubs as health-promoting settings has been acknowledged for almost a decade (Donaldson & Finch, 2012; Geidne et al., 2013b; Kokko et al., 2013), because (1) they reach a large population, across socio-economic levels and across life stages, (2) they enhance the physical, psychological, mental and social health of their participants through sport participation and physical activity practices (Eime et al., 2013; Oja et al., 2015; Rhodes et al., 2017), and (3) their informal educational nature, due to voluntary participation, provides opportunities for tailored health promotion, through daily sporting activities (Kokko, 2014).

There is wide variation in sports clubs around the world, with different national-level (e.g. different sports systems, including the role of the state) and club-level (e.g. sports discipline, club size and/or participants—children and adolescents or adults or all ages) characteristics (Balish et al., 2015; Ibsen et al., 2016). Still, some universal commonalities can be found, which help to define sports clubs in the present chapter. Sports clubs are typically nonprofit (volunteer), grassroot-level actors that organize sporting activities for particular target groups at the local level (Breuer et al., 2015). For children and adolescents, sports clubs are settings in which they (regularly) participate in sports, while coaches and other adults can not only be participants, but also contribute to through their actions, as volunteers or parents (Kokko et al., 2013; Van Hoye et al., 2020a). In addition, sports clubs have in common 'the provision of opportunities for competition and sports practice, while some can also be considered social organizations, promoting social welfare and health' (Donaldson & Finch, 2012). In other words, organizing sport practice and competition is the core business of sports clubs (Kokko, 2014). Therefore, when considering integrating health promotion into sports clubs, it is important to (1) recognize the core business of sports clubs, (2) identify a link between the core business and health promotion, and (3) use the language and terminology commonly used in sports.

11.2.2   History and Development

Health promotion in sport-related settings began in the mid-1990s when some first actions took place in Australia. At that time, tobacco sponsorship and advertising in sports settings were prohibited in Australia and replaced by equivalent health-related products and services (Corti et al., 1995), and the effectiveness of this sponsorship and advertising at sports venues targeting people's health behaviours were studied (Giles-Corti et al., 2001). In Australia, an alcohol-use prevention programme in sports clubs—the Good Sports Program—was launched in 2000 in the State of Victoria. Today, this programme has spread to other states. The programme shares the principles of the setting approach and has been proven effective (Eime et al., 2008; Rowland et al., 2012a, 2012b). More recently, several research groups are working on areas such as sports participation and physical activity (Eime et al., 2008), nutrition and food (Kelly et al., 2008, 2011), sports organizations' capacity-building strategies (Casey et al., 2012a; Casey et al., 2009, 2012b) and sports injury prevention research (Donaldson et al., 2013, 2004).

In Europe, the application of the setting-based approach in sports clubs started in the early 2000s, when Kokko and colleagues developed the standards for health-promoting sports clubs (HPSC) (Kokko et al., 2006). Thereafter, Kokko et al. (Kokko, 2014; Kokko et al., 2009, 2013) published the theoretical grounds for the setting-based approach and a measurement tool known as the HPSC Index (Kokko et al., 2009, 2011). Around the same time, in Sweden, the alcohol policies of sports clubs were studied (Geidne et al., 2013a), as was the collaboration between clubs and external stakeholders (Geidne et al., 2013b). In Belgium, sports clubs' motives and barriers to health promotion were in focus (Meganck et al., 2014,

2016). In France, the health promotion activities of coaches were examined (Van Hoye et al., 2015, 2016a, b), while in Ireland, a Healthy Club concept was created (Lane et al., 2017, 2020). More recent developments are presented throughout the chapter.

11.2.3 The Framework and Fundamentals

Taking into account that the application of the setting-based approach is very diverse, depending on the type of setting and the people available at a certain time and place (Kokko et al., 2013), its application to sport clubs needed a specific model and definitions. A setting-based approach in a sports club setting means recognizing the whole system, i.e. the different levels and various determinants (at each level), and the influence of the preconditions at each level on the next level and its actors. Within sports clubs, the setting-based approach has been underpinned by two categorizations (levels and determinants). Three levels of sports club activities identified (Johnson et al., 2019) (Fig. 11.1) are the (1) macro-level, related to the club's policies and operation regulations on health promotion; (2) meso-level, encompassing the guidance and support given to coaches and staff by club officials and management; and (3) micro-level, incorporating the health promotion activities and support given to participants by coaches. It should be noted that the relationship between different levels of a club and its participants is reciprocal; i.e. the club shapes and affects coach-level activities and further individuals, and the participants shape and affect how the coach and club function and develop (Van Hoye et al., 2020a). Alongside these internal actors, external actors like the local community,

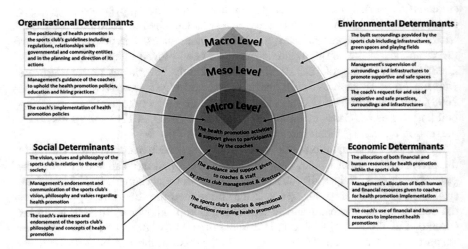

Fig. 11.1 Health-promoting sports clubs model. (Source: Adapted with permission from Johnson et al., 2019)

public authorities, and health and sport organizations also support the health promotion capacity (time, money, people, policies) and readiness of a sports club (Geidne et al., 2013b).

Regarding the levels within a single sports club, the key question for health promotion is 'what kind of preconditions and aims do the macro and meso-levels set out for the micro-level and its actors' (Kokko, 2014). Four types of health determinants have been defined for each level: social, cultural/organizational, environmental and economic (Johnson et al., 2019). Furthermore, five indicators that have been identified to signal a sports club are health-promoting (Van Hoye et al., 2020a). Sports clubs are encouraged to (1) have an approach embracing all club actions, which extend beyond promoting only one health topic; (2) involve all levels—participants, parents, coaches, management, volunteers, etc.—in their health promotion actions and decision-making; (3) involve external partners and the community in their health promotion actions and decision-making; (4) be conscious that promoting health within the club is a continuous, iterative process; and (5) base actions on needs, acknowledging the limitations of a 'one-size-fits-all' approach.

Whenever working with a setting that does not have health issues as core business, despite the provision of physical activity, a health determinant, the setting involvement in HP and HP activity organization as part of daily routine are not always explicit. For example, if a club has not previously undertaken health promotion activities, it would make sense to start with basic level actions (e.g. a passive education model, as outlined below). Three different stages have been defined for sports clubs to become health-promoting settings (Kokko et al., 2013). The first stage is a passive education model, where the club is a vehicle for individual-centred health promotion targeting a specific risk behaviour (e.g. alcohol consumption), implemented by external experts not related to sport, targeting a specific audience (club members) in the club environment. The second stage, the club-based education stage, requires an active engagement of sport clubs by recognizing the club that can play a role in the heath of individual sport participants. In this case, participants and coaches are targeted through specific training. The third stage, the club society development stage, has a primary goal of modifying the setting by changing collective norms and club culture towards HP, as well as the organization of sports clubs to support health promotion actions.

The previous text has explained the principles of the setting-based health promotion work within sports clubs. However, the setting-based approach also recognizes the relationship between other settings/actors outside a club setting. Closely related to and influencing the sports club setting are the different regional support systems (which can vary in different countries) across economic, educational and administrative contexts. Other actors include sponsors and partners, and municipalities or regional councils (often responsible for city planning and sports facilities etc.) (Geidne et al., 2013b). It is important that HPSCs undertake their activities within a community and develop relationships with other settings as their participants spend their lives going in and out of different settings (Dooris, 2004). In addition, it is worthwhile to consider crossing the boundaries between settings or finding the boundary spaces to be able to cooperate on joint problems with other settings

(McCuaig et al., 2020). In this socio-ecological approach, it is also important to balance the top-down managerial input with bottom-up club engagement (Dooris, 2006). A study of the support sports clubs' need to promote health in France revealed nine action areas (Johnson et al., 2020): tools for health promotion; communication tools; stakeholder training courses; diagnostics and financing; awareness and mobilization; advocacy; policies and methods; sharing; and networking, communication and dissemination. In other words, sports clubs need recognition and advocacy of their role in health promotion, and tools and support to promote health.

A literature review identified that three interventions have been evaluated rigorously to produce evidence of effective health-promoting sports clubs, but also highlighted that the application of a setting-based approach in sports clubs is often poor, at a single level and principally targeting participants (McFadyen et al., 2018). An exemplar programme was identified in Ireland, where health promotion was targeted at all three organizational levels and focused on several health behaviours (see Case in Box 11.1) (Geidne et al., 2019). In the example, interventions target several groups with multicomponent and multilevel (inside and outside the sport club including participants, coaches, officials, federations or healthcare workers) actions and a community and inter-sectoral dimensions (crossing both health and sport expertise).

> **Box 11.1 Case 1: GAA Healthy Club, Ireland**
> The GAA Healthy Club Project (Lane et al., 2017) was established to harness and formalize health promotion activities in GAA clubs. This project is based on the health-promoting sports clubs' approach. The intervention was led by key actors at national and regional level of the sport and health sector, and advises clubs to (1) develop a plan, which includes policies and/or actions plans; (2) recruit partners to assist in delivering the initiative; (3) identify an activity-focused specifically on behaviour change; and (4) assess any impact on the club, physically and culturally.

11.2.4   Current Situation

In 2016, a study on international research about health-promoting sports clubs (Kokko et al., 2016) provided six case studies from five countries (Australia, Finland, Sweden, Belgium and Ireland). The main conclusion was that research and practice are moving slowly from health promotion initiatives in sports clubs to an understanding of a health-promoting sports club.

Evidence of the effectiveness of the setting-based model is a challenge (Dooris, 2006), in terms of identifying both process and outcomes, as well as unexpected results. A recent literature review (McFadyen et al., 2018) was conducted to determine the effectiveness of strategies to improve the implementation of policies, practices or programmes in sporting organizations. Only three studies met the criteria:

(1) to improve implementation of policies, practices or programmes targeting one or more health risk, and (2) having a control group. Two studies focused on nutrition issues and one on alcohol policies and practices. Each study showed an improvement on at least one measure of policy or practice implementation. Despite these positive results, the authors (McFadyen et al., 2018) conclude that the evidence base underpinning the effectiveness of health-promoting sports clubs is lacking.

As studies with controlled groups were lacking, another review (Geidne et al., 2019) focused on published articles describing or evaluating health promotion interventions within sports clubs. A total of 58 studies were included. This literature review showed several gaps in studying health promotion in sports clubs: half of the papers came from Australia, and only one came from Asia and Africa, respectively. Half of the studies targeted sport participants directly and did not identify or focus on a specific population. The majority of the studies targeted men and principally team sports, limiting the knowledge base. The review analysed 33 unique interventions, mostly delivered at the intrapersonal level (29 studies), with only two working at all levels. Moreover, 35 studies did not use any specific theoretical background, indicating that setting-based approach is not implemented properly in sports clubs so far.

The literature review also qualitatively analysed the key strategies (see Box 11.2) described within the included studies, to provide empirical evidence to theoretical statements provided by Kokko (Kokko, 2013).

Box 11.2 14 Strategies to Implement Health-Promoting Sports Clubs

1. Determine club previous experience in HP, organizational readiness, rationale and club sense of endorsement for engaging in HP in your club
2. Turn health promotion aims into a written form, with positive messages, adapted to sport language, culture and HP representation of club, taking social inequalities into account.
3. Consider socio-ecological and the sports clubs' sense of belonging enhancing strategies to define the most relevant HP aims
4. Consider the financial (subsidize, sponsorship), human (volunteer time, staff turnover) and capacity-building resources to invest in the health promotion development work
5. Use role models and experts to lead the development process
6. Use a bottom-up approach in HP interventions, applied at the three levels (micro, meso, macro), based on recognition and reward system, as well as trust and shared interest between all participants
7. Collaborate with other agencies (clubs, health agencies and practitioner), by building common culture (trust, recognition, shared time) and processes for collaboration (clear roles, shared experiences, contract specification, evaluation of results, power balance between partners)
8. Evaluate the cost, the time, the accessibility and the enjoyment in regard to feasibility of health promotion aims regularly

9. Create a clear implementation plan (for routine and event organization), including the target population and funding mechanisms, establishing core objectives, infrastructure, coordinator, key process, taking sustainability issues into actions

10. Base internal on a single clear, explicit and inclusive message, visible to the community and partners, enhancing sports clubs' sense of ownership

11. Motivate coaches regarding HP implementation, by fostering interpersonal relationship (humour, support, encouragement), autonomy, a sense of ownership, and by taking coaches' capacity to handle situations, career opportunities and development into account

12. Educate coaches by varying support and strategies, using a participatory approach and focusing on the specificity of their population

13. Monitor health promotion activities in daily practice using a small win philosophy and evaluating effects not only at short terms

14. Integrate practice evaluation into HP policies, to help refine future planning and policies

To better operationalize health-promoting sports clubs, the 14 strategies in Box 11.2 need to be implemented. We are aware that sports clubs may not fulfil all the guidelines, but they should strive for them in a way that makes sense to their particular organization. The real challenge is to develop integrated, not separate health promotion initiatives into sports club settings. Based on the findings of preceding reviews, workshops with sport and health promotion stakeholders transformed these 14 evidence-based strategies into 55 intervention components (Van Hoye et al., 2020a).

11.2.5 Evaluation: A Challenge in Sports Club Settings?

Comprehensive evaluation tools for setting-based health promotion are limited in setting-based work overall (Dooris, 2004; Poland et al., 2009). This is also the case within health-promoting sports clubs, although a few suggestions have been proposed. Two Delphi studies have been undertaken to identify the indicators of health promotion within sport clubs; only one of these has led to a validation process of a measurement tool. Beyond this, another evaluation tool has been developed and tested. The first Delphi study (Kokko et al., 2006) was based on the Ottawa Charter and identified 22 standards of health promotion in sports clubs to build the Health Promotion in Sport Clubs index (HPSC). The index was then used to collect data amongst a sample of Finnish officials and coaches (Kokko et al., 2009). This measurement tool has also been used with officials and coaches in Finland (Kokko et al., 2011, 2015) and the officials in Belgium (Meganck et al., 2014), and a modified version was used with clubs in Ireland (Lane et al., 2017) and with coaches in France (Van Hoye et al., 2015, 2016b, 2018, 2020b).

The second Delphi study was conducted in Australia on health promotion objectives relevant to determine what sports clubs needed to develop healthy sporting environments for children (Kelly et al., 2014). The standards were related to seven health-promoting themes, such as healthy eating and alcohol management. These standards have not been directly used to evaluate the health promotion status of sport clubs. The evaluation tool developed is the Health Promotion in Sport Assessment Tool (HP-SAT), which aims to capture sport-related policies, practices and organizational capacity by directly questioning state sport organizations (Casey et al., 2011). It has been validated using a test–retest reliability method and included a general organizational capacity section and nine dimensions, such as smoke-free environment, responsible serving of alcohol, sun protection, welcoming and inclusive environment, and violence in sport (Casey et al., 2011).

In 2020, a new measurement tool has been developed with the perspective shifting from a national to international focus (Johnson et al., 2019). This novel evaluation tool—i.e. the e-PROSCeSS scale—combines the three levels of sports clubs (micro, meso and macro) and the four types of determinants for the health-promoting sports club. The scale is comprised of 23 macro-level items, 20 meso-level items and 19 micro-level items. Validation studies are currently underway in France (Johnson et al., 2022) and Sweden.

11.2.6   Future Direction

The research around health-promoting sports clubs is emerging. The application of the setting-based approach within sports clubs is taking its first steps and sports clubs are still at the stage of promoting health in clubs, rather than being health-promoting sports clubs (Geidne et al., 2019). The key challenge from a practical perspective is to identify and demonstrate why sports clubs should invest in health promotion. A simple answer is because it helps them achieve their core business! In other words, supporting sports clubs' members' healthy eating, positive climate, sleep and rest, respect and fair play, and community involvement will lead to decreased dropout of sport, as well as support individual sport performance. At the same time, it is important to acknowledge that health promotion is unlikely to become a priority for sports clubs—but doing something is better than doing nothing.

The approach needs to be spread internationally, especially in Asia, Africa and America, where only a few studies have been identified. Nevertheless, research is moving forward, with a grounded theoretical basis (Van Hoye et al., 2020a), cross-sectional studies across Europe and Australia (Kokko et al., 2016), development of controlled interventions (McFadyen et al., 2018) and identification of key leverage for health promotion (Geidne et al., 2019), as well as an intervention framework (Van Hoye et al., 2020a). Moreover, tools have been developed for sports clubs (Johnson et al., 2019) and state organizations (M. Casey et al., 2011) to measure health-promoting sports club activity. However, there are still many opportunities to develop setting-based health promotion in sports clubs. This can include steps to (1) develop a universal definition of a health-promoting sports club, (2) gather evidence on how sports clubs' benefit from investing in health promotion, (3) identify the specific outcomes from using the setting-based approach with sports clubs, (4) understand how the setting-based work can be appropriately evaluated and (5) identify how to create and implement feasible and effective interventions to support sports clubs to become health-promoting sports clubs.

References

Balish, S., Rainham, D., & Blanchard, C. (2015). Community size and sport participation across 22 countries. *Scandinavian Journal of Medicine & Science in Sports, 25*(6), e576–e581.

Breuer, C., Hoekman, R., Nagel, S., & van der Werff, H. (2015). *Sport clubs in Europe*. Springer.

Casey, M., Harvey, J., Eime, R., & Payne, W. (2011). The test-retest reliability of a health promotion assessment tool in sport. *Annals of Leisure Research, 14*(4), 304–324.

Casey, M., Harvey, J., Eime, R., & Payne, W. (2012a). Examining changes in the organisational capacity and sport-related health promotion policies and practices of State Sporting Organizations. *Annals of Leisure Research, 15*(3), 261–276.

Casey, M. M., Payne, W. R., & Eime, R. M. (2009). Building the health promotion capacity of sport and recreation organisations: A case study of Regional Sports Assemblies. *Managing Leisure, 14*(2), 112–124.

Casey, M. M., Payne, W. R., & Eime, R. M. (2012b). Organisational readiness and capacity building strategies of sporting organisations to promote health. *Sport Management Review, 15*(1), 109–124.

Corti, B., Holman, C. D. J., Donovan, R. J., Frizzell, S. K., & Carroll, A. M. (1995). Using sponsorship to create healthy environments for sport, racing and arts venues in Western Australia. *Health Promotion International, 10*(3), 185–197.

Donaldson, A., Borys, D., & Finch, C. F. (2013). Understanding safety management system applicability in community sport. *Safety Science, 60*, 95–104.

Donaldson, A., & Finch, C. F. (2012). Sport as a setting for promoting health. *British Journal of Sports Medicine, 46*(1), 4–5.

Donaldson, A., Forero, R., Finch, C. F., & Hill, T. (2004). A comparison of the sports safety policies and practices of community sports clubs during training and competition in northern Sydney, Australia. *British Journal of Sports Medicine, 38*(1), 60–63.

Dooris, M. (2004). Joining up settings for health: A valuable investment for strategic partnerships? *Critical Public Health, 14*(1), 49–61.

Dooris, M. (2006). Healthy settings: Challenges to generating evidence of effectiveness. *Health Promotion International, 21*(1), 55–65.

Eime, R. M., Payne, W. R., & Harvey, J. T. (2008). Making sporting clubs healthy and welcoming environments: A strategy to increase participation. *Journal of Science and Medicine in Sport, 11*(2), 146–154.

Eime, R. M., Young, J. A., Harvey, J. T., Charity, M. J., & Payne, W. R. (2013). A systematic review of the psychological and social benefits of participation in sport for children and adolescents: Informing development of a conceptual model of health through sport. *International Journal of Behavioral Nutrition and Physical Activity, 10*(98), 16.

Geidne, S., Kokko, S., Lane, A., Ooms, L., Vuillemin, A., Seghers, J., et al. (2019). *Health promotion interventions in sports clubs: Can we talk about a setting-based approach? A systematic mapping review* (p. 1090198119831749). Health Education & Behavior.

Geidne, S., Quennerstedt, M., & Eriksson, C. (2013a). The implementation process of alcohol policies in eight Swedish football clubs. *Health Education, 113*(3), 196–215.

Geidne, S., Quennerstedt, M., & Eriksson, C. (2013b). The youth sports club as a health-promoting setting: An integrative review of research. *Scandinavian Journal of Public Health, 41*(3), 269–283.

Giles-Corti, B., Clarkson, J. P., Donovan, R. J., Frizzell, S. K., Carroll, A. M., Pikora, T., & Jalleh, G. (2001). Creating smoke-free environments in recreational settings. *Health Education & Behavior, 28*(3), 341–351.

Ibsen, B., Nichols, G., Elmose-Østerlund, K., Breuer, C., Claes, E., Disch, J., et al. (2016). *Sports club policies in Europe: A comparison of the public policy context and historical origins of sports clubs across ten European countries.* University of Southern Denmark.

Johnson, S., Van Hoye, A., Donaldson, A., Lemonnier, F., Rostan, F., & Vuillemin, A. (2020). Building health-promoting sports clubs: A participative concept mapping approach. *Public Health, 188*, 8–17.

Johnson, S., Vuillemin, A., Geidne, S., Kokko, S., Epstein, J., & Van Hoye, A. (2019). Measuring health promotion in sports club settings: A modified delphi study. *Health Education & Behavior, 47*, 78–90. https://doi.org/10.1177/1090198119889098

Kelly, B., Baur, L. A., Bauman, A. E., King, L., Chapman, K., & Smith, B. J. (2011). Food and drink sponsorship of children's sport in Australia: Who pays? *Health Promotion International, 26*(2), 188–195.

Kelly, B., Chapman, K., King, L., Hardy, L., & Farrell, L. (2008). Double standards for community sports: Promoting active lifestyles but unhealthy diets. *Health Promotion Journal of Australia, 19*(3), 226–228.

Kelly, B., King, L., Bauman, A. E., Baur, L. A., Macniven, R., Chapman, K., & Smith, B. J. (2014). Identifying important and feasible policies and actions for health at community sports clubs: A consensus-generating approach. *Journal of Science and Medicine in Sport, 17*(1), 61–66. https://doi.org/10.1016/j.jsams.2013.02.011

Kokko, S. (2013). Guidelines for youth sports clubs to develop, implement, and assess health promotion within its activities. *Health Promotion Practice, 15*, 373–382.

Kokko, S. (2014). Sports clubs as settings for health promotion: Fundamentals and an overview to research. *Scandinavian Journal of Public Health, 42*(15 suppl), 60–65.

Kokko, S., Donaldson, A., Geidne, S., Seghers, J., Scheerder, J., Meganck, J., et al. (2016). Piecing the puzzle together: Case studies of international research in health-promoting sports clubs. *Global Health Promotion, 23*(1_suppl), 75–84.

Kokko, S., Green, L. W., & Kannas, L. (2013). A review of settings-based health promotion with applications to sports clubs. *Health Promotion International, dat046*.

Kokko, S., Kannas, L., & Villberg, J. (2006). The health promoting sports club in Finland—A challenge for the settings-based approach. *Health Promotion International, 21*(3), 219–229.

Kokko, S., Kannas, L., & Villberg, J. (2009). Health promotion profile of youth sports clubs in Finland: Club officials' and coaches' perceptions. *Health Promotion International, 24*(1), 26–35.

Kokko, S., Kannas, L., Villberg, J., & Ormshaw, M. (2011). Health promotion guidance activity of youth sports clubs. *Health Education, 111*(6), 452–463.

Kokko, S., Villberg, J., & Kannas, L. (2015). Health promotion in sport coaching: Coaches and young male athletes' evaluations on the health promotion activity of coaches. *International Journal of Sports Science & Coaching, 10*(2–3), 339–352.

Lane, A., Murphy, N., Donohoe, A., & Regan, C. (2017). Health promotion orientation of GAA sports clubs in Ireland. *Sport in Society, 20*(2), 235–243.

Lane, A., Murphy, N., Donohoe, A., & Regan, C. (2020). A healthy sports club initiative in action in Ireland. *Health Education Journal, 76*(6).

McCuaig, L., Carroll, T., Geidne, S., & Okade, Y. (2020). *The interdisciplinary challenge.* School Physical Education and Teacher Education: Collaborative Redesign for the 21st Century.

McFadyen, T., Chai, L. K., Wyse, R., Kingsland, M., Yoong, S. L., Clinton-McHarg, T., et al. (2018). Strategies to improve the implementation of policies, practices or programmes in sporting organisations targeting poor diet, physical inactivity, obesity, risky alcohol use or tobacco use: A systematic review. *BMJ Open, 8*(9), e019151. https://doi.org/10.1136/bmjopen-2017-019151

Meganck, J., Scheerder, J., Thibaut, E., & Seghers, J. (2014). Youth sports clubs' potential as health-promoting setting: Profiles, motives and barriers. *Health Education Journal, 74*, 531–543.

Meganck, J., Seghers, J., & Scheerder, J. (2016). Exploring strategies to improve the health promotion orientation of Flemish sports clubs. *Health Promotion International, 32*(4), 681–690.

Oja, P., Titze, S., Kokko, S., Kujala, U. M., Heinonen, A., Kelly, P., et al. (2015). Health benefits of different sport disciplines for adults: Systematic review of observational and intervention studies with meta-analysis. *British Journal of Sports Medicine, 49*(7), 434–440.

Poland, B., Krupa, G., & McCall, D. (2009). Settings for health promotion: An analytic framework to guide intervention design and implementation. *Health Promotion Practice, 10*(4), 505–516.

Rhodes, R. E., Janssen, I., Bredin, S. S., Warburton, D. E., & Bauman, A. (2017). Physical activity: Health impact, prevalence, correlates and interventions. *Psychology & Health*, 1–34.

Rowland, B., Allen, F., & Toumbourou, J. W. (2012a). Association of risky alcohol consumption and accreditation in the 'Good Sports' alcohol management programme. *Journal of Epidemiology and Community Health, 66*(8), 684–690.

Rowland, B., Allen, F., & Toumbourou, J. W. (2012b). Impact of alcohol harm reduction strategies in community sports clubs: Pilot evaluation of the Good Sports program. *Health Psychology, 31*(3), 323.

Skille, E. Å. (2010). Competitiveness and health: The work of sport clubs as seen by sport clubs representatives-a Norwegian case study. *International Review for the Sociology of Sport, 45*(1), 73–85.

Van Hoye, A., Heuzé, J.-P., Larsen, T., & Sarrazin, P. (2016b). Comparison of coaches' perceptions and officials guidance towards health promotion in French sport clubs: A mixed method study. *Health Education Research, 31*(3), 328–338.

Van Hoye, A., Heuzé, J.-P., Meganck, J., Seghers, J., & Sarrazin, P. (2018). Coaches' and players' perceptions of health promotion activities in sport clubs. *Health Education Journal, 77*(2), 169–178.

Van Hoye, A., Heuzé, J.-P., Van den Broucke, S., & Sarrazin, P. (2016a). Are coaches' health promotion activities beneficial for sport participants? A multilevel analysis. *Journal of Science and Medicine in Sport, 19*(12), 1028–1032.

Van Hoye, A., Johnson, S., Geidne, S., Donaldson, A., Rostan, F., Lemonnier, F., & Vuillemin, A. (2020a). The health promoting sports club model: An intervention planning framework. *Health Promotion International*. https://doi.org/10.1093/heapro/daaa093

Van Hoye, A., Johnson, S., Geidne, S., & Vuillemin, A. (2020b). Relationship between coaches' health promotion activities, sports experience and health among adults. *Health Education Journal, 79*(7).

Van Hoye, A., Sarrazin, P., Heuzé, J.-P., & Kokko, S. (2015). Coaches' perceptions of French sports clubs: Health-promotion activities, aims and coach motivation. *Health Education Journal, 74*(2), 231–243.

11.3   Healthy Stadia

Matthew Philpott

11.3.1   Introduction

Over the last 15 years, the potential for using sports venues—from small amateur clubs through to national stadia—as health-promoting settings has started to be realized. This not only benefits local communities, but also can contribute to achieving the corporate objectives of the clubs and stadia involved (Conrad & White, 2015).

Sports stadia play iconic roles amongst fans and in the communities they are located, capable of engaging large numbers of people both in the stadia and in the surrounding area. In addition, the demographic and age group of fans visiting stadia—largely middle-aged, working-class males—often exhibit higher levels of unhealthy behaviours and associated noncommunicable diseases such as obesity, cardiovascular disease, some types of cancer, type 2 diabetes and mental health issues. However, both professional and amateur sports clubs are in an almost unique position to harness the power and loyalty engendered by their badge/brand when engaging fans, with sports stadia and their teams able to positively influence the behaviour of fans, including health-related behaviours.

11.3.2   Healthy Stadia Definition and Background

During the early to mid-2000s, a number of pioneering sports stadia in the North West of England worked with the regional cardiovascular disease prevention charity Heart of Mersey, to trial several health promotion initiatives (Lloyd-Williams et al., 2008). This setting-based approach emphasized the potential for sports venues to develop policies and interventions promoting healthier lifestyles across three cross-cutting themes: healthier stadium environments for fans and non-matchday visitors (e.g. smoke-free environments); healthier club workforces (e.g. bike to work schemes); and healthier populations in local communities (e.g. child obesity interventions). During this trial, the following working definition of a 'healthy stadium' was established in 2005:

> 'Healthy Stadia are …..those which promote the health of visitors, fans, players, employees and the surrounding community… places where people can go to have a positive healthy experience playing or watching sport' (Crabb & Ratinckx, 2005).

11.3.3   A European Dimension

In 2006, a proposal for a 'Sports Stadia and Community Health' project by Heart of Mersey was supported by the European Commission. This project worked with a group of partners in Finland, Greece, Italy, Latvia, Ireland, Poland, Spain and the

UK. They were tasked with piloting the healthy stadia concept with sports venues in four European countries and developing guidelines to enhance the rollout of healthy stadia initiatives (Drygas et al., 2013). A primary outcome from this project was the founding of a 'European Healthy Stadia Network' to share good practice and emerging research amongst clubs, stadium operators, sport governing bodies, public health practitioners and academic institutions. The European Healthy Stadia Network (hereon Healthy Stadia) is now a successful social enterprise based in the UK with over 300 members, with long-term partnerships established with both public health and sports stakeholders such as the World Heart Federation and UEFA (UEFA, 2019).

11.3.4 Current Practices and Policy Change

Healthy Stadia may be considered a leader in advocating for sports stadia, clubs and sports governing bodies to develop health-promoting sports settings. There has been a groundswell in healthy stadia practices, policies and research over the last 10 years, something that applies to a wide number of sports and different European settings. There is now a genuine recognition amongst clubs, governing bodies of sport and— perhaps, most importantly—agencies commissioning health interventions, that sports settings offer a unique opportunity for both population-level approaches to improving public health (e.g. smoke-free sports environments) and interventions attempting to change the individual behaviours of target groups (e.g. addressing low levels of physical activity and sedentary behaviour in male football fans) (Wyke et al., 2019).

Part of Healthy Stadia's role is to capture current good practices and to disseminate these case studies across its network of members and to decision-makers with sports governing bodies. For certain themes, examples of good practice are expanded upon through practical guidelines intended to help sports organizations develop policies and practices as part of the healthy stadia agenda. This includes guidelines on active travel to sports stadia (2014), on developing smoke-free and tobacco-free sports venues (2016), and on healthier catering to be published in 2021 (see: https://healthystadia.eu/stadium-support/).

Healthy Stadia is UEFA's social responsibility partner for health within its 2017–2021 portfolio and works closely with Europe's football governing body and national associations across a range of health issues. Tobacco control and sports stadia are an area that has seen considerable success in terms of advocacy and policy change. Healthy Stadia has worked closely with UEFA since 2012 to ensure tobacco-free environments at club competition finals, and the European football championships (EURO) in 2012, 2016 and the delayed 2020 finals, which will now be held in the summer of 2021. Supported by tobacco-free guidance and training documents published in 2016 (Viggars et al., 2019), Healthy Stadia has launched a major programme of work advocating for all European sports venues to be smoke-free by 2025 through its Tobacco-Free Stadia Declaration.

11.3.5   Where Next? Developing the Evidence Base

For the healthy stadia agenda to be fully realized, particularly amongst commissioning agencies within local and national governments, it is vital that a rigorous evidence base is developed. This will demonstrate the impact that both population-level and individual behaviour change programmes developed through sports settings can have on public health outcomes. Although many 'community' or 'social' programmes attached to sports clubs have included process evaluation in their health projects, it is rare to find evaluation of a project's health outcomes and long-term impact (Parnell et al., 2017). Therefore, it is imperative that clubs, sports governing bodies and league administrators partner with academic partners to design and evaluate programmes and projects. This will address the lack of 'in-house' expertise and capacity within sports organizations to develop an evidence base to demonstrate the impact and cost-effectiveness of using sports settings to deliver public health programmes.

There is a growing number of pioneering clubs, sports governing bodies and tournament hosts developing research partnerships with universities, integrating insight, programme design and evaluation techniques into their work (Krustrup & Parnell, 2019). Hopefully, a robust evidence base will continue to emerge over the next 5 years. This will help both commissioning agencies and stadium/club management justify continued investment in health-promoting policies and practices through stadium settings.

References

Conrad, D., & White, A. (Eds.). (2015). *Sports-based health interventions: Case studies from around the world*. Springer.

Crabb, J., & Ratinckx, L. (2005). *The healthy stadia initiative*. North West Public Health Team, Department of Health (UK).

Donaldson, A., & Finch, C. F. (2012). Sport as a setting for promoting health. British journal of sports medicine, 46(1), 4–5.

Drygas, W., et al. (2013). Good practices and health policy analysis in European sports stadia: Results from the 'Healthy Stadia' project. *Health Promotion International, 28*(2), 157–165.

Johnson, S., Vuillemin, A., Epstein, J., Geidne, S., Donaldson, A., Tezier, B., ... & Van Hoye, A. (2022). French validation of the e-PROSCeSS questionnaire: stakeholder perceptions of the health promoting sports club. Health Promotion International. https://academic.oup.com/heapro/advance-article-abstract/doi/10.1093/heapro/daab213/6513385

Krustrup, P., & Parnell, D. (Eds.). (2019). *Football as medicine: Prescribing football for global health promotion*. Routledge.

Lloyd-Williams, F., et al. (2008). Delivering a cardiovascular disease prevention programme in the United Kingdom: Translating theory into practice. *European Journal of Public Health, 18*(4), 357–359.

Parnell, D., Curran, K., & Philpott, M. (2017). *Healthy stadia: An insight from policy to practice* (pp. 181–186). Routledge.

UEFA. (2019). Football and Social Responsibility report 2018/19. Retrieved from https://www.uefa. com/MultimediaFiles/Download/uefaorg/General/02/64/11/33/2641133_DOWNLOAD.pdf.

Viggars, M., Curran, K. M., & Philpott, M. (2019). *Tobacco-free stadia: A case study at the 2016 UEFA European Championships in France*.

Wyke, S., et al. (2019). The effect of a programme to improve men's sedentary time and physical activity: The European Fans in Training (EuroFIT) randomised controlled trial. *PLoS Medicine, 16*(2), e1002736.

Chapter 12
Digital Environment and Social Media as Settings for Health Promotion

Diane Levin-Zamir, Isabella C. Bertschi, Evelyn McElhinney, and Gill Rowlands

12.1 Background

The settings approach to health promotion reminds us that a setting is where people live, love, work, learn, and play. Throughout the world, the digital development has transformed the way in which people are creating and utilizing the digital world for the same purposes as they do other settings. Thus, increasingly digital opportunities are involving people globally in their health. Beginning with the rise of the Internet decades ago, and continuing through the development of social media and even virtual settings, the digital world has reshaped the traditional definition of health-promoting settings and thus should be considered, explored, and analyzed for its contribution to health promotion (Levin-Zamir & Bertschi, 2018).

The challenges for making optimal use of the digital environment for health gave rise to the need for acknowledging the skills needed for optimizing the use of digital resources for health. Thus, the definition of eHealth literacy, now often called digital

D. Levin-Zamir (✉)
School of Public Health, University of Haifa, Haifa, Israel

Department of Health Education and Promotion, Clalit Health Services, Tel Aviv, Israel
e-mail: diamos@zahav.net.il

I. C. Bertschi
Department of Psychology, Clinical Psychology for Children/Adolescents & Couples/Families, University of Zurich, Zurich, Switzerland
e-mail: isabella.bertschi@uzh.ch

E. McElhinney
Department of Nursing and Community Health, School of Health and Life Sciences, Glasgow Caledonian University, Glasgow, Scotland
e-mail: evelyn.mcelhinney@gcu.ac.uk

G. Rowlands
Population Health Sciences Institute, Newcastle University, Newcastle upon Tyne, UK
e-mail: gill.rowlands@newcastle.ac.uk

© Springer Nature Switzerland AG 2022
S. Kokko, M. Baybutt (eds.), *Handbook of Settings-Based Health Promotion*,
https://doi.org/10.1007/978-3-030-95856-5_12

health literacy, was initially defined as "the ability to seek, find, understand and appraise health information from electronic sources, and apply the knowledge gained to addressing or solving a health problem" (Norman & Skinner, 2006). Yet, as in any other setting, the risk for health-compromising influences exists in the digital environment as well. Thus, the digital environment as a health-promoting setting requires a more updated definition of digital health literacy that also entails critical and interactive skills. People who are digitally health literate are more empowered to have a more active role in promoting their health throughout the life course.

While eHealth digital ecosystem includes an abundance of digital opportunities and resources for health (information, apps, devices, digital health records, and more), this chapter will highlight three specific areas of interest regarding digital settings and health—the Internet, social media, and Health-Promoting 3D Social Virtual Worlds and Social Virtual Reality.

12.2 Health Promotion, Health Literacy, and Internet

This section explores health promotion, health literacy, and the Internet. It starts with relevant definitions, explores inequalities in digital access and skills, and explores the benefits and potential harms of Internet-based health information. Finally, it describes how the development of digital health literacy could improve equity of access and widen the health promotion benefits of the Internet, while also promoting people skills to protect themselves from harmful health information.

12.2.1 Definitions

Acknowledging that health promotion is the process of enabling people to take control over, and to improve their health (World Health Organization, 1986) and that health is a resource for everyday life, and is a positive concept emphasizing social and personal resources as well as physical capacities, health literacy can be defined as being "linked to literacy and entailing people's knowledge, motivation and competences to access, understand, appraise and apply health information in order to make judgements and take decisions in everyday life concerning healthcare, disease prevention and health promotion to maintain or improve quality of life during the life course" (Sorensen et al., 2012). Health literacy is one of the three key elements for health promotion; the others being good governance for health and healthy cities (World Health Organization, 2016).

Increasingly, the Internet and other IT-based sources of information, such as mobile phone applications, are being used as sources of health information. "Accessing, understanding, appraising and applying" information from the Internet requires additional capacities to those required for health literacy in other spheres of life, leading to the emergence of the term "digital health literacy." Digital health literacy has been defined as "the ability to seek, find, understand, and appraise health information from electronic sources and apply the knowledge gained to assessing and solving a health problem" (Norman & Skinner, 2006), although the concept is now being to include skills to "promote health to maintain or improve quality of life during the life course" and to evaluate aspects such as reliability and relevance (van der Vaart & Drossaert, 2017). Most recently, the MPOHL HLS19 survey has defined Digital health literacy as "the ability to search for, access, understand, appraise, validate and apply online health information, the ability to formulate and express questions, opinions, thoughts, or feelings when using digital devices" (The HLS19 Consortium of the WHO Action Network on Health Literacy MPOHL 2021)

12.2.2   The Digital Divide

There are marked geographical and sociodemographic variations in access to the Internet and in digital skills. The proportion of the population using the Internet to search for health information in the European Union ranges from 74% in the Netherlands to 49% in Romania (2014). Across all 28 EU countries, 32% of people use the Internet to search for health information once a month or more, while 41% of people state they have never used the Internet for this purpose (2014). Within countries, there are both age-related and socioeconomic gradients. In 2015, the percentage of the population who had never used the Internet (for any purpose) was 32% in people aged 65 years and older compared with 1% of people aged 16–24 years, and 55% of people with no formal qualifications had never used the Internet compared with just 2% of those with degree-level qualifications (Hirst, 2015). Poor health is more prevalent in those who are socioeconomically disadvantaged and in older people (CSDH, 2008), the digital divide thus risks exacerbating these sociodemographic inequalities in health.

12.2.3   Promoting Health Through the Internet

The increasing availability of health information on increasingly sophisticated digital platforms is, generally, seen as a positive development, supporting individual choice, empowerment, and knowledge; "'Digital health' (is)…empowering us to better track, manage and improve healthcare…reduce inefficiencies in healthcare delivery, improve access, reduce costs, increase quality, and make medicine more personalized" (Eurobarometer, 2014). Over half of health-related Internet searches are made to gather information to promote health or to prevent illness (2014). Studies have shown health promotion benefits of digital health information across a range of areas such as increasing levels of physical activity (Peymann et al., 2018), reducing harmful alcohol consumption (Linke et al., 2007), and sexual health (Bailey et al., 2015). The contribution of digital health resources when used appropriately and in conjunction with the healthcare system has been shown to be associated with improved health outcomes (Levin-Zamir & Bertschi, 2019).

An interesting development in digital health promotion is "digital storytelling," where disadvantaged or vulnerable communities such as rural and indigenous peoples (Cueva et al., 2015; Fletcher & Mullett, 2016), vulnerable youth, (DiFulvio et al., 2016; Fletcher & Mullett, 2016), and minority ethnic groups (DiFulvio et al., 2016; Briant et al., 2016) engage in a group-based process to create and share narrative accounts of life events.

Participants described a range of benefits including increased health knowledge, empowerment and self-esteem, social support, and sense of community. It is possible, therefore, that digital storytelling can help to bridge the "digital divide" for currently digitally disenfranchised groups.

12.2.4 Drawbacks to Health Promotion Information on the Internet

While increasing availability of health and health promotion information on the Internet is generally seen as positive, some drawbacks have been identified. The term "healthism" was coined by Crawford (Crawford, 1980) and has come to be seen as a "socio-cultural phenomenon … characterized by high health awareness and expectations, information-seeking, self-reflection, high expectations, distrust of doctors and scientists, healthy and often 'alternative' lifestyle choices, and a tendency to explain illness in terms of folk models of invisible germ-like agents and malevolent science" (Greenhalgh & Wessely, 2004). The ease with which opinions and evidence can be spread via the Internet can lead to the dissemination of inaccurate and, sometimes, dangerous information. An example is the anti-vaccination movement, which has led to a reduction in vaccination rates for infectious diseases such as measles, with the resultant risk of higher infection rates and epidemics (Bosely, 2019).

12.2.5 The Importance of Digital Health Literacy

Digital health literacy has much to offer in maximizing the health promotion opportunities brought through the Internet and in reducing the risks of inaccurate and misleading information. While digital access and digital skills are lower in socio-economically deprived, marginalized, and older age groups (Hirst, 2015), programs to build digital skills in such groups have had success. The "Widening Digital Participation Programme," led by the Tinder Foundation (now the Good Things

Foundation) (Tinder Foundation, 2016), and funded by NHS England, engaged with older people, socioeconomically deprived and excluded groups to run locally embedded projects to promote digital engagement for health. The program aimed to be self-sustaining through training local "champions" who would then go on to train others. Over the 3 years of the program, over 200,000 people were trained and an additional 380,000 people reached. Over half of learners went on to find information on the Internet about health conditions, symptoms, or tips for staying healthy (2016a). Widening digital participation not only means that those at higher risk of lower levels of health and higher levels of illness have access to information for health, but also that techniques such as "digital storytelling" can be promoted to build not only health knowledge but also community engagement, empowerment and esteem.

A key aspect of digital health literacy is the capacity to critically appraise information to determine not only its relevance and importance to an individual or community, but also its provenance, and hence its likely accuracy and reliability. Little research has been undertaken in this area so far, but useful pointers can be gleaned from the work of Wharf Higgins and Begoray, who developed an intervention for adolescents that developed skills to critically evaluate advertising messages. (Begoray et al., 2013). Developing ways to build similar skills in individuals and communities in relation to critically appraising information on the Internet has potential to counteract false information that can damage health and reduce the effectiveness of health promotion. This has come to the forefront in particular, during the COVID-19 pandemic where infodemics have been of particular concern (Okan et al., 2020).

12.2.6 Section Summary

The Internet provides great opportunities for health promotion, with availability of information tailored to peoples' needs, available at times most convenient for them. The development of digital health literacy, in parallel with increasing access to those most at need, has the potential to increase health and health knowledge and empower individuals and communities. A crucial aspect of digital health literacy is the capacity to identify and evaluate potentially incorrect or harmful information; more resources and focus should be applied to address the current gap in knowledge and practice, and the definition of digital health literacy expanded to reflect the full range of capacities required for health in a digital world.

12.3 Social Media as a Setting for Health Promotion

Since the rise of Web 2.0 in the early years of the twenty-first century, scholars and professionals have discussed the utility of adopting social media technology for health promotion. A prominent quote underlined the importance for health promoters to become involved with this novel technology: "Imagine there is a centre that the vast majority of (…) people go to most days of the week for several hours a day. (…) [P]eople at this centre are seeking health related and wellbeing information, but there are no health promotion workers" (Centre for Health Promotion, Women's and Children's Health Network, 2012, S. 8). Since the quote was published, health promotion workers have started to work at those centers, and more and more scientific evidence about their experience becomes available.

The purpose of this section is to introduce readers to the definition and characteristics of social media, to theoretically explore their potential for settings-based health promotion and to present an overview of research findings of health promotion initiatives that implemented social media features. Some critical issues to be considered in research and practice will accompany the outlook.

12.3.1 Definition and Characteristics of Social Media

Various attempts at defining and/or categorizing social media have been undertaken, for example by Kaplan and Haenlein (2010), Ellison and Boyd (2013), and Nesi et al. (2018). The difficulties in agreeing on one definition are rooted in two main factors: Both existing and new formats commonly referred to as "social media" are rapidly developing, and the forms of communication facilitated by social media services are similar to those enabled by other technologies (Obar et al., 2012; Obar & Wildman, 2015). Commonalities identified in definitions of social media can be summarized as follows: Social media are Web 2.0 Internet-based applications, they feed primarily on user-generated content, the use of social media requires a user profile, and the connection of user profiles leads to creation of social networks (Obar & Wildman, 2015). Popular social media with high numbers of active users are Facebook, YouTube, WhatsApp, Facebook Messenger, WeChat, or Instagram, but also Wikipedia or Skype, for instance, can be considered social media.

12.3.2 Theoretical Considerations Regarding Social Media as Settings for Health Promotion

As is the case with media in general, the principal motive for considering social media for health promotion purposes is their ubiquity in people's daily lives (e.g., Gold et al., 2012; Johns et al., 2017). Social media have the potential to establish a route of access to a vast number of citizens. Some authors argue that additionally, social media offer the opportunity to engage traditionally hard to reach populations in health promotion efforts (e.g., Norman, 2012). In addition to their wide reach, social media are an attractive arena for health promotion due to their capacity to mobilize and pool social resources for health (Jane et al., 2018; McElhinney et al.,

2018). Social media enable interpersonal communications that can be considered mediators of behavior adoption and change. Perceived and actual social support can be fostered by social media, e.g., through provision of informational resources, access to emotional support in the form of positive feedback, and a sense of belonging, or by providing positive role models. Social media thus represent "a hybrid channel for intervention delivery with the benefit of both mass media (e.g., wide reach) and interpersonal communication (e.g., personalized messages ...)" (Chou et al., 2012, S. e12).

From a practical perspective, these two points make it seem worthwhile to conceptualize social media as a setting for health promotion. The question remains whether theoretically, social media should be considered a setting for health promotion. By analyzing key features of definitions of a setting and a settings approach to health promotion, medical sociologists identified several arguments in favor of conceptualizing social media as a setting for health promotion, e.g., the possibility to reach target audiences directly in their everyday digital environment, the presence of a clear structure of the setting, or the high frequency of social interactions in social media. However, several factors warrant caution on the matter. For instance, it remains unclear whether structural elements of social media actually influence health and well-being, or whether users can influence some of those structural elements (Loss et al., 2014). Although theoretically it remains unclear whether social media are settings for health promotion, the authors concluded that they are "too important a communicative social venue to be completely neglected by health promoters" (p. 169).

12.3.3   Overview of Studies Reporting the Use of Social Media for Health Promotion Purposes

The aforementioned potentials of social media for health promotion have been taken up in practice, and some preliminary evidence on the effectiveness of social media for health promotion has been published. An earlier systematic review on the use of Web 2.0 technology for health promotion (Chou et al., 2012) reported that several feasibility and intervention studies on the topic had been published. The most investigated platforms were social networking sites, both in their Web and in mobile versions. The addressed health topics ranged from broad mental health promotion to interventions for maintaining sexual health or the promotion of physical activity and healthy eating. A review of 42 studies on the use of social networking sites (SNS) in health promotion (Balatsoukas et al., 2015) reported on the effectiveness of social media for health promotion purposes. Although the randomized controlled trials (RCTs) that were reviewed did not show a clear effect of social media use on objectively measured behavior change, evidence from pilot studies suggested that interventions including SNS could affect self-reported and measured behavior. Similarly, a review on social media in pediatric health (Hamm et al., 2014) stated that most conclusions regarding the utility of social media drawn in studies were positive, although statistical significance was hardly ever reached for outcome measures in trials. One meta-analysis reported a slight positive effect of the influence of SNS on individual health behavior change (Laranjo et al., 2015), solidifying the review findings summarized here.

A review by Condran et al. (2017) suggested that health promotion using social media could also target outcomes at levels of analysis other than the intrapersonal: Initiatives showed a potential to establish health-promoting social norms and, at a community level, to promote behaviors that are related to these established social norms, e.g., HIV testing. Generally, the most important mediator for effectiveness as measured by behavior change was social support. The possibility for information sharing or peer pressure as other key features of SNS does not seem to have an equal impact on outcomes (Balatsoukas et al., 2015). The development of a social support network was also identified as the key feature of social media in pediatric health promotion. User experience and thus acceptance rates were particularly good when the intervention facilitated the development of such a support network (Hamm et al., 2014). There is some evidence that suggests the effectiveness of social media for health promotion, but conclusions are only tentative to date.

The limited conclusiveness of existing evidence is mostly attributed to two factors. Social media was most often described as one component of a complex intervention, making it difficult to isolate the effects of the social media component (Hamm et al., 2014; Jane et al., 2018; Laranjo et al., 2015). Besides the difficulties to isolate social media-specific effects of health promotion programs, several studies have criticized that only about half of the studies reported on their use of theory when developing health-promoting social media interventions (Hamm et al., 2014; Korda & Itani, 2013; Laranjo et al., 2015). This is critical as review evidence clearly suggests that extensive use of theory is associated with an increase in effect sizes of Internet-based health interventions (Webb et al., 2010).

Overall, evidence on the effectiveness of social media as a setting for health promotion cannot be considered conclusive (yet). Several factors support the positive outlook that predominated the discourse when social media were first taken up in health promotion, but more research is needed.

12.3.4   Social Media and the COVID-19 Pandemic

As the world faces a pandemic that challenges the public and health experts alike, health care and disease prevention are the focal points. As such, health promotion efforts are critically important to control a global pandemic as they enable people to increase control over their health and its determinants (Van den Broucke, 2020). The pandemic has caused public health experts to (re)consider the role social media are playing in promoting health, including preventing disease. As is supported by theoretical work on the role of social media in epidemic response, social media have potentially conflicting functions that can either enhance or undermine public health efforts during health crises (Schillinger et al., 2020). On the one hand, the large-scale spread of information and particularly misinformation around COVID-19, strongly enabled by social media, has caused some to call out an "infodemic" (World Health Organization, 2020). Misinformation about COVID-19 has confused the general public and healthcare providers, as is evidenced in collections of individual cases from around the world (see, e.g., Tasnim et al., 2020). Consequently, it is key to develop health communication strategies that take into account the particularities of social media as a setting for health promotion and disease prevention (e.g., Mhei Mheidly and Fares 2020). On the other hand, preliminary evidence also points to the beneficial contributions of social media for public health during the COVID-19 pandemic. For instance, higher social media exposure was associated with higher perception of severity of COVID-19 and with higher perceived control or intention to carry out preventive measures in medical students (Lin et al., 2020). Furthermore, social media use frequency (but not use time) significantly predicted preventive behaviors around COVID-19 in young Chinese (Li & Liu, 2020). Further research is needed to thoroughly evaluate the influence of social media on the COVID-19 pandemic and to derive lessons learned for future uptake of social media as a setting for health promotion.

12.3.5   Conclusions and Outlook

Settings-based health promotion addresses the "setting" in two ways: The setting is used as a "place" where a health promotion initiative can be implemented, and the structure of the setting itself is targeted to make it more conducive to health (Dooris et al., 1998; Poland et al., 2009; Whitelaw et al., 2001). Looking at social media in health promotion, mainly the former aspect has been taken up. Programs to promote physical activity or sexual health, for instance, have implemented characteristic features of social media such as discussion forums or video and audio uploads. Evidence on the effectiveness is still inconclusive, but promising. We will close this section of the chapter by summarizing some of the key factors to consider in research and practice in order for social media to fulfill their potential as settings for health promotion.

Using a settings-based approach to health promotion requires sound knowledge of the setting to be addressed. Regarding social media, the danger is for health promoters to implement programs where they consider it useful without careful analysis of patterns of use. For example, Hamm et al. (2014) state: "[O]utreach strategies may be more effective if efforts are made up-front to identify the tools that the target audience is already using and tailor the intervention accordingly, rather than expect the group to find and adopt new technologies that have been developed" (p. 13). If health promotion agents fail to identify the setting, the setting will not support their efforts to promote health.

Furthermore, researchers are challenged to propose novel evaluation designs that take into account the rapid development of technology (Norman, 2012). Health promotion experts should partner with ICT specialists to implement evaluation strategies that continuously inform software development (Chou et al., 2012). Novel metrics measuring user engagement and usability should be registered alongside more traditional outcomes that measure program effectiveness (Neiger et al., 2012, 2013). In conclusion, considering social media as settings for health promotion goes way beyond sharing the number of steps one has walked during the day or creating a profile page for a health center. It should rather be considered as one more step toward a democratization of health and citizen empowerment to actively engage in their health. As Norman (2012) states: "[W]hether social media "works" in producing positive health outcomes will constantly be a negotiated idea as the media changes along with the messages and audiences, requiring equally large changes in the mindsets of health promoters, funders and policy makers to adapt to this new reality" (p. 5).

12.4 Health-Promoting 3D Social Virtual Worlds and Social Virtual Reality

Social Virtual Worlds (VWs), for example, Second Life, are online 3D multiuser virtual environments (MUVE). People access these worlds by downloading a viewer and creating an avatar, the virtual self. Avatars can be humanoid, animal, or a fantasy creature. See Fig. 12.1—Avatars.

For the purpose of this section of the chapter, the term physical world (PW) will be used to represent the world people are situated in. The virtual world (VW) will

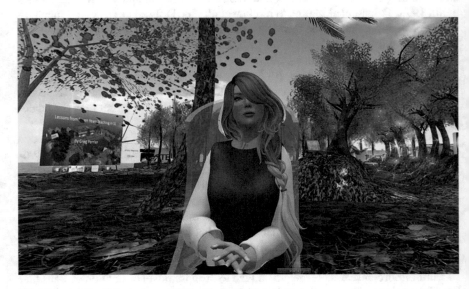

Fig. 12.1 Avatar. (Source: Second Life, Linden Lab)

represent where the person's avatar is situated. The use of the term "real world" will not be used as this may contribute to the impression that the meaning of interactions or attitudes and behavior enacted in the VW has no real meaning, value, or influence in the PW.

Just as in the PW, activities, such as socializing, shopping, role play, dancing, attending group meetings, conferences, and accessing health information, can all be undertaken in VWs. Avatars can "chat" to, and interact with, other avatars in the VW either privately via instant messaging (IM) or with other avatars in close proximity through local text chat or voice (not private, but can only be seen or heard by avatars in close proximity), or collectively across a group of users of the VW (not private, seen/accessed by all avatars in the group) (Blascovich & Bailenson, 2011). Similar to the PW, as people move through the VW via their avatar, the environment reacts to the proximity of objects to the avatar position, changing the view of the VW (for example, objects and people, appear closer or more distant, and the view and movement of the avatar are blocked by people and buildings). This spatial cognition, realism of the environment, continuous sensory stimuli, and reaction of the environment to interactions by the user can influence and increase people's feelings of immersion and presence in the VW setting (Lombard & Ditton, 1997; Witmer & Singer, 1998; McLeod et al., 2014). This immersion and social presence contribute to positive health assets such as feelings of belonging, social connection, community (McElhinney, 2015), and sense of place identity (Relph, 2007; Twigger-Ross, 2013), which are important to well-being. During the COVID-19 pandemic, the use of VWs and in particular Second Life has increased, as reported by the CEO of Linden Labs. This was noted, in particular, in countries and states where lockdown or stay-at-home policies were in place (Kariuki, 2020), further highlighting the value of these "places" for maintaining health and well-being, and reducing social isolation.

Additionally, the recent development of more affordable immersive social virtual reality (VR) headsets and social platforms, for example, AltspaceVR (https://altvr. com/), VR chat (https://www.vrchat.net/), and Virbela (https://www.virbela.com/), has increased the use for health promotion and behavior change beyond laboratory settings, where VR research had traditionally been undertaken (Rothbaum et al., 2010; Blascovich & Bailenson, 2011). In VR, the user views the world through a headset and the environment is viewed using a first-person view, where the person sees the world as if viewing it through their eyes. The user may see partial body parts such as animated hands; however, normally, there is no virtual self-visible. However, in new social multiuser VR, other people in the VR environment see each person as an avatar and the user can present themselves as an avatar meaning they now see their virtual self in the environment, similarly to VWs. Interestingly, many people access these areas without a headset, essentially turning the setting into a 3D social VW. Therefore, whether viewing with a headset or via the computer screen, similar psychological processes as discussed earlier in the context of VWs are experienced by the user of social VR. Despite this, there are still issues with cost of computers which are powerful enough to run the software required for mainstream use, or use by people when and if they require access at home. This may be negated by recent developments in standalone/untethered VR which has meant studies with members of the public outside the laboratory setting are increasing. Recent studies have shown benefits for improving health literacy (Saab et al., 2019) and reducing pain (Mallari et al., 2019), and a recent systematic review of 82 studies (Jerdan et al., 2018) found positive health benefits to subjective well-being and mental health outcomes.

12.4.1   Health Promotion and Behavior via VWs and VR

Several VW health studies undertaken using multiple methodology and methods have reported positive health benefits. Kamel Boulos and Toth-Cohen (2009) surveyed 135 avatars who had accessed VW sexual health games, healthcare talks, weblinks, and health information videos embedded in VW interactive objects. They found over 80% of participants reported information as useful or very useful, 39% reported learning something new and, most importantly, 16% said the information would change their behavior in the PW, with 36% reporting possible change in behavior.

Subsequent studies have compared face-to-face (f2f) health interventions with VW interventions. Johnston et al. (2012) compared the use of a VW and a previously validated face-to-face (f2f) 12-week weight loss program focusing on classes on nutrition, movement, healthy habits, and a support group. Fifty-two participants, from the USA, completed the study, with 38 in the VW group and 24 in the f2f group. The participants in the VW were able to choose and manipulate their avatar throughout the study and most mimicked their PW appearance making changes to their shape as they lost weight in the PW. Health information in the VW was available via games (see Fig. 12.2, which shows a similar nutrition game developed by The VITAL Lab, Ohio University), interactive objects, and the avatar was able to participate in group physical activity (seeing their avatar on a treadmill, exercise bike, roller skating), enabling tracking of their health changes. VW peer support was also available via support groups based in VW social environments (beach, swimming pool). Findings indicated that the VW was as effective for weight loss as the f2f group. Additionally, the VW group made improvements on all measures of behavioral change, 70% of the VW group reported better results than previous f2f interventions. A subsequent longitudinal study by Sullivan et al. (2013) compared f2f versus a VW weight loss and maintenance program in the USA. Twenty overweight females were randomized to either 3 months in the VW (weight loss) with 6 months f2f (weight maintenance) or a 9-month VW program (weight loss and maintenance). Findings showed a higher weight loss in the f2f group. However, the VW group had greater weight maintenance and consumed more fruit and vegetables and, interestingly, recorded more steps on a pedometer than the f2f group. Similar to Johnston et al.'s study, the VW-only group had the advantage of instantly interacting with the program tools, allowing repeated practice of skills, receiving instant automated feedback, and access to social support, all important features of

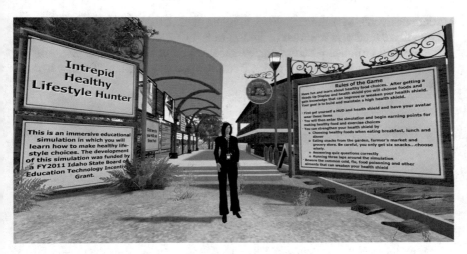

Fig. 12.2 Nutrition game. (Source: Second Life, Linden Lab)

encouraging learning and maintaining behavior (Dewey, 1910/1997, Bandura, 1998). Similar findings have been reported in several other studies investigating weight loss programs via a VW (Siddiqi et al., 2011; Ruiz et al., 2012; Morie & Chance, 2011; Mitchell et al., 2014; Behm-Morawitz et al., 2013; Nosek 2011).

Across these studies, explanations of findings were deemed to be due to the immersive environment, embodiment of the avatar, and the ability to model behavior and see changes to avatar weight in relation to weight loss in the PW, suggesting support for the Proteus Effect discussed by Yee et al. (2007) and Yee et al. (2009) where it was found that viewing an avatar as the virtual self, promoted embodiment and led to positive PW behavior change. Several authors have also supported this in previous and subsequent VW health studies (Fox & Bailenson, 2009; Behm-Morawitz, 2013, McLeod et al. 2014, Ahn and Fox 2017, McElhinney, 2015, McElhinney et al., 2018). Paul et al. (2022) study during the first year of the COVID-19 pandemic also found increased psychological resilience to COVID-19 due to the Proteus Effect in users of SVWs.

Other areas where better or equivalent health outcomes have been achieved using validated offline interventions delivered in VWs are addiction treatment (Gorini et al., 2008), self-esteem enhancement for women with disabilities (Nosek et al., 2011), mind-body relaxation (Hoch et al., 2012), social anxiety (Yuen et al., 2013), and virtual therapy. Similar findings are being reported through out of laboratory VR particularly in areas of mental health and well-being and exercise (Hsieh et al., 2018).

Several studies have also found VWs can offer people with long-term health conditions or disabilities a "place" to take part in social activities that interest them, or which they cannot do in the PW as well as a place to practice social skills, life skills, build friendships, seek peer support, have fun, or take part in work, education, and volunteering (Boellstorff & Davis, 2018 (movie by http://www.draxtor.com/

ourdigitalselves/), McElhinney, 2015, Galliers et al., 2017). Additionally, using an able-bodied avatar was reported in studies to be exciting and fun, protected people from negative attitudes based on appearance, which was often experienced in the PW (Davis, 2013; McElhinney, 2015; Boellstorff & Davis, 2018). Similar benefits are emerging from social VR.

12.4.2   Virtual Nature

Another interesting area being explored in VWs and VR is the restorative health benefits of virtual nature. Edward Wilson defines biophilia as "the innate tendency to focus on life and lifelike processes" (Wilson, 1984 p. 1). He particularly focused on human interaction with nature and argues that humans are genetically biased to experience positive mental well-being after interacting with nature. He terms this the biophilia hypothesis (Wilson, 1984; Kellert & Wilson, 1995). Thomas (2013, p. 12) argued that when we use metaphors of nature and scenes of virtual nature within technology, we create "the innate attraction to life and lifelike processes as they appear in technology" and terms this Technobiophilia. Interestingly, several VW studies (McElhinney, 2015; Jones et al., 2018) and VR studies (Valtchanov et al., 2010) have reported restorative health benefits from virtual nature similar to health benefits reported in PW nature such as reduced anxiety and stress, feeling relaxed, improved subjective well-being, and distraction from pain (Ulrich et al., 1991; Ulrich, 1999; Rampton, 2013; Guisset-Martinez et al., 2013). This is an interesting area for future public health settings research especially for use with people who cannot access or are restricted to access in the PW. This is particularly pertinent in times of "lockdown" during the COVID-19 pandemic, where people may be restricted in access (time or travel) to areas of nature, leading to a detrimental effect on mental health and well-being.

12.4.3   Conclusion

Arguably, it has been shown through multiple studies that immersive VWs and VR particularly in a social context can positively influence health and well-being and are important settings for health promotion (Davis, 2013, Gilbert et al., 2013, Delemere 2014, Stendal & Balandin, 2015, Kleban & Kaye, 2015, McElhinney, 2015, Boellstorff & Davis, 2018, McElhinney et al., 2018). In the majority of these studies, there were very few negative health outcomes reported. Where people did have a negative experience, they often blocked, reported, or changed their avatar. This is not to say that these "places" are utopia; however, they do provide an engaging immersive avatar-based health promotion settings where health interventions can be implemented, as well as giving access to peer-led social support and education using a participatory asset-based network approach.

12.5   Summary and Implications for Future Action

As described in this chapter, the digital world has emerged as a setting that provides enormous opportunity for health promotion, applying a systems approach. As seen in the examples presented, it is relevant for the individual, the family, organizations, and societies globally. Future action needs to focus on research in a variety of areas including, for example, the role of the digital environment in empowerment for health at all levels. In addition, the role of policy and regulation must be considered in an arena where the lack of policy and regulation was the conceptual basis for its development. Finally, the role of digital settings joined up with other health-promoting settings should be explored more specifically, including an understanding of the potential symbiosis for promoting health.

References

Ahn, S. J., & Fox, J. (2017). Immersive virtual environments, avatars, and agents for health. In *Encyclopedia of health and risk message design and processing*. Oxford University Press.

Bailey, J., Mann, S., Wayal, S., Hunter, R., Free, C., Abraham, C., & Murray, E. (2015). *Sexual health promotion for young people delivered via digital media: A scoping review. Sexual health promotion for young people delivered via digital media: A scoping review*. NIHR Journals Library.

Balatsoukas, P., Kennedy, C. M., Buchan, I., Powell, J., & Ainsworth, J. (2015). The role of social network technologies in online health promotion: A narrative review of theoretical and empirical factors influencing intervention effectiveness. *Journal of Medical Internet Research, 17*(6), e141.

Bandura, A. (1998). Health promotion from the perspective of social cognitive theory. *Psychology and Health, 13*(4), 623–649.

Begoray, D., Wharf Higgins, J., Harrison, J., & Collins-Emery, A. (2013). Adolescent reading/viewing of advertisements. Understandings from transactional and positioning theory. *Journal of Adolescent & Adult Literacy, 57*, 121–130.

Behm-Morawitz, E. (2013). Mirrored selves: The influence of self-presence in a virtual world on health, appearance, and well-being. *Computers in Human Behavior, 29*(1), 119–128.

Blascovich, J., & Bailenson, J. (2011). *Infinite reality: Avatars, eternal life, new worlds, and the dawn of the virtual revolution*. William Morrow.

Boellstorff, T., & Davis, D. (2018). Our Digital Selves: My Avatar is me Documentary Draxtor Despres https://www.youtube.com/watch?time_continue=2&v=GQw02-me0W4

Bosely, S. (2019, December). Measles cases at highest for 20 years in Europe, as anti-vaccine movement grows. *Guardian*.

Briant, K. J., Halter, A., Marchello, N., Escareno, M., & Thompson, B. (2016). The power of digital storytelling as a culturally relevant health promotion tool. *Health Promotion Practice, 17*, 793–801.

Centre for Health Promotion, Women's and Children's Health Network. (2012). *"Where they hang out": Social media use in youth health promotion. An analysis on a literature review and survey of the youth sector in South Australia*. Department of Health, Government of South Australia, Adelaide.

Chou, W. S., Prestin, A., Lyons, C., & Wen, K. (2012). Web 2.0 for health promotion: Reviewing the current evidence. *American Journal of Public Health, 103*, e9–e18. https://doi.org/10.2105/AJPH.2012.301071

Condran, B., Gahagan, J., & Isfeld-Kiely, H. (2017). A scoping review of social media as a platform for multi-level sexual health promotion interventions. *Canadian Journal Human Sexuality.* https://doi.org/10.3138/cjhs.261-A1

Crawford, R. (1980). Healthism and the medicalization of everyday life. *International Journal of Health Services, 10,* 365–388.

CSDH. (2008). Closing the gap in a generation: Health equity through action on the social determinants of health. *Final Report of the Commission on Social Determinants of Health.* Geneva: World Health Organization.

Cueva, M., Kuhnley, R., Revels, L., Schoenberg, N. E., & Dignan, M. (2015). Digital storytelling: A tool for health promotion and cancer awareness in rural Alaskan communities. *International Journal Circumpolar Health, 74,* 28781.

Davis, Z. D. (2013). Exploring the influence of avatar performance on individuals with Parkinson's disease. In T. Boellstorff (Ed.), *People with disabilities in virtual worlds—Selected Papers of Internet Research, 14.0, 2013* (p. 6). Association of Internet Researchers (AOIR).

Delemere, F. (2014). People with disabilities in virtual worlds: Not just a game! In N. S. Halifax (Ed.), *Our new leisure society: Abstracts from the 14th Canadian Congress on Leisure Research* (pp. 1–4). Canadian Association for Leisure Studies.

Dewey, J. (1910, reprinted 1997). How We Think. Mineola, NY: Courier Corporation.

Difulvio, G. T., Gubrium, A. C., Fiddian-Green, A., Lowe, S. E., & Del Toro-Mejias, L. M. (2016). Digital storytelling as a narrative health promotion process: Evaluation of a Pilot Study. *International Quarterly Community Health Education, 36,* 157–164.

Digital Health. (n.d.) [Online]. Edinburgh: The Digital Health and Care Institute. Retrieved 30 April, 2019, from http://dhi-scotland.com/about-dhi/.

Dooris, M., et al. (1998). The settings-based approach to health promotion. In A. D. Tsouros, G. Dowding, J. Thompson, & M. Dooris (Eds.), *Health promoting universities: Concept, experience and framework for action* (pp. 21–32). WHO Regional Office for Europe.

Ellison, N. B., & Boyd, D. M. (2013). Sociality through social network sites. In W. H. Dutton (Ed.), *The Oxford handbook of Internet studies.* Oxford University Press.

Eurobarometer, F. (2014). European citizens' digital health literacy. A report to the European Commission.

Fletcher, S., & Mullett, J. (2016). Digital stories as a tool for health promotion and youth engagement. *Canadian Journal of Public Health, 107,* e183–e187.

Fox, J. and Bailenson, J.N., (2009). Virtual Self-Modeling: The Effects of Vicarious Reinforcement and Identification on Exercise Behaviors. *Media Psychology. 12*(1), pp. 1-25.

Galliers, J. R., Wilson, S., Marshall, J., Talbot, R., Devane, N., Booth, T., Woolf, C., & Greenwood, H. (2017). Experiencing EVA Park, A Multi-User Virtual World For People With Aphasia. ACM Transactions on Accessible Computing, (18) (PDF) Experiencing EVA Park, a Multi-User Virtual World for People with Aphasia. Retrieved 26 January, 2021, from https://www.researchgate.net/publication/320260063_Experiencing_EVA_Park_a_Multi-User_Virtual_World_for_People_with_Aphasia.

Gilbert, R. L., et al. (2013). Psychological Benefits of Participation in Three-dimensional Virtual Worlds for Individuals with Real-world Disabilities. *International Journal of Disability, Development and Education., 60*(3), 208–224.

Gold, J., Pedrana, A. E., Stoove, M. A., Chang, S., Howard, S., Asselin, J., & y Hellard, ME. (2012). Developing health promotion interventions on social networking sites: Recommendations from The FaceSpace Project. *Journal of Medical Internet Research, 14*(1), e30.

Gorini, A., Gaggioli, A., Vigna, C., & Riva, G. (2008). A second life for eHealth: Prospects for the use of 3-D virtual worlds in clinical psychology. *Journal of Medical Internet Research, 10(3), e21.*

Greenhalgh, T., & Wessely, S. (2004). 'Health for me': A sociocultural analysis of healthism in the middle classes. *British Medical Bulletin, 69,* 197–213.

Guisset-Martinez, M., Villez, M., & Coupry, O. (2013). Gardens: Outdoor living spaces for the wellbeing of people with Alzheimer's and their entourage. Study Report Foundation Mederic Alzheimer. Retrieved 1 May, 2019, from fondation-mederic-alzheimer.org.

Hamm, M. P., Shulhan, J., Williams, G., Milne, A., Scott, S. D., & Hartling, L. (2014). A systematic review of the use and effectiveness of social media in child health. *BMC Pediatrics, 14*(1), 1–15.

Hirst, D. (2015). *Mind the gap: The digital divide and digital inclusion* [Online]. The Royal Statistical Society and the American Statistical Association. Retrieved 30 April, 2019, from https://www.statslife.org.uk/science-technology/2445-mind-the-gap-the-digital-divide-and-digital-inclusion.

Hoch, D. B., Watson, A. J., Linton, D. A., Bello, H. E., Senelly, M., Milik, M. T., et al. (2012). The feasibility and impact of delivering a mind-body intervention in a virtual world. *PLoS One, 7*(3), e33843.

Hsieh, C.-C., Lin, P.-S., Hsu, W.-C., Wang, J.-S., Huang, Y.-C., Lim, A.-Y., & Hsu, Y.-C. (2018). The Effectiveness of a virtual reality-based tai chi exercise on cognitive and physical function in older adults with cognitive impairment. *Dementia Geriatric Cognitive Disorders, 46*, 358–370. https://doi.org/10.1159/000494659

Jane, M., Hagger, M., Foster, J., et al. (2018). Social media for health promotion and weight management: A critical debate. *BMC Public Health, 18*, 932. https://doi.org/10.1186/s12889-018-5837-3

Jerdan, S. W., Grindle, M., van Woerden, H. C., & Kamel Boulos, M. N. (2018). Head-mounted virtual reality and mental health: Critical review of current research serious games. *Journal of Medical Internet Research, 6*(3), e14. https://doi.org/10.2196/games.9226

Johns, D. J., Langley, T. E., & Lewis, S. (2017). Use of social media for the delivery of health promotion on smoking, nutrition, and physical activity: A systematic review. *The Lancet, 390*, S49. https://doi.org/10.1016/S0140-6736(17)32984-7

Johnston, J. D., Massey, A. P., & DeVaneaux, C. (2012, January). Innovation in weight loss intervention programs: An examination of a 3D virtual world approach. In *2012 45th Hawaii international conference on system sciences* (pp. 2890–2899). IEEE.

Jones, J. K., Farley, H., & Murphy, A. (2018). Virtual worlds as restorative environments. In S. Gregory & D. Wood (Eds.), *Authentic virtual world education: Facilitating cultural engagement and creativity* (pp. 45–59). Springer Singapore.

Kamel Boulos, M. N., & Toth-Cohen, S. (2009). The University of Plymouth Sexual Health SIM experience in Second Life®: Evaluation and reflections after 1 year. *Health Information & Libraries Journal, 26*(4), 279–288.

Kaplan, A. M., & Haenlein, M. (2010). Users of the world, unite! The challenges and opportunities of Social Media. *Business Horizon, 53*, 59–68. https://doi.org/10.1016/j.bushor.2009.09.003

Kellert, S. R., & Wilson, E. O. (1995). *The biophilia hypothesis*. Island Press.

Kleban, C., & Kaye, L. K. (2015). Psychosocial impacts of engaging in Second Life for individuals with physical disabilities. *Computers in Human Behavior, 45*, 59–68.

Korda, H., & Itani, Z. (2013). Harnessing social media for health promotion and behavior change. *Health Promotion Practice, 14*, 15–23. https://doi.org/10.1177/1524839911405850

Kariuki, D., (2020) Pandemic spurs Second Life usage, book club, lower non–profit prices –8th April 2020, Hypergrid Business: Available online via https://www.hypergridbusiness.com/2020/04/second-life-sees-increase-inusers-during-coronavirus-pandemic/accessed 14/2/2022.

Laranjo, L., Arguel, A., Neves, A. L., et al. (2015). The influence of social networking sites on health behavior change: A systematic review and meta-analysis. *Journal of American Medical Informatics Association, 22*, 243–256. https://doi.org/10.1136/amiajnl-2014-002841

Levin-Zamir, D., & Bertschi, I. (2018). Media health literacy, eHealth literacy, and the role of the social environment in context. *International Journal for Environmental Research for Public Health, 15*(8), 1643.

Levin-Zamir, D., & Bertschi, I. (2019). Media health literacy, eHealth literacy, and health behavior across the lifespan: Current progress and future challenges (Chapter 18). In Okan,

Bauer, Levin-Zamir, Pinheiro, & Sorensen (Eds.), *International handbook of health literacy* (pp. 275–290). Research, Policy and Practice across the Lifespan, Policy Press.

Lin, Y., Hu, Z., Alias, H., & Wong, L. P. (2020). Influence of mass and social media on psychobehavioral responses among medical students during the downward trend of COVID-19 in Fujian, China: Cross-sectional study. *Journal of Medical Internet Research, 22*(7), e19982. https://doi.org/10.2196/19982

Linke, S., Murray, E., Butler, C., & Wallace, P. (2007). Internet-based interactive health intervention for the promotion of sensible drinking: Patterns of use and potential impact on members of the general public. *Journal of Medical Internet Research, 9*, e10.

Li, X., & Liu, Q. (2020). Social media use, eHealth literacy, disease knowledge, and preventive behaviors in the COVID-19 pandemic: Cross-sectional study on Chinese netizens. *Journal of medical Internet research, 22*(10), e19684.

Lombard, M. & Ditton I, T (1997). At the heart of it all: The concept of presence. Journal of Computer-Mediated Communication. 3(2), pp. 0.

Loss, J., Lindacher, V., & Curbach, J. (2014). Online social networking sites—A novel setting for health promotion? *Health & Place, 26*, 161–170. https://doi.org/10.1016/j.healthplace.2013.12.012

Mallari, B., Spaeth, E. K., Goh, H., & Boyd, B. S. (2019). Virtual reality as an analgesic for acute and chronic pain in adults: A systematic review and meta-analysis. *Journal of Pain Research, 12*, 2053.

McElhinney, E. (2015). *Living in 3D social VWs and the influence of health literacy, health behavior and wellbeing.* Unpublished thesis, Glasgow Caledonian University.

McElhinney, E., Kidd, L., & Cheater, F. M. (2018). Health literacy practices in social virtual worlds and the influence on health behaviour. *Global Health Promotion, 25(4), 34–47.* https://doi.org/10.1177/1757975918793334

McLeod, P. L., Liu, Y., & Axline, J. E. (2014). When your second life comes knocking: Effects of personality on changes to real life from virtual world experiences. *Computers in Human Behaviour, 39*, 59–70.

Mhei Mheidly, N., & Fares, J. (2020). Leveraging media and health communication strategies to overcome the COVID-19 paniinfodemic. *Journal of Public Health Policy, 41*(4), 410–420. https://doi.org/10.1057/s41271-020-00247-w

Mitchell, S. E., Mako, M., Sadikova, E., Barnes, L., Stone, A., Rosal, M. C., & Wiecha, J. (2014). The comparative experiences of women in control: Diabetes self-management education in a virtual world. *Journal of Diabetes Science and Technology, 8*(6), 1185–1192.

Morie, J. F., & Chance, E. (2011). Extending the reach of health care for obesity and diabetes using virtual worlds. *Journal of Diabetes Science and Technology, 5*(2), 272–276.

Morie, J.F. & Chance, E., (2011). Extending the Reach of Health Care for Obesity and Diabetes Using Virtual Worlds. *Journal of Diabetes Science and Technology, 5*(2), pp. 272–276.

Neiger, B. L., Thackeray, R., Burton, S. H., Giraud-Carrier, C. G., & Fagen, M. C. (2013). Evaluating social media's capacity to develop engaged audiences in health promotion settings: Use of Twitter metrics as a case study. *Health Promotion Practice, 14*(2), 157–162.

Neiger, B. L., Thackeray, R., Van Wagenen, S. A., Hanson, C. L., West, J. H., Barnes, M. D., & Fagen, M. C. (2012). Use of social media in health promotion: Purposes, key performance indicators, and evaluation metrics. *Health Promotion Practice, 13*(2), 159–164.

Nesi, J., Choukas-Bradley, S., & Prinstein, M. J. (2018). Transformation of adolescent peer relations in the social media context: Part 1—A theoretical framework and application to dyadic peer relationships. *Clinical Child Family Psychology Review, 21*, 267–294. https://doi.org/10.1007/s10567-018-0261-x

Norman, C. D., & Skinner, H. A. (2006). eHealth literacy: Essential skills for consumer health in a networked world. *Journal of Medical Internet Research, 8*, e9.

Norman, C. D. (2012). Social media and health promotion. *Global Health Promotion, 19*, 3–6. https://doi.org/10.1177/1757975912464593

Nosek, M. A., Whelen, S. R., Hughes, R. B., Porcher, E., Davidson, G., & Nosek, T. M. (2011). Self-esteem in second life: An in World group intervention for women with disabilities. *Journal of Virtual Worlds Research, 4*(3).

Obar, J. A., & Wildman, S. (2015). Social media definition and the governance challenge: An introduction to the special issue. *Telecommunication Policy, 39*, 745–750. https://doi.org/10.1016/j.telpol.2015.07.014

Obar, J. A., Zube, P., & Lampe, C. (2012). Advocacy 2.0: An analysis of how advocacy groups in the United States perceive and use social media as tools for facilitating civic engagement and collective action. *Journal of Information Policy, 2*, 1–25. https://doi.org/10.5325/jinfopoli.2.2012.0001

Okan, O., Bollweg, T. M., Berens, E. M., Hurrelmann, K., Bauer, U., & Schaeffer, D. (2020). Coronavirus-related health literacy: A cross-sectional study in adults during the COVID-19 infodemic in Germany. *International Journal of Environmental Research and public health, 17*(15), 5503.

Peymann, N., Rezai-rad, M., Tehrani, H., Gholian-aval, M., Vahedian-shahroodi, M., & Heidarian Miri, H. (2018). Digital Media-based Health Intervention on the promotion of Women's physical activity: A quasi-experimental study. *BMC Public Health, 18*, 134.

Poland, B., Krupa, G., & McCall, D. (2009). Settings for health promotion: An analytic framework to guide intervention design and implementation. *Health Promotion Practice, 10*, 505–516. https://doi.org/10.1177/1524839909341025

Rampton, L., (2013). *Landscape design for everyday wellness*. Master of Landscape Architecture, The University of Manitoba. Retrieved 2 April, 2019, from http://mspace.lib.umanitoba.ca/xmlui/handle/1993/19390.

Relph, E., (2007). Spirit of place and sense of place in virtual realities. Techné: *Research in Philosophy and Technology, 10*(3), pp. 17–25.

Rothbaum, B. O., Rizzo, A., & Difede, J. (2010). Virtual reality exposure therapy for combat-related posttraumatic stress disorder. *Annals of the New York Academy of Sciences., 1208*(1), 126–132.

Ruiz, J. G., et al. (2012). Using anthropomorphic avatars resembling sedentary older individuals as models to enhance self-efficacy and adherence to physical activity: Psychophysiological correlates. *Studies in Health Technology and Informatics., 173, 405–411.*

Saab, M. M., Landers, M., Cooke, E., Murphy, D., & Hegarty, J. (2019). Feasibility and usability of a virtual reality intervention to enhance men's awareness of testicular disorders (E-MAT). *Virtual Reality, 23*(2), 169–178.

Schillinger, D., Chittamuru, D., & Ramírez, A. S. (2020). From "infodemics" to health promotion: A novel framework for the role of social media in public health. *American Journal of Public Health, 110*(9), 1393–1396. https://doi.org/10.2105/AJPH.2020.305746

Siddiqi, S., Mama, S. K., & Lee, R. E. (2011). Developing an obesity prevention intervention in virtual worlds: The international health challenge in Second Life. *Journal for Virtual Worlds Research, 3*(3), 3–26. https://doi.org/10.4101/jvwr.v3i3.809

Sorensen, N. K., Van Den Broucke, S., Fullam, J., Doyle, G., Pelikan, J., Slonska, Z., Brand, H., & Consortium Health Literacy Project, E. (2012). Health literacy and public health: A systematic review and integration of definitions and models. *BMC Public Health, 12, 80.*

Stendal, K., & Balandin, S. (2015). Virtual worlds for people with autism spectrum disorder: A case study in Second Life. *Disability & Rehabilitation., 1–8.* https://doi.org/10.3109/0963828 8.2015.1052577

Sullivan, D. K., Goetz, J. R., Gibson, C. A., Washburn, R. A., Smith, B. K., Lee, J., et al. (2013). Improving weight maintenance using virtual reality (Second Life). *Journal of Nutrition Education and Behavior, 45*(3), 264–268.

Tasnim, S., Hossain, M. M., & Mazumder, H. (2020). Impact of rumors and misinformation on COVID-19 in social media. *Journal of Preventive Medicine and Public Health, 53*(3), 171–174. https://doi.org/10.3961/jpmph.20.094

The HLS19 Consortium of the WHO Action Network M-POHL (2021). *International Report on the Methodology, Results, and Recommendations of the European Health Literacy Population Survey 2019-2021 (HLS19) of M-POHL*. Austrian National Public Health Institute, Vienna.

Thomas, S. (2013). *Technobiophilia: Nature and Cyberspace*. Bloomsbury.

Tinder Foundation. (2016). *Health & Digital: Reducing inequalities, improving society. An evaluation of the Widening Digital Participation programme*. UK: (now the Good Things Foundation).

Twigger-Ross, C., (2013). DR6: How will environmental and place based change affect notions of identity in the UK over the next 10 years - Future Identities: Changing identities in the UK–the next 10 years. Collingwood Environmental Planning.

Ulrich, R. S. (1999). *Effects of gardens on health outcomes: Theory and research* (pp. 27–86). Therapeutic Benefits and Design Recommendations.

Ulrich, R. S., et al. (1991). Stress recovery during exposure to natural and urban environments. *Journal of Environmental Psychology, 11*(3), 201–230.

Valtchanov, D., Barton, K. R., & Ellard, C. (2010). Restorative effects of virtual nature settings. *Cyberpsychology, Behavior and Social Networking, 13*(5), 503–512.

Van den Broucke, S. (2020). Why health promotion matters to the COVID-19 pandemic, and vice versa. *Health Promotion International, 35*(2), 181–186. https://doi.org/10.1093/heapro/daaa042

Van Der Vaart, R., & Drossaert, C. (2017). Development of the digital health literacy instrument: Measuring a broad spectrum of health 1.0 and health 2.0 skills. *Journal of Medical Internet Research, 19*, e27.

Webb, T., Joseph, J., Yardley, L., & Michie, S. (2010). Using the Internet to promote health behavior change: A systematic review and meta-analysis of the impact of theoretical basis, use of behavior change techniques, and mode of delivery on efficacy. *Journal of Medical Internet Research, 12, e4*. https://doi.org/10.2196/jmir.1376

Whitelaw, S., Baxendale, A., Bryce, C., Machardy, L., Young, I., & Witney, E. (2001). 'Settings' based health promotion: A review. *Health Promotion International, 16*(4), 339–353.

Wilson, E. O. (1984). *Biophilia*. Harvard University Press.

Witmer, B. G., & Singer, M. J. (1998). Measuring presence in virtual environments: A presence questionnaire. *Presence, 7*(3), 225–240.

World Health Organization. (1986). The Ottawa Charter for Health Promotion. *First international conference on health promotion*, Ottawa.

World Health Organization. (2016). *What is health promotion?* [Online]. Retrieved 30 April, 2019, from https://www.who.int/features/qa/health-promotion/en/.

World Health Organization. (2020). *Novel Coronavirus (2019-nCoV)*. Situation Report—13. WHO. https://www.who.int/docs/default-source/coronaviruse/situation-reports/20200202-sitrep-13-ncov-v3.pdf?sfvrsn=195f4010_6.

Yee, N., Bailenson, J. N., & Ducheneut, N. (2009). The proteus effect: Implications of transformed digital self-representation on online and offline behavior. *Communication Research, 36*(2), 285–312.

Yee, N., Bailenson, J. N., Urbanek, M., Chang, F., & Merget, D. (2007). The unbearable likeness of being digital: The persistence of nonverbal social norms in online virtual environments. *Cyberpsychology & Behavior, 10*(1), 115–121.

Yuen, E. K., Herbert, J. D., Forman, E. M., Goetter, E. M., Comer, R., & Bradley, J. C. (2013). Treatment of social anxiety disorder using online virtual environments in second life. *Behavior Therapy, 44*(1), 51–61.

Chapter 13
Emerging Settings

Michelle Baybutt, Sami Kokko, Alana Crimeen, Evelyne de Leeuw, Emma Tomalin, Jo Sadgrove, and Ursula Pool

13.1 Introduction

As has been set out in the book so far, the settings-based approach has been developed at local, national and international levels spanning over the past 30 years, but arguably with quite a limited range of settings initiatives. In Part I, this book presented both the theoretical grounds and practical principles for settings-based health promotion, and Part II, so far, has focused on long- and/or well-established settings initiatives. In this final chapter of Part II, we refer to 'emerging settings' because the case studies set out below are either new or in the early stages of development, not currently widespread and perhaps not yet considered to have an international focus. However, we acknowledge that a variety of terms have been used to describe the development of settings—such as whether they are traditional, e.g. schools and cities, or non-traditional, e.g. sports clubs and prisons; legitimate, formal/informal, and 'less obvious' (Kickbusch, 1995, p. 25 cited in Poland et al., 2000). Many settings have flourished by being supported through formal networks at local, national,

M. Baybutt (✉) · U. Pool
Healthy and Sustainable Settings Unit, School of Community Health and Midwifery,
University of Central Lancashire, Preston, Lancashire, UK
e-mail: mbaybutt@uclan.ac.uk; upool1@uclan.ac.uk

S. Kokko
Research Center for Health Promotion, Faculty of Sport and Health Sciences,
University of Jyväskylä, Länsi-Suomi, Finland
e-mail: sami.p.kokko@jyu.fi

A. Crimeen
School of Built Environment, Faculty of Arts, Design and Architecture, University of New South Wales (UNSW), and the Centre for Health Equity Training, Research & Evaluation (CHETRE), part of the Centre for Primary Health Care and Equity, University of New South Wales, Sydney, Australia
e-mail: a.crimeen@unsw.edu.au

© Springer Nature Switzerland AG 2022
S. Kokko, M. Baybutt (eds.), *Handbook of Settings-Based Health Promotion*,
https://doi.org/10.1007/978-3-030-95856-5_13

and European levels as have been discussed in previous chapters that have focused on schools, universities, workplaces, prisons and sports clubs for example.

The most long-lasting and widespread settings initiatives internationally are schools and cities, which are also formal institutional structures of societies (see also Chaps. 1, 5 and 6). Historically, settings-based work has been limited, with traditional setting initiatives and new initiatives tending to be overlooked (Kokko et al., 2014). Dooris (2013) has argued that in order to respond to societal changes and address inequalities, the settings approach needs to be extended into non-traditional and non-institutional settings. However, these other less formally recognised settings have generally struggled to receive the momentum required to secure the resources and support they need to become more widespread and formalised.

Internationally, there are a wide range of settings that could be referred to as emerging or non-traditional such as healthy marketplaces (Moy, 2001), health-promoting general practice (Watson, 2008), beauty salons (Linnan & Ferguson, 2007), farms as settings for health promotion (Thurston & Blundell-Gosselin, 2005) and healthy islands (Galea et al., 2000), which are not discussed as part of the more recognised settings that form previous chapters in Part II of this book. Still, it is worth noting that some settings have more potential than are currently noticed. For example, sports clubs have strong potential due to their wide reach and informal educational nature and the fact that most of the clubs are non-profit associations belonging to the voluntary and civic sector (Kokko et al., 2014). Almost any setting could have the potential to become a health-promoting setting. If using the guiding definition set out by Wenzel (1997) whereby a setting is a socially and culturally defined geographical and physical area of factual social interaction and a socially and culturally defined set of patterns to be performed while in the setting, it is more a question of willingness of a setting and how to apply settings-based health promotion principles introduced in Chap. 2.

Green et al. (2000, p. 25) have highlighted the potential weakness of settings as being those who can be 'reached' versus those who can't, raising the issue of some settings (e.g., workplaces and schools) being more 'legitimate' than others (e.g., bingo halls and nightclubs). More so, Dooris (2009, p. 32) questioned how relevant the settings approach is to addressing inequalities and inclusion when it has tended

E. de Leeuw
Centre for Health Equity Training, Research & Evaluation (CHETRE), Part of the UNSW Australia Research Centre for Primary Health Care & Equity, A Unit of Population Health, South Western Sydney Local Health District, NSW Health, A member of the Ingham Institute, Liverpool Hospital, University of New South Wales, Sydney, Australia
e-mail: e.deleeuw@unsw.edu.au

E. Tomalin
Centre for Religion and Public Life, School of Philosophy, Religion and History of Science, University of Leeds, Leeds, West Yorkshire, UK
e-mail: E.tomalin@leeds.ac.uk

J. Sadgrove
Centre for Religion and Public Life, University of Leeds, Leeds, West Yorkshire, UK
e-mail: j.e.m.sadgrove@leeds.ac.uk

to neglect less defined settings. Earlier in the book, Chap. 10 focused on prisons, arguing that they are legitimate places to intervene to address risky health behaviours and positively influence wider public health beyond the prison and in the wider community post-release. This important setting has the potential to address health inequalities yet there is relatively little practical guidance to enable prisons to become more health promoting. Conversely, Chap. 12 sets out a convincing argument for digital and social media being an important contemporary setting. Woodall and Rowlands (2021) refer to the 'virtual world' as part of a second wave of environments whereby engaging with the 'online setting' can offer significant benefits in terms of reach and engagement.

It is important to differentiate between a health-promoting setting and health promotion in the setting. The latter may involve aspects of health promotion that are carried out as part of the normal activities of the setting (Watson, 2008); however, often the setting itself is passive, only allowing external experts to enter and act whereas the former takes a more comprehensive, systems-level and coordinated approach whereby the position of the setting is active and willing to develop its activities (Kokko et al., 2014).

It is also important to note that there is a diversity of activity happening under the banner of what is variously labelled settings-based health promotion, health-promoting settings, healthy settings and settings for health (Kokko et al., 2014; Dooris, 2006). In academia, there is a debate on how 'health promoting' or 'healthy' settings initiatives should be labelled and which concept should be used (e.g., Kokko et al., 2014). Either way, currently the term 'healthy' setting is used in the same way as 'health promoting' setting. For practice, more important than the label is to fit the concept used into the particular setting and the needs and aims of the initiative. For example, in terms of language, practitioners will be less likely to use the words 'healthy' or 'health-promoting' settings rather, they will refer to specific settings - for example, 'a healthy or health promoting workplace'. A healthy workplace programme will have the settings approach in the background even if the terminology of healthy setting or settings approach is not used. It is often the case that the concept of 'healthy' or 'health promoting' may not even be visible in the title of the programme or the related activities in the setting. Indeed, it is generally accepted to use the language of a particular setting and to tailor it to the usual business activities of that setting.

The continued relevance of the settings approach today remains evident 30 years after the Ottawa Charter and as demonstrated below with how the case studies reflect continued changes in society. The case studies set out fresh perspectives, new innovations and renewed efforts to develop the settings-based approach in settings that are responding to contemporary health challenges. The development of healthy airports with actions through intersectoral governance approaches; places of worship as 'nested' settings and central in communities; and the paradox of health and the coast for developing healthy coastal communities in the UK, particularly following the COVID-19 pandemic, illustrate the multi-layered and complex nature of context when applying the settings approach.

13.2   Case Study 1: Healthy Airports

Alana Crimeen and Evelyne de Leeuw

13.2.1   Background and Context: Airports, Cities and Public Health

Airports, and the aviation industry more generally, are not necessarily seen as settings for health. Both negatively influence communities by changing and disrupting the natural and built environments in many ways, such as creating noise and air pollution, prioritising unhealthy mobility patterns and contributing to climate change (Passchier et al., 2000). All of which can result in serious population health impacts. Despite these problems, airports are still desirable city features for governments and private organisations due to their relationship with economic growth, tourism, city status and global connectivity (Conventz & Thierstein, 2015; Knippenberger, 2010). Airports have increasingly diversified core businesses around the physical runways and terminals, including freight and transportation networks and real estate for industry and commercial centres. There are complex models for airport development, where airports are imagined, planned and operated as types of metropolitan or urban centres, with close relationships to the cities around them (Freestone & Baker, 2011). Forms of these include the airport city, the aerotropolis and airport corridors. This planning approach, combined with rapid urbanisation, means airports that were once separate from cities are being subsumed into the urban area, or airports are now being specifically developed or expanded within city boundaries (Forsyth, 2014).

Airports alter and influence the physical, social and economic factors of the regions in which they are located, which we recognise as determinants of health. As airports become more entangled with urban living, conflicts with human health occur across larger populations. Despite city and airport planners considering airports more like cities than separate or independent infrastructure, public health responses to airports have largely focused on health protection measures. Public health typically limits its aviation gaze to reducing the negative environmental, physical, social and psychological impacts of issues such as aviation related pollution and disruption. This work is important, but a broader health promotion perspective is warranted to engage with the urban influence of airports.

13.2.2   Current Situation: A Greenfields Airport

In 2015, development of a new international airport for Sydney, Australia, commenced. Keeping with contemporary airport design, the Western Sydney Airport (WSA) will be an aerotropolis, with a 30-min city around the airport complex

(Western Sydney Planning Partnership, 2020). This has created significant changes to the longer-term regional planning for Sydney and aims to support urban growth in the Western Sydney region (Greater Sydney Commission, 2018).

This airport development has initiated a closer examination of the urban airports by local health organisations. Aiming for proactive engagement, the Centre for Health Equity Training, Research and Evaluation (CHETRE) (a joint academic unit under the Population Health department of the South Western Sydney Local Health District and the University of New South Wales) undertook multiple streams of airport-related research and development activities. Projects included participating in an independent peer review of the Environmental Impact Statement for the WSA and conducting a Health Impact Assessment with community partners (Haigh et al., 2020; Hirono et al., 2017; Western Sydney Regional Organisation of Councils, 2015). Both works highlighted concerns for negative health impacts and contained suggestions for the mitigation and improvement of health-related features of the airport.

A third stream of work, inspired by Healthy Cities and Healthy Regions developments elsewhere, considers the airport region as a setting for health. This work culminated in a 'Healthy Airports' report (de Leeuw, Crimeen, et al., 2018). Drawing from Healthy Cities and contemporary healthy urban planning approaches, it described unique features of airport regions, impacted populations and created a definition of the Healthy Airport region (Crimeen et al., 2019). Eleven potential dimensions of Healthy Airports were proposed, spanning concepts including public participation, form and design, economy, ecosystems, heritage and public health and sick care services (de Leeuw, Crimeen, et al., 2018).

13.2.3   The Future: A Healthy Airport?

Improvement programmes for airports are already a feature for the industry. The aviation industry and airports are a globe-spanning network of industry groups and stakeholders, some more rigorously regulated than others, and with divergent interests. Across this complex network, airport corporations and aviation actors are implementing activities with numerous goals. They include aspirations of environmental and economic sustainability, community development and social responsibility. At the highest level, the United Nations agency for Aviation, the International Civil Aviation Organisation (ICAO), has adopted a range of the UN Sustainable Development Goals and undertakes urban, health and environmental-related airport improvement projects (ICAO, 2018a, 2018b). In some instances, Health Impact Assessments are being conducted on airports to supplement the Environmental Impact Assessment processes (Haigh et al., 2020). Within private networks and individual airports, there are a range of diverse airport-led partnership projects covering topics such as citizen science, local employment commitments, transport connectivity and community engagement projects (IAU Île-de-France, 2018). These projects address issues that urban health practitioners would recognise as determinants of health. However, a systematic appraisal of such social, political and commercial determinants and their impact on health is generally absent.

The ongoing global pandemic has highly disrupted the airport industry, creating interesting circumstances for health and airports, as more focused attention shifts to the role of airports in the community, demonstrating clearly the intersection of glocal and local (the glocal) challenges airports experience with respect to public health. Resources are being invested to create health protective airport terminals, largely through approaches to infectious disease control. This is resulting in partnerships being built at both high levels (WHO and ICAO) and local levels between airports and local, state, and national public health organisations. As the situation evolves, public health approaches relative to air travel, and airports, evolve simultaneously (The Lancet Infectious Diseases, 2020). What this looks like for health in airports more broadly, and in the longer term, is unclear.

13.2.4 Next Steps

Airport development and operations are sophisticated processes, requiring a multitude of technical specialities. Health (as opposed to disease control) is generally absent from the core considerations in this area. Healthy Airports initiated a roadmap towards more fully developing airports as settings for health, but thinking up, developing and implementing settings for health is not an easy task. Both Healthy Cities and Health Promoting Schools took decades to be established, and the tenets of virtually all settings for health are consistently challenged. Authoritative declarations and statements may help, e.g., the Yanuca Declaration on Healthy Islands (de Leeuw, Martin, & Waqanivalu, 2018; WHO, 2015) or the Shanghai Statement on Healthy Cities (WHO, 2017). Currently, airports are far from such global agreement. This is not just because they are such complex glocal environments, but also because the governance of airports and the aviation industry is challenging. Many different players, and their 'consumers' (the passengers, workers and local communities impacted by the industry), are severely underrepresented in these governance systems (Hirono et al., 2017).

In the context of airport's rapid and continuing growth into urban areas, it seems important that a model operational framework for taking account of health with and by airports is developed, tested and disseminated for trial. We could take inspiration from some other benchmarks in the healthy settings family, e.g., the Healthy Cities' Twenty Steps (WHO, 1997) or Health Promoting Hospitals and Healthcare Systems Core Strategies (Pelikan et al., 2005). The COVID-19 pandemic may have provided a window of opportunity where many of the actors in the complex governance system around airports and aviation have been alerted to the challenges and opportunities around health promotion (rather than disease and risk) (Macilree & Duval, 2020). With an appropriately scoped research programme, glocal strategy and support from the health promotion community, airports may well become healthier in the twenty-first century.

13.3   Case Study 2: Places of Worship as Healthy Settings in the UK

Emma Tomalin and Jo Sadgrove

13.3.1   Background and Context: Places of Worship

Places of worship have received very little attention in the literature about healthy settings (Corcoran et al., 2013; Tomalin et al., 2019). This is despite evidence that they can play an important role in the health of their congregations or membership, as well as the wider community. First, participation in the regular religious activities at places of worship, such as prayer or meditation, can have a positive impact on people's well-being and mental health (Nooney & Woodrum, 2002; Ridge et al., 2008) and religious leaders sometimes integrate health messages into their sermons or prayers (Tomalin et al., 2015). Second, places of worship often directly engage in self-initiated public health-related activities, such as churches organising pastoral teams to take part in home visits to reduce loneliness, the hosting of traditional medical practitioners in Hindu temples or the Dementia Friendly Gurdwara Project in Bradford (Dementia Friendly Gurudwaras Project, 2014; Tomalin et al., 2015; Tomalin & Sadgrove, 2016). Finally, collaborations between places of worship and external public health actors are common, including blood pressure and diabetes testing carried out by local health professionals (Boltri et al., 2008; Ghouri, 2005). Places of worship may also play a role in promoting attitudes and activities that act against good health outcomes, such as healing rituals to cure people of HIV/AIDS in Pentecostal churches or other faith settings where people might be encouraged to pray for a cure to an illness rather than visit a doctor (Tomalin et al., 2015). Moreover, places of worship may not always be the best spaces within which to address issues around sexuality and sexual health. Places of worship are gendered spaces which can limit their utility to pursue women's health issues or those of sexual minorities.

13.3.2   What Is the Current Situation?

Activities relating to health promotion in places of worship are largely ad hoc and uncoordinated. There is next to no academic research that examines the potential to develop a healthy settings approach in places of worship and no guidelines for places of worship to become healthy settings. However, statutory public health actors in the UK are increasingly seeking engagement with faith actors to achieve their goals. This 'turn to faith' is evidenced in a recent report from Public Health England, which has the remit to 'protect and improve the nation's health and well-being and reduce health inequalities' (Public Health England, 2016). It states that

> *Public Health England understands the importance of faith in shaping the health and care*
> *decisions of many people, and recognises that providing appropriate community care is*
> *likely to require collaboration with faith leaders and Places of Worship* (Public Health
> England, 2016).

This 'turn to faith' is a response to the needs of increasingly pluralistic societies. This has led to calls for a 'new wave of development in public health and health promotion' (Hanlon et al., 2012, p. 235) where, as Hanlon et al. argue, 'the future practitioner will need to understand how different worldviews are profoundly influential in shaping the ways in which all of us understand and act in the world' (2012, p. 236). However, this also reflects a shift from models of health care that focus on biomedical approaches to social models where 'a perspective of health is realised that embraces all aspects of human experience and places health fully in the dynamic interplay of social structures and human agency' (Yuill et al., 2010, p. 11; Marmot, 2005). Finally, in the UK we need to consider the role that neoliberal welfare reforms since the 1980s, and the austerity agenda pursued by the government in response to the 2008 recession, have played in this 'turn to faith' to fill gaps in government service provision (Kus, 2006; Farnsworth & Irving, 2018).

13.3.3 The Future: Recognising Places of Worship as a Healthy Setting

Corcoran et al. assert that 'religious organisations and faith groups have often been able to engage in important roles in health…and thus have potential as a health promotion setting' (2013, p. 121). Moreover, they may 'allow access to some populations that traditional health promotion efforts may not reach, including specific ethnic groups and older people who may be traditionally low users of health care' (2013, p. 122). However, it cannot be assumed that places of worship will necessarily be interested in becoming healthy settings. In our research, we have encountered the perception amongst some religious leaders and community members that public health actors are expecting places of worship to do their work for them and for free, when they lack the time and resources to do this, particularly since health and wellbeing is not their core business (Tomalin et al., 2015).

13.3.4 Next Steps

Places of worship present a diverse set of institutions, not all of which will have the interest or capacity to engage significantly with the healthy settings approach. However, many are already working towards becoming healthy settings, via the health benefits of participating in religious activities or through specific health-related initiatives that are instigated by the place of worship itself. It is recommended that when public health actors wish to engage with places of worship, for instance to promote a healthy settings approach, that they communicate their reasons for wishing to engage and are clear about what resources they can offer to a joint project. This is to mitigate suspicions on the part of faith leaders that public health actors are primarily interested in instrumentalising places of worship to meet public health ends. In order for collaborations to be successful and sustainable, places of worship need to take ownership of any public health work they engage in. It cannot be assumed that all religious leaders see themselves as having a responsibility to their members' health needs. Therefore, in seeking engagement it is important to consider building on health-related work that places of worship are already undertaking in order to find mutual grounds for collaboration.

13.4 Case Study 3: Emerging Settings: Healthy Coastal Communities

Ursula Pool

13.4.1 Background: The Paradox of Health and the Coast

Many of Britain's once vibrant seaside towns are in a state of decline. While not all coastal communities are affected equally, these areas are more likely than inland communities to suffer from higher than average social, economic, and health problems. The economic gap (in terms of average wages) between coastal and non-coastal communities is growing, and coastal communities face issues such as outward migration of young people, ageing populations, transitory populations, low-quality housing and geographical isolation (Corfe, 2017). These conditions are associated with poorer public health profiles, particularly for mental health.

In the past, however, these coastal locations were the places considered to be the most healthy. Sea bathing became popular in the eighteenth century; it was encouraged by doctors for health reasons, based on the supposed recuperative powers of sea water (Foley, 2016). During the nineteenth century, seaside resorts were developed and became popular. As improved transport links improved and leisure time increased, pleasure overtook health as the driving force behind people visiting the coast in growing numbers (Walton, 1983). This was still seen as a healthy leisure option, however, and the sea (along with other aquatic environments including lakes, spas and springs) has long been associated with health and well-being. There is now evidence to support these ideas, with a growing body of research showing that exposure to aquatic environmental features can be beneficial to health and well-being, and that living by the coast is also associated with positive health outcomes.

For example, a study (Wheeler et al., 2012) based on census data for England, which looked at data for more than 48 million people, found that the number of people reporting good health was 1.13% points higher in urban coastal communities compared with urban communities further away from the coast (this was after adjustment for potential confounding variables such as age, gender, green space density and socioeconomic factors). The study also found that that the association between good health and coastal proximity was strongest in the most deprived areas, with the strength of association decreasing with decreasing deprivation.

Seaside towns thus seem to embody a contradiction: From one perspective, their coastal setting is associated with disadvantage and illness; from another perspective, it is associated with health and well-being. The question, then, is how to develop an approach that is tailored to the place-based problems of coastal communities, while also harnessing their place-based resources to improve health and well-being.

13.4.2   Today: How Can This Paradox Be Resolved?

A number of initiatives have recently been developed with the potential to begin to transform deprived seaside towns into healthy coastal communities. For example, in the UK, the Blue New Deal (Balata, 2016; Balata & Vardakoulias, 2016) aims to introduce social and environmental goals into key coastal industries. The strategy is based on five areas, all rooted in characteristics of coastal settings. These are sustainable fishing, sustainable tourism, renewable energy, innovative coastal management and re-connecting people with nature. The underlying rationale is to balance economic and social needs with environmental considerations: recognising the interconnections between these areas makes it possible to engineer an upward spiral where the areas are reciprocally benefiting and improving—in direct contrast to the downward spiral of decline seen in some coastal communities.

Further afield, the Blue Zone Project (Buettner & Skemp, 2016) arose from research based on the observation that several coastal populations round the world were unusually long-lived and healthy (Poulain et al., 2013). These populations (Ikaria, in Greece; Nicoya, in Costa Rica; Okinawa, in Japan; Sardinia, in Italy) were all located in coastal settings. Dan Buettner, founder of the Blue Zone Project, studied these locations (along with Loma Linda in California, home to a community of around 9000 Seventh-Day Adventists, who share health and longevity characteristics with other Blue Zone populations) in order to derive principles based on common features of the lifestyles in these settings. This is a different approach from the Blue New Deal mentioned above, as the principles are not dependent on living in a coastal community; rather, they are derived from healthy communities which happen to be coastal. Buettner came up with nine principles, including moving naturally; developing a sense of purpose; incorporating some kind of mindfulness or means of dissipating stress; not overeating; eating mostly plants; moderate alcohol consumption; belonging to a (faith-based) community; keeping family networks close; maintaining committed, small social networks of friends. These can be simplified into the four categories of outlook, diet, activity and connections (Roundtable on Health, 2015) and are currently being implemented in a number of locations, both coastal and inland.

13.4.3   What Is the Future for Healthy Coastal Communities?

Combining the two initiatives described above provides a potential route forward for healthy coastal communities. While the Blue Zone formula, inspired by the healthiest coastal communities, describes what can be done at the community level working with individuals, the Blue New Deal provides a framework within which to do it; linking community and policy and tailored to the particular problems faced in British coastal towns. This could be implemented in practice when developing each of the five areas in the Blue New Deal, by ensuring (via evidence of what works, along with community consultation) that the four overarching Blue Zone categories are considered and incorporated in a manner that maximises well-being. Coastal communities provide an example of the interconnectedness of the fate of the environment, the economy and public health in a particular setting—all of these need to be included in a coherent strategy that enables them to be reciprocally beneficial and sustainable.

References

Dementia Friendly Gurudwaras Project (2014) *A Toolkit to making your Local Gurudwara Dementia Friendly*. Retrieved from https://dementiafriendlygurudwaras.files.wordpress.com/2012/06/dementia-friendly-gurudwaras-toolkit.pdf.

Balata, F. (2016). Shaping a new deal for coastal communities. *Renewal: A Journal of Labour Politics, 24*(2), 84–89.

Balata, F., & Vardakoulias, O. (2016). *Turning back to the sea: A blue new deal to revitalise coastal communities*, New Economics Foundation, London. Retrieved from https://neweconomics.org/2016/11/turning-back-to-the-sea/.

Boltri, J. M., Davis-Smith, M., Okosun, I. S., Seale, J. P., & Foster, B. (2008). Translation of the National Institutes of Health Diabetes Prevention Program in African American Churches. *Journal of the National Medical Association, 103*(3), 194–202.

Buettner, D., & Skemp, S. (2016). Blue Zones: Lessons from the world's longest lived. *American Journal of Lifestyle Medicine, 10*(5), 318–321.

Conventz, S., & Thierstein, A. (2015). *Airports, cities and regions*. Routledge. https://doi.org/10.4324/9780203798829

Corcoran, N., Bone, A., & Everett, C. (2013). Using settings. In N. Corcoran (Ed.), *Communicating health: Strategies for health promotion* (pp. 112–113). Sage.

Corfe, S. (2017). *Living on the edge: Britain's coastal communities*. Social Market Foundation.

Crimeen, A., de Leeuw, E., & Freestone, R. (2019). Towards a health promotion paradigm for airport development. *Cities & Health*. https://doi.org/10.1080/23748834.2019.1585701

de Leeuw, E., Crimeen, A., Freestone, R., Jalaludin, B., Sainsbury, P., Hirono, K., & Reid, A. (2018). *Healthy airports*. Centre for Health Equity Training, Research and Evaluation (CHETRE).

de Leeuw, E., Martin, E., & Waqanivalu, T. (2018). *Healthy Islands. Oxford textbook of nature and public health: The role of nature in improving the health of a population* (p. 285).

Dooris, M. (2009). Holistic and sustainable health improvement: The contribution of the settings-based approach to health promotion. *Perspectives in Public Health, 129*(1), 29–36.

Dooris, M. (2006). Health promoting settings: Future directions. *IUHPE-Promotion and Education Vol XIII, 1*.

Dooris, M. (2013). Expert voices for change: Bridging the silos – towards healthy and sustainable settings for the 21st century. Health & Place, 20, 39-50.

Farnsworth, K., & Irving, Z. (2018). Austerity: Neoliberal dreams come true? *Critical Social Policy, 38*(3), 461–481.

Foley, R. (2016). *Healing waters: Therapeutic landscapes in historic and contemporary Ireland*. Routledge.

Forsyth, P. (2014). *Air capacity for Sydney. Expanding airport capacity in large urban areas*. International Transport Forum, OECD Publishing.

Freestone, R., & Baker, D. (2011). Spatial planning models of airport-driven urban development. *Journal of Planning Literature, 26*, 263–279.

Galea, G., Powis, B., & Tamplin, A. T. (2000). Healthy Islands in the Western Pacific—International settings development. *Health Promotion International., 15*(2), 169–177.

Ghouri, N. (2005). Health fair in a mosque: Putting policy into practice. *Public Health, 119*, 197–201.

Greater Sydney Commission. (2018). *Greater Sydney region plan: A metropolis of three cities*. State of New South Wales.

Green, L.W., Poland, B.D., Rootman, I. (2000). The settings approach to health promotion. In B.D. Poland, L.W. Green, I. Rootman (Eds.) Settings for health promotion: Linking theory and practice (pp. 1-43). London: Sage.

Haigh, F., Fletcher-Lartey, S., Jaques, K., Millen, E., Calalang, C., de Leeuw, E., Mahimbo, A., & Hirono, K. (2020). The health impacts of transformative infrastructure change: Process matters as much as outcomes. *Environmental Impact Assessment Review, 85*, 106437. https://doi.org/10.1016/j.eiar.2020.106437

Hanlon, P., Carlisle, S., Hannah, M., Lyon, A., & Reilly, D. (2012). A perspective on the future public health: An integrative and ecological framework. *Perspectives on Public Health, 132*(6), 313–319.

Hirono, K., Haigh, F., Jaques, K., Fletcher-Lartey, S., Millen, E., & Calalang, C. (2017). *Is anyone listening? A Health impact assessment of the Western Sydney Airport community engagement process*. Liverpool, NSW: Centre for Health Equity Training, Research and Evaluation, part of the Centre for Primary Health Care and Equity, Faculty of Medicine, UNSW Sydney.

IAU Île-de-France. (2018). *Sustainable airport areas: Guidelines for decision makers*. France, Paris Region Urban Planning and Development Agency.

International Civil Aviation Organisation, (2018a). *Aviation and Urbanisation*. Retrieved from https://www.icao.int/ESAF/aviation-urbanism/Pages/default.aspx.

International Civil Aviation Organisation, (2018b). *ICAO and the United Nations Sustainable Development Goals*. Retrieved from https://www.icao.int/about-icao/aviation-development/Pages/SDG.aspx.

Kickbusch. (1995). Cited in Poland et al, 2000.

Knippenberger, U. (2010). *Airports in Cities and Regions: Research and Practise: 1st International Colloquium on Airports and Spatial Development, Karlsruhe, 9th–10th July 2009*, KIT Scientific Publishing.

Kokko, S., Green, L. W., & Kannas, L. (2014). A review of settings-based health promotion with applications to sports clubs. *Health Promotion International, 29*(3), 494–509.

Kus, B. (2006). Neoliberalism, institutional change and the Welfare State: The case of Britain and France. *International Journal of Comparative Sociology, 47*(6), 488–525.

Linnan, L. A. and Ferguson, Y.O. (2007) Beauty Salons: A Promising Health Promotion Setting for Reaching and Promoting Health Among African American Women. Health Education & Behavior, Vol. 34 (3): 517-530 DOI: 10.1177/1090198106295531.

Macilree, J., & Duval, D. T. (2020). Aeropolitics in a post-COVID-19 world. *Journal of Air Transport Management, 88*, 101864.

Marmot, M. (2005). Social determinants of health inequalities. *The Lancet., 365*(9464), 1099–1104.

Moy, G. G. (2001). Healthy marketplaces: An approach for ensuring food safety and environmental health. *Food Control, 12*, 499–504.

Nooney, J., & Woodrum, E. (2002). Religious coping and church-based social support as predictors of mental health outcomes: Testing a conceptual model. *Journal for the Scientific Study of Religion, 41*(2), 359–368.

Passchier, W., Knottnerus, A., Albering, H., & Walda, I. (2000). Public health impact of large airports. *Reviews on Environmental Health, 15*(1–2), 83–96.

Pelikan, J. M., Dietscher, C., Krajic, K., Nowak, P., Groene, O., & Garcia-Barbero, M. (2005). 18 core strategies for health promoting hospitals (HPH). In O. Groene & M. Garcia-Barbero (Eds.), *Health promotion in hospitals: Evidence and quality management* (pp. 46–63). World Health Organization.

Poland, B. D., Green, L. W., & Rootman, I. (Eds.). (2000). *Settings for health promotion.* Sage.

Poulain, M., Herm, A., & Pes, G. (2013). The Blue Zones: Areas of exceptional longevity around the world. *Vienna Yearbook of Population Research, 11*(1), 87–108.

Public Health England (2016). *Faith at end of life: A resource for professionals, providers and commissioners working in communities.* Retrieved from https://www.stgeorges.nhs.uk/wp-content/uploads/2017/01/Faith-at-end-of-life.pdf.

Ridge, D., Williams, I., Anderson, J., & Elford, J. (2008). Like a prayer: The role of spirituality and religion for people living with HIV in the UK. *Sociology of Health & Illness, 30*(3), 413–428.

Roundtable on Population Health Improvement; Board on Population Health and Public Health Practice; Institute of Medicine. Business Engagement in Building Healthy Communities: Workshop Summary. Washington (DC): National Academies Press (US). (2015, May 8). *Lessons from the Blue Zones®.* Retrieved from https://www.ncbi.nlm.nih.gov/books/NBK298903/.

The Lancet Infectious Diseases. (2020). Air travel in the time of COVID-19. *The Lancet Infectious Diseases, 20*(9), 993. https://doi.org/10.1016/S1473-3099(20)30647-2

Tomalin, E., Sadgrove, J., & Summers, R. (2019). Health, Faith and Therapeutic Landscapes: Places of worship as Black, Asian and Minority Ethnic (BAME) public health settings in the United Kingdom. *Social Science and Medicine.*

Tomalin, E., & Sadgrove, J. (2016) *Places of Worship as Minority Ethnic Public Health Settings in Bradford.* Retrieved from http://www.faithaction.net/resources/.

Tomalin, E., Sadgrove, J., & Russell, A. (2015). *Places of Worship as Minority Ethnic Public Health Settings in Leeds.* Retrieved from http://www.leeds.gov.uk/docs/Places%20of%20Worship%20as%20Minority%20Public%20Health%20Settings%20in%20Leeds.pdf.

Thurston, W. E. and Blundell-Gosselin, H. J. (2005) The farm as a setting for health promotion: results of a needs assessment in South Central Alberta. Health & Place Volume 11, Issue 1, 31-43 doi:10.1016/j.healthplace.2004.01.001.

Western Sydney Planning Partnership. (2020). *Draft Aerotropolis Precinct Plan.* NSW Government.

Walton, J. K. (1983). *The English seaside resort. A social history 1750–1914.* Leicester University Press.

Watson, M. (2008). Going for gold: The health promoting general practice. *Quality in Primary Care, 16*, 177–185.

Western Sydney Regional Organisation of Councils. (2015). *Review of Western Sydney Airport Draft Environmental Impact Statement Sydney.* Parsons Brinckerhoff Australia.

Wenzel, E. (1997) A comment on settings in health promotion. Internet Journal of Health Promotion. https://checkpoint.url-protection.com/v1/url?o=http%3A//ldb.org/setting.htm&g=ZmIwOTE5ZjU5OGNmMWNkMw==&h=OTUxNGI1Y2I2MGQ4NzFlZTEzZWE5YjZkYj

BkMDBhNWM1NjBlNDM5YjFjNDk1ZTExZTU1ZDBkZTdhOTg2NTgxNA==&p=Y3Ax ZTp1Y2xhbmxpdmU6Y2hlY2twb2ludDpvZmZpY2UzNjVfZW1haWxxX2VtYWlsOjAyM GY1YmQxN2I2ODhhODdkMzAyZWJhYTNjMDY5M2Y5OnYx (accessed 10 May 2021).

Wheeler, B. W., White, M., Stahl-Timmins, W., & Depledge, M. H. (2012). Does living by the coast improve health and wellbeing? *Health & Place, 18*(5), 1198–1201.

Woodall, J., & Rowlands, S. (2021). In R. Cross, L. Warwick-Booth, S. Rowlands, J. Woodall, I. O'Neil, & S. Foster (Eds.), *Health promotion. Global principles and practice*. CABI.

World Health Organization. (1997). *Twenty steps for developing a healthy cities project* (No. EUR/ ICP/HSC 644 (2)). Copenhagen: WHO Regional Office for Europe.

World Health Organization. (2015). 2015 Yanuca Island Declaration on health in Pacific island countries and territories: Eleventh Pacific Health Ministers Meeting, 15–17 April 2015.

World Health Organization. (2017). Shanghai consensus on healthy cities 2016. *Health Promotion International, 32*(4), 603–605.

Yuill, C., Crinson, I., & Duncan, E. (2010). *Key concepts in health studies*. Sage Publications.

Part III
Gaia—The Ultimate Setting for Health Promotion

Chapter 14
Gaia and the Anthropocene: The Ultimate Determinant of Health

Trevor Hancock

Take a look around you. Chances are you are in a building in a city or town. Globally, we are 55% urbanized; North America, Latin America and the Caribbean are the most highly urbanized region at more than 80%, followed by Europe (74%), Oceania (68%), Asia (approximately 50%) and Africa (43%) (UN Department of Economic and Social Affairs, 2018). In North America, people spend about 90% of their time indoors (Leech et al., 1996; Klepeis et al., 2001). But look a bit further. Where is your built environment located? We are all situated within a regional and ultimately a global ecosystem, within which we spend 100% of our time. It is the ultimate setting, our only home—and thus the ultimate determinant of our health.

The Earth provides us—and the myriad species with whom we share the Earth—a set of vitally important ecosystem goods and services: air, water, food, fuel, materials, waste detoxification and disposal, protection from UV radiation and a generally stable climate—at least for the past 11,000 years of the Holocene. These are the ecological determinants of our health, and they are even more fundamental to our health—and indeed to our very survival—than the social determinants of health, with which they interact (Hancock et al., 2015).

In this and the next chapter (Chap. 15), I will first explore Gaia—the Earth, our home—as a living entity in its own right; as the ultimate determinant of our health, it is the ultimate setting for health promotion. This is followed by an examination of the Anthropocene, a new geologic epoch that is replacing the Holocene. As its name implies, this new epoch is human-created; we have become a force of nature equal to or greater than natural forces.

These changes in turn are driven by the socio-cultural phenomenon of a globalized twenty-first-century industrial and post-industrial/digital age, with a focus on progress understood largely as growth in material and financial wealth. But

T. Hancock (✉)
School of Public Health and Social Policy, University of Victoria, Victoria, BC, Canada
e-mail: Thancock@uvic.ca

© Springer Nature Switzerland AG 2022
S. Kokko, M. Baybutt (eds.), *Handbook of Settings-Based Health Promotion*,
https://doi.org/10.1007/978-3-030-95856-5_14

human-driven global ecological changes threaten our health and the stability and perhaps even survival of our societies.

In Chap. 15, I turn from an examination of the problem to a discussion of potential solutions, which require us to take a socio-ecological approach to health, recognizing public health as a branch of human and social ecology. What we might call "Health promotion 2.0" (Hancock, 2015) needs to integrate both social and ecological sustainability and justice. We need to help imagine and then create a future where governance is focused not on unsustainable—and thus unattainable—growth in material prosperity, but on sustainable, equitable human development. Among other things, this calls for a new economic system, which we might call an economics for well-being. These concepts fit well with the Geneva Charter for Well-being (WHO, 2021), the product of the 10th Global Conference on Health Promotion in December 2021. The Charter calls for the creation of well-being societies "committed to achieving equitable health now and for future generations without breaching ecological limits". Importantly, the first rwo of five action areas are to "Value, respect and nurture planet Earth and its ecosystems" and "Design an equitable economy that serves human development within planetary and local ecological boundaries".

I will close by discussing the work I and others are doing to re-think one of the key healthy settings approaches—healthy cities and communities. What would our cities and communities be like if we had to live within the natural limits of the Earth, with an ecological footprint equivalent to one planet's worth of biocapacity and resources—while at the same time maintaining a high quality of life and good health for all? We might call it "Healthy Cities 2.0" (Hancock, 2018). How might we make that happen?

14.1 Gaia: The Earth—Is Our Home

Gaia was the name the Ancient Greeks gave to the Earth goddess, Mother Earth. But the concept of the Earth as our Mother is much older, perhaps as old as humanity itself. It is preserved today in some form in Indigenous and many other traditions around the world and is even included in something as modern as the recent Ecuador Constitution, which recognizes and protects the rights of Pacha Mama (Mother Earth) (Boyd, 2012). The Indigenous Peoples' Statement for Planetary Health and Sustainable Development developed at the IUHPE Global Health Promotion Conference in Rotorua, Aotearoa New Zealand in 2019, states:

> "Core features of Indigenous worldviews are the interactive relationship between spiritual and material realms, intergenerational and collective orientations, that Mother Earth is a living being – a 'person' with whom we have special relationships that are a foundation for identity, and the interconnectedness and interdependence between all that exists, which locates humanity as part of Mother Earth's ecosystems alongside our relations in the natural world" (IUHPE, 2019).

The concept has also been widely used in recent decades in many "new age" groups that have sought a set of beliefs and values more commensurate with an holistic and perhaps spiritual understanding of our relationship with the Earth.

The Earth is not only our Mother, it is also our home—our only home, a point brought home to us in dramatic fashion in 1968 with the first photos of the Earth from moon orbit; it quite literally changed our view of ourselves and of the Earth. Despite the fantasies of Elon Musk and others who want to colonize Mars and beyond, it is the only home we will ever have. There are no other livable planets within our reach, so we must live here on Earth, and within the limits of Earth's ability to nurture life—all life, not just humanity but the entire web of life of which we are a part, and upon which we depend, which means we must understand the Earth in all its complexity, its limits and our place within it.

14.1.1   Gaia as a Living Organism, and Earth System Science

In recent years, the concept of Gaia has also been given a scientific interpretation: Gaia was the name that planetary scientist James Lovelock (1972) gave to his hypothesis that the Earth itself is a living entity:

> [The] "concept of the Earth as a very large living creature, Gaia, several giga-years old who has moulded the surface, the oceans, and the air to suit her and for the very brief time we have been part of her, our needs."

Lovelock's understanding of Gaia as a living system did not come from the widespread and deep cultural myths of the Earth as our Mother, but from thinking about "just how well suited is the environment of Earth for life" (Lovelock, 1972) and how we would identify life on other planets. He has also referred to his Gaia Theory as Earth System Science, which is defined by the Earth System Science Partnership (consisting of four international global change research programmes) as:

> "The study of the Earth System, with an emphasis on observing, understanding and predicting global environmental changes involving interactions between land, atmosphere, water, ice, biosphere, societies, technologies and economies." (Earth System Science Partnership, 2001).

A very important point here is that the Earth System is not seen as simply a natural ecosystem, but as a system that includes both natural (land, atmosphere, water, ice, biosphere) and social (societies, technologies and economies) components.

Worryingly, the Amsterdam Declaration (2001) noted— more than 20 years ago:

> "In terms of some key environmental parameters, the *Earth System has moved well outside the range of the natural variability exhibited over the last half million years at least*. The nature of changes now occurring simultaneously in the Earth System, their magnitudes and rates of change are unprecedented."

Since then, the situation has significantly worsened, with worrisome implications for health and social well-being, as will be discussed later.

14.1.2   Gaia: The Ultimate Determinant of Our Health

There are many factors that affect the health of populations, from sub-atomic particles and radiation (e.g., UV radiation from the sun, radon gas in rocks in some parts of the world) to molecules (hormones, chemical pollutants) and on up through our genes to cellular, physiological and organ system functions, mental processes and functions. Beyond our bodies lie the social realms of family, peers, community and society with all the social, economic and cultural factors of gender, age, ethnicity, indigeneity, income, education and so on. Then, there are the physical realms of our built environments (home, school, work, neighbourhood, city) and the natural environment, both locally and—ultimately—globally.

But arguably, the most fundamental determinants of health are what we have come to call the ecological determinants of health (Hancock et al., 2015). We need air, water and food to survive, as do all other species, each in their own way. We can last a few minutes without oxygen, a few days at most without water, a few weeks at most without food. We and other species also depend upon the stratospheric ozone layer to protect us from the sun's UV radiation, and natural cycles to replace water and nutrients and to remove and decompose wastes.

But unlike other species, we humans also depend upon fuels to heat our dwellings, cook our food and—in this industrial age—power our societies, and materials to build our homes, tools and all our goods and infrastructure. And we have developed civilization—agriculture, cities and all that goes with these developments—within the relatively warm and stable climate of the Holocene over the past 11,000 years. All of this comes from nature, as a package of what are sometimes called ecosystem goods and services, which WHO's Director General described as

> "the ultimate foundations of life and health, even though in modern societies this fundamental dependency may be indirect, displaced in space and time, and therefore poorly recognized" (Foreword in WHO, 2005)

14.1.3   Gaia as the Ultimate Setting for Health Promotion

One way to think of a setting is that it is both a physical place and a social space—it is where our physical and social environments intersect and interact at significant "nodes" in our lives. Those nodes include home, school, workplace, institutional settings such as hospitals and prisons, our neighbourhoods, towns and cities.

So is the Earth—Gaia—a setting? We should recall that Earth System Science understands that the Earth "behaves as a single, self-regulating system comprised of physical, chemical, biological and human components" (Earth System Science Partnership, 2001). Clearly, then, the Earth can be considered a setting, in that it is a significant node in our lives, it is both a physical place and a social space and that these components interact, and it is the ultimate determinant of our health—which makes it the ultimate setting for health promotion. The implications of this understanding for health promotion and health promoters will be discussed in this chapter and in Chap. 15.

14.2   Welcome to the Anthropocene

I noted in the previous section that human civilization as we know it evolved following the last Ice Age, during the 11,000-year warm interglacial period known as the Holocene. But we are leaving the Holocene and entering a new geologic epoch, the Anthropocene (Steffen et al., 2011; Waters et al., 2016; Gaffney & Steffen, 2017). As its name suggests—*anthropos* being the ancient Greek term for human—it is the age of humans. But note, this is not called the Anthropocene because it is about or for us, but because it is caused by us, the result of human activity.

The term in its modern sense is new—it was proposed by Nobel prize-winning chemist Paul Crutzen at a meeting of the Scientific Committee of the International Geosphere-Biosphere Program (IGBP)—because the phenomenon is new: Crutzen and Stoermer (2000) noted:

> "Considering . . . (the) major and still growing impacts of human activities on earth and atmosphere, and at all, including global, scales it seems to us more than appropriate to emphasize the central role of mankind in geology and ecology by proposing to use the term 'anthropocene' for the current geological epoch."

Note that they see it in both geological and ecological terms, to which I would add that it is also important to see it as a socio-cultural phenomenon. In this section, I will discuss these three aspects of the Anthropocene and the profound health implications of these massive eco-social changes.

(For a succinct but powerful introduction to the Anthropocene, see the 3.5-min video produced for the "Planet Under Pressure" conference in London in 2012; available at https://www.youtube.com/watch?v=fvgG-pxlobk)

14.2.1   The Anthropocene as a Geological Phenomenon

Geological ages are identified by the International Commission on Stratigraphy, based on the signals they leave in the planet's rocks, which are technically called chrono-stratigraphic units: (Williams et al., 2016). Perhaps the most famous of these is the layer of iridium at the Cretaceous–Tertiary (K–T) boundary that marks the impact of the asteroid 65 million years ago that triggered the extinction of the dinosaurs, the fifth and most recent "Great Extinction" that life on Earth has experienced.

Modern human presence on Earth has been apparent in the geologic strata for hundreds of thousands of years, dating back to the presence of stone tools in the Palaeolithic Age (three million to about 11,000 years ago). But until comparatively recently, the geologic record showed only "mere human presence and localized influences on various environments" However, since the mid-twentieth century, there has been growing evidence of "significant human influence upon several key global biogeochemical cycles, with attendant influences on the climate system." (Williams et al., 2016).

This led the International Commission on Stratigraphy to create an Anthropocene Working Group (AWG) in 2009. The AWG has noted the presence of unique human markers in new stratigraphic layers: These include new human-created materials (concrete, plastic, glass, pure aluminium, radioactive materials from fallout, persistent organic pollutants (s)), marked changes in levels of important chemicals as a result of human activity (carbon dioxide, nitrogen, phosphorus) and a shift in fossil assemblages.

Emblematic of the sixth Great Extinction we are triggering, we have dramatically reduced the biomass of both land and marine mammals and roughly halved fish and plant biomass; "the present-day biomass of wild land mammals is approximately sevenfold lower" than it was 50,000 years ago, before we started wiping out the large land mammals (Bar-On et al., 2018). As a result, we now outweigh wild animals tenfold (Bar-On et al., 2018); future palaeontologists will see that we humans make up about one third of the mass of all land vertebrates and our domesticated species make up almost all of the remainder, with wild species now comprising less than 5% (Waters et al., 2016; Zalasiewicz, 2016).

In May 2019, the AWG voted 88% in favour of treating the Anthropocene as "a formal chrono-stratigraphic unit" with a base "around the mid-twentieth century of the Common Era" (International Commission on Stratigraphy, 2019).

14.2.2   The Anthropocene as an Ecological Phenomenon

The stratigraphic changes that signal the Anthropocene as a geological phenomenon are markers of the global ecological changes that human activity has created. Of these, the best known is climate change, which has been described by the two Lancet Commissions on climate change and health as "the biggest global health threat of the 21st century" (Costello et al., 2009) and as posing "an unacceptably high and potentially catastrophic risk to human health" (Watts et al., 2015).

But it is much more than climate change, important though that is. Other global scale ecological changes we are creating—all of which have important health implications (Hancock et al., 2015)—include the following:

- Acidifying the oceans;
- Changing the great cycles of life (e.g., water, carbon, nitrogen and phosphorus);
- Polluting entire ecosystems with POPs (many of which are endocrine disruptors), heavy metals and plastic and other nano-particles;
- Using renewable resources at unsustainable rates (e.g., freshwater, forests, fisheries, soils and farmlands);

- Depleting some key non-renewable resources (e.g., fossil fuels, some minerals);
- Creating a sixth Great Extinction.

Moreover, we are creating these changes all at the same time, and they often interact—and often in ways that amplify their effects. The scale and breadth of the ecological changes now underway are well captured in three key indicators:

- **Planetary Boundaries:** We are now approaching and in some cases have crossed estimated planetary boundaries that constitute the margins of a "safe operating space" for humans. Of ten key earth systems, we have moved into a zone of high risk for 2 of them (nitrogen and phosphorus flows and for species extinctions); are in a zone of increasing risk for three others (climate system change, land system change and ocean acidification) and do not know the boundary of risk for three others ("novel entities," which are persistent organic pollutants (POPs), heavy metals, nano-particles and GMOs; atmospheric aerosol loading; functional biodiversity), although it has recently been suggested that we have crossed the planetary boundary for novel entities (Persson et al., 2022); only in two systems—freshwater use and stratospheric ozone depletion—are we sure we are in a safe zone—see Fig. 14.1 (Steffen et al., 2015a).
- **The Ecological Footprint:** The ecological footprint (EF) converts human resource demands and waste production into a common metric—the number of hectares of bio-productive land it would take to replace the resource or absorb

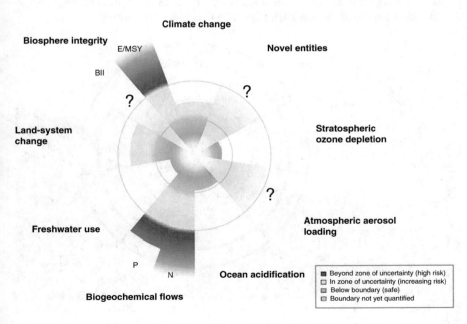

Fig. 14.1 Crossing Planetary Boundaries. (*Source*: Steffen et al. (2015a). Reprinted with permission from AAAS)

the wastes. It is not an exact measure; for example, POPs are not included, since no method to convert their impact to a land equivalent has been found.

- Often expressed as the number of Earths we require, we surpassed the Earth's bio-productive capacity in about 1970. Currently (not really current, this is 2016 data, the most recent available), "humans use as much ecological resources as if we lived on 1.75 Earths" (Global Footprint Network, 2019), which is clearly unsustainable—and more than half that global EF is due to carbon emissions (Fig. 14.2).
- But high-income countries (HICs) on average used 3.6 times the available biocapacity of 1.7 gha per person, far more than their fair share. So if the entire planet were to live the way HICs live, we would need another 2 or 3 planets; if we all lived as Americans, Canadians, and Australians live (5 planets' worth), we would need 4 more Earths (Global Footprint Network, 2019).
- Yet we all know that we only have one planet, so—as will be discussed later—we have to learn to live in a healthy way with an ecological footprint of just one planet. For HICs as a whole, this will require about a 70% reduction, while for the USA, Canada, and Australia, it requires an 80% reduction in the footprint.
- **The Living Planet Index:** Produced every 2 years by the World Wide Fund for Nature (WWF), the Living Planet Index (LPI) measures trends in the populations of vertebrate species (mammals, birds, reptiles, amphibians and fish) in terrestrial, marine and freshwater ecosystems around the world. Their 2020 report, with data only up to 2016, covers 20,811 populations of 4392 species. It shows an overall global decline in the abundance of monitored vertebrate populations of 68% between 1970 and 2016 (Fig. 14.3)—a mere 46 years! (WWF, 2020).

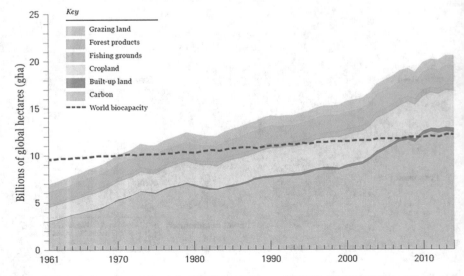

Fig. 14.2 Global Ecological Footprint, 1961–2014. (*Source*: WWF—World Wide Fund for Nature (2018) Living Planet Report—2018: Aiming Higher, © 2018 WWF—All rights reserved)

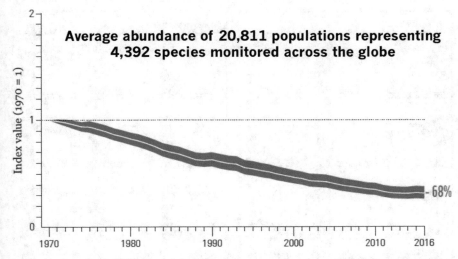

Fig. 14.3 Living Planet Index, 1970–2016. (*Source*: WWF—World Wide Fund for Nature (2020) Living Planet Report—2020—Bending the curve of biodiversity loss. © 2020 WWF—All rights reserved)

Moreover, things may be moving at a much faster rate than was feared, and we may be reaching a point of no return, at least with respect to climate change, where we risk triggering "tipping cascades" that could make the process essentially irreversible. (Lenton et al., 2019—and see section below on the Anthropocene as an existential threat.)

14.2.3   The Anthropocene as a Sociocultural Phenomenon

While the Anthropocene is at one level simply a geological marker of the changes we are creating in global ecosystems, another way to understand it is that it is a metaphor for the human-driven changes in global ecological systems. It can be seen as shorthand for our global socioeconomic and technological systems and the underlying values and beliefs that drive our current development path.

The forces that drive these changes are threefold; population growth, economic growth and technological power. We have seen a massive—although globally uneven—expansion in the human population, in our wealth and material demands and in the power of our technology, all driven by a belief in progress as continued growth in material wealth. However, this ignores the reality that we live within a finite geophysical and ecological system—the Earth. As Kenneth Boulding, at one time President of both the American Economic Association and the American Association for the Advancement of Science, noted:

"Anyone who believes exponential growth can go on forever in a finite world is either a madman or an economist" (US Congress, 1973, p. 248).

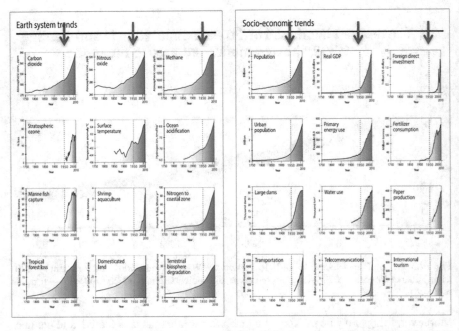

Fig. 14.4 The Great Acceleration. (*Source*: Steffen, Will; Broadgate, Wendy; Deutsch, Lisa; Gaffney, Owen and Ludwig, Cornelia (2015a). The trajectory of the Anthropocene: The Great Acceleration The Anthropocene Review 2(1) 81–98)

Not only has the change been massive in its scale, the rate of change in a wide variety of both socioeconomic and natural systems also has been very rapid in recent years. As noted earlier, the AWG has suggested the starting time for the Anthropocene is the mid-twentieth century, which coincides with what Steffen et al. (2015b) call "The Great Acceleration." As shown in Fig. 14.4, around this time (1950 is marked in red in all the charts), there was a dramatic surge in a wide array of social and economic system indicators, and a concomitant (but negative) surge in a range of natural system indicators.

So the Anthropocene is not just a geological marker of the changes we are creating in global ecosystems; it also is an indicator of the scale of human activity—we are, after all, the *anthropos* in the Anthropocene—and the accelerating rate of change, and thus serves as a warning of the present and future impacts of these changes on human and other life forms.

14.2.4 The Anthropocene as an Existential Threat

> "If the present growth trends in world population, industrialization, pollution, food production, and resource depletion continue unchanged, the limits to growth on this planet will be

reached sometime within the next 100 years. The most probable result will be a sudden and uncontrollable decline in both population and industrial capacity." (Meadows et al., 1972)

Troublingly, the statement above is not a recent one but is 50 years old at the time of writing; it comes from the Club of Rome's 1972 report *"The Limits to Growth."* A group of MIT systems scientists reported their results from an early World System computer model with which they investigated five major trends of global concern: Accelerating industrialization, rapid population growth, widespread malnutrition, depletion of non-renewable resources, and a deteriorating environment.

While savagely attacked by traditional economists, corporations, and governments, at the time, it seems they were correct, as recent evidence confirms. Turner (2008) looked back at their original scenarios and the actual record since then and concluded that:

> "Thirty years of historical data compare favourably with key features of a business-as-usual scenario called the 'standard run' scenario which results in collapse of the global system midway through the 21st century."

He later updated his examination of *The Limits* and concluded again that the business-as-usual scenario "aligns well with historical data that has been updated in this paper" (Turner, 2014).

More than a decade ago, the Board of the UN's Millennium Ecosystem Assessment, in summarizing this major UN report, stated:

> "At the heart of this assessment is a stark warning. Human activity is putting such strain on the natural functions of Earth that the ability of the planet's ecosystems to sustain future generations can no longer be taken for granted." (Millennium Ecosystem Assessment, 2005)

Since then, the situation has generally worsened, and there has been a flurry of sobering reports about the severity of our situation. People are beginning to openly raise the question as to whether these global ecological changes—and particularly climate change—pose an existential threat to humanity, and thus of course to health.

- Steffen et al. (2018) explore what they call "tipping elements"—sub-systems within the climate system that contribute to global warming and that can exhibit "tipping point behavior in which the feedback process becomes self-perpetuating after a critical threshold is crossed." Alarmingly, they conclude:

> "the Earth System may be approaching a planetary threshold that could lock in a continuing rapid pathway toward much hotter conditions—Hothouse Earth. . . . The impacts of a Hothouse Earth pathway on human societies would likely be massive, sometimes abrupt, and undoubtedly disruptive."

In a later paper, Lenton et al. (2019) conclude:

> "If damaging tipping cascades can occur and a global tipping point cannot be ruled out, then this is an existential threat to civilization."

- In a report for the Australian independent think tank Breakthrough (aka the National Centre for Climate Restoration), the authors—one of whom was formerly an international oil, gas and coal industry executive and chairman of the Australian Coal Association—found:

"Human-induced climate change is an existential risk to human civilisation: an adverse outcome that will either annihilate intelligent life or permanently and drastically curtail its potential, unless carbon emissions are rapidly reduced." (Spratt & Dunlop, 2018)

- In commenting on the summary report of the global assessment of Biodiversity and Ecosystem Services by the Intergovernmental Science-Policy Platform on Biodiversity and Ecosystem Services (IPBES), Sir Robert Watson, the chair of IPBES, stated:

  "The health of ecosystems on which we and all other species depend is deteriorating more rapidly than ever. We are eroding the very foundations of our economies, livelihoods, food security, health and quality of life worldwide." (Watson, Sir Robert, 2019)

Clearly, these statements are very worrying, and they are not popular; nobody likes to think or talk about bad news, whether it be a diagnosis of cancer at an individual level or an existential threat to humanity. This reluctance is well-illustrated in a paper from the Institute of Leadership and Sustainability (IFLAS) at the University of Cumbria in the UK (Bendell, 2018). The author, a Professor of Sustainability Leadership for many years, has concluded that we face "an inevitable near term social collapse due to climate change" and that this calls for "deep adaptation." However, he reports that the paper was rejected by a peer-reviewed journal in part because a reviewer did not want to dishearten readers.

Then, in December 2020, in a speech on the state of the planet, Antonio Guterres, the UN Secretary General, put it bluntly:

"the state of the planet is broken. Humanity is waging war on nature. This is suicidal." (Guterres, 2020)

while Bradshaw et al. (2021) believe "future environmental conditions will be far more dangerous than currently believed" and that we are underestimating the challenges we face and failing to take the necessary actions to avoid "a ghastly future."

14.2.5 Inequity in the Anthropocene

Thus far, I have been exploring the overall impact of human activity on the planet. But it is especially important in talking about "we," "us" and "ourselves" that we recognize that the people of Earth are not one equally responsible, homogeneous population. It is not the entire population that is responsible for the ecological problems we face; rather, as is always the case, there are winners and losers—and as is also always the case, those who reap the benefits are not those who bear the costs.

In its final report, the WHO Commission on the Social Determinants of Health (2008) pointed to the roots of health inequalities in the unequal distribution of power, wealth and resources. We see the same causes and the same effects with respect to the Anthropocene. The dominant development model comes from and is directly or indirectly imposed by high-income countries (HICs). These HICs have

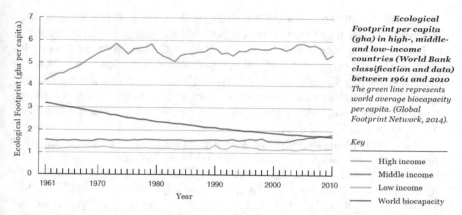

Fig. 14.5 Inequality in the Ecological Footprint, 1961–2010. (*Source*: WWF—World Wide Fund for Nature (2014) Living Planet Report © 2014 WWF—All rights reserved)

the longest life expectancies, the largest GDPs and the largest ecological footprints today (Fig. 14.5).

For example, the International Resource Panel (2017) reports that global resource use more than tripled between 1970 and 2017, "with high-income countries consuming ten times more per person than low-income countries." That level of consumption is accompanied by high levels of pollution; it is estimated that between them the USA and the EU will have contributed almost half (46%) of temperature increase resulting from overall Kyoto GHG emissions by 2100, excluding the land use, land use change and forestry sectors—and 36% if they are included (Rocha et al., 2015, Tables 2 and 3, p's 14 and 15).

Moreover, high-income people within all countries have a larger EF than low-income countries and people. Kenner (2015) examined data from several countries (USA, Japan, China, UK and France) on the expenditure patterns of the richest 10% of the population by income and found, not surprisingly perhaps, that they "spend more than each of the income deciles below them on private transport and on meat." In fact, in the USA, the top decile accounted for 23% of all household expenditure. More broadly, Berthe and Elie (2015) summarized a 2008 OECD review as finding "most studies conclude that consumption behaviour-related environmental pressure increases with household income," including "waste, recycling, transportation choices and domestic use of energy and water."

Not surprisingly, this is also true of carbon emissions. The World Inequality Report 2022 (Chancel et al., 2021) found that globally the people who are the "top 10% of emitters are responsible for close to 50% of all emissions, while the bottom 50% produce 12% of the total". This is also true across regions. The same report found that the top 10 percent of emitters in North America emitted 7 times that of the bottom 50 percent per person, and more than twice that of the top 10 percent in Europe.

In Canada, the EF of the richest 10% of the population in 2002 (based on income) was nearly 2.5 times larger than that of the poorest 10% (Mackenzie et al., 2008). In fact, the per person footprint of the richest 10% of Canadians in 2002 was 25% greater than that of the country with the largest footprint in 2009. When it comes to carbon emissions by Canadians, Chancel et al. (2021) report that since 1990 "the bottom 50% and middle 40% have reduced their emissions by 3.5 and 4.5 tonnes respectively per person, [while] emissions of the top 10% have increased by around 4 tonnes per person".

Thus, wealthy countries and wealthy people are responsible for generating most of the harm we are doing to the Earth. But the burden of those problems will be borne unequally, with the wealthy generally benefitting and the poor generally suffering the consequences, which is why the World Inequality Report 2022 (Chancel et al., 2021) concludes "Large inequalities in [carbon] emissions suggest that climate policies should target wealthy polluters more".

Not surprisingly, the inequality is also reflected in the Living Planet Index (Fig. 14.6); HICs actually had a 10% increase in their LPIs from 1970 to 2010, while middle-income countries (MICs) saw a decline of 18% and low-income countries (LICs) experienced a 58% reduction in their LPI.

Some of the increase of the LPI in the HICs may be because they had already experienced a large reduction in their wildlife during the nineteenth and early twentieth century as they industrialized, urbanized and grew wealthier, and in the mid- to late twentieth century began to invest in pollution reduction, habitat protection and species conservation. But it also seems likely that they were protecting their own biodiversity while increasing their wealth and ecological footprint by exploiting the resources of MICs and LICs, which would account for the dramatic declines in those countries.

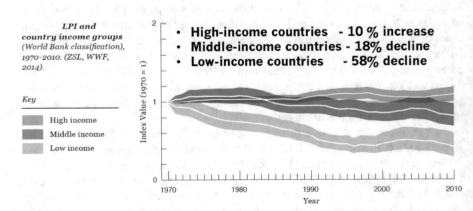

Fig. 14.6 Inequality in the Living Planet Index, 1961–2010. (*Source*: WWF—World Wide Fund for Nature (2014) Living Planet Report © 2014 WWF—All rights reserved)

14.3   Summary

The Earth is our Mother, our only home, and through the provision of a fundamental set of life support systems—air, water food, materials, fuels and so on—the ultimate determinant of our health. But the Earth is not simply an inert platform on which we live, in some way separate from us; it is a complex dynamic system involving inter-actions between land, atmosphere, water, ice, biosphere, societies, technologies and economies. The Earth is thus an eco-social system, both a physical place and a social space, which makes it a setting, in fact, the ultimate setting for health promotion.

But we are creating massive and rapid changes in the Earth systems of which we are a part and upon which we depend for our health and well-being, indeed our very existence. Rapid increases in population, wealth and technology, especially since the mid-twentieth century, have combined to make humanity a force of nature. We are heating the planet, acidifying its oceans, polluting its food chains, depleting its resources and causing a new Great Extinction. These changes, collectively known as the Anthropocene, are arguably the greatest threat to health we face in the twenty-first century.

But the term "we" is misleading. In reality, it is high-income people and high-income countries that cause most of the problems, while low-income people and countries bear much of the burden and shoulder many of the costs. This compounds existing inequalities in health. So any attempt to improve the health of the popula-tion in the twenty-first century and reduce inequalities in health, both locally and globally, needs to come face to face with the Anthropocene, and the human social and economic systems and underlying values that drive it.

References

Bar-On, Y. M., Phillips, R., & Milo, R. (2018). The biomass distribution on Earth. *PNAS, 115*, 6506–6511.

Bendell, J. (2018). *Deep adaptation: A map for navigating climate tragedy* (IFLAS Occasional Paper 2). Institute of Leadership and Sustainability (IFLAS), University of Cumbria, UK. Retrieved from http://www.lifeworth.com/deepadaptation.pdf.

Berthe, A., & Elie, L. (2015). Mechanisms explaining the impact of economic inequality on envi-ronmental deterioration. *Ecological Economics, 116*, 191–200.

Boyd, D. (2012). *The right to a healthy environment: Revitalizing Canada's constitution Vancouver*. UBC Press.

Bradshaw, C., Ehrlich, P. R., Beattie, A., et al. (2021). Underestimating the challenges of avoiding a ghastly future. *Front. Conserv. Sci., 1*, 615419. https://doi.org/10.3389/fcosc.2020.615419

Chancel, L., Piketty, T., Saez, E., Zucman, G. et al. (2021). *World Inequality Report* 2022 World Inequality Lab. Available at https://wir2022.wid.world/ Accessed 11 February 2022

Costello, A., Abbas, M., Allen, A., et al. (2009). Managing the health effects of climate change. *Lancet, 373*, 1693–1733.

Crutzen, P. J., & Stoermer, E. F. (2000). The 'Anthropocene'. *International Geosphere-Biosphere Program Newsletter, 41*, 17–18.

Earth System Science Partnership. (2001). *Amsterdam declaration on earth system science.* Retrieved January 30, 2020, from http://www.igbp.net/about/history/2001amsterdamdeclarationonoonearthsystemscience.4.1b8ae20512db692f2a680001312.html.

Gaffney, O., & Steffen, W. (2017). *The Anthropocene equation, The Anthropocene Review.* https://doi.org/10.1177/2053019616688022

Global Footprint Network. (2019). *National footprint accounts: Ecological footprint and biocapacity* (Data Year 2016). Retrieved January 29, 2020, from https://www.footprintnetwork.org/.

Guterres, A. (2020). *The State of the Planet* (UN Secretary-General's address at Columbia University, 2 December 2020). Retrieved from https://www.un.org/sg/en/content/sg/statement/2020-12-02/secretary-generals-address-columbia-university-the-state-of-the-planet-scroll-down-for-language-versions.

Hancock, T. (2015). Population health promotion 2.0: An eco-social approach to public health in the Anthropocene. *Canadian Journal of Public Health, 106*(4), e252–e255. https://doi.org/10.17269/CJPH.106.5161

Hancock, T. (2018). Healthy Cities 2.0: Transitioning towards 'One Planet' cities (Key challenges facing 21st century cities, Part 3). *Cities & Health, 1*(3). https://doi.org/10.1080/23748834.2018.1526659

Hancock, T., Spady, D. W., & Soskolne, C. L. (Eds.). (2015). *Global change and public health: Addressing the ecological determinants of health: The report in brief.* Canadian Public Health Association. Retrieved from www.cpha.ca/sites/default/files/assets/policy/edh-brief.pdf.

International Commission on Stratigraphy (2019) *Working group on the 'Anthropocene'—Results of binding vote by AWG subcommission on quaternary stratigraphy.* Retrieved May 21, 2019, from http://quaternary.stratigraphy.org/working-groups/anthropocene/.

International Resource Panel. (2017). *Assessing global resource use: A systems approach to resource efficiency and pollution reduction* (Summary for Policy Makers) United Nations Environment Programme, Nairobi, Kenya.

IUHPE. (2019). *Waiora–indigenous peoples' statement for planetary health and sustainable development.* Retrieved from https://www.iuhpe2019.com/PicsHotel/iuhpe/Brochure/Indigenous%20Statement%20for%20Plenary%20Revised.pdf.

Kenner, D. (2015). *Inequality of overconsumption: The ecological footprint of the richest.* GSI Working Paper 2015/2. Cambridge: Global Sustainability Institute, Anglia Ruskin University.

Klepeis, N. E., et al. (2001). *The National Human Activity Pattern Survey (NHAPS): A resource for assessing exposure to environmental pollutants.* Lawrence Berkeley National Laboratory.

Leech, J. A., Wilby, K., McMullen, E., & Laporte, K. (1996). The Canadian human activity pattern survey: Report of methods and population surveyed. *Chronic Diseases in Canada, 17*(3/4), 118–123.

Lenton, T., Rockström, J., Gaffney, O., Rahmstorf, S., Richardson, K., et al. (2019). Climate tipping points—Too risky to bet against. *Nature, 575*, 592–595.

Lovelock, J. E. (1972). Gaia as seen through the atmosphere. *Atmospheric Environment, 6*, 579–580.

Mackenzie, H., Messinger, H., & Smith, R. (2008). *Size matters: Canada's ecological footprint, by income.* Canadian Centre for Policy Alternatives.

Meadows, D., Meadows, D., Randers, J., & Behrens, W. (1972). *The limits to growth.* Universe Books.

Millennium Ecosystem Assessment. (2005). *Living beyond our means: Natural assets and human well-being.* Island Press. Retrieved from https://www.millenniumassessment.org/documents/document.429.aspx.pdf.

Persson, L., Almroth, B. M. C., Collins, C. D. et al. (2022). Outside the Safe Operating Space of the Planetary Boundary for Novel Entities *Environmental Science & Technology, 56*(3) 1510–1521. https://doi.org/10.1021/acs.est.1c04158

Rocha, M., et al. (2015). *Historical responsibility for climate change—From countries emissions to contribution to temperature increase.* Climate Analytics and Potsdam Institute for Climate

Impact Research. Retrieved July 5, 2019, from https://climateanalytics.org/media/historical_ responsibility_report_nov_2015.pdf.

Spratt, D., & Dunlop, I. (2018). *What lies beneath: The understatement of existential climate risk.* Breakthrough - National Centre for Climate Restoration.

Steffen, W., Broadgate, W., Deutsch, L., Gaffney, O., & Ludwig, C. (2015b). The trajectory of the Anthropocene: The great acceleration. *The Anthropocene Review, 2*(1), 81–98.

Steffen, W., Grinevald, J., Crutzen, P., et al. (2011). The Anthropocene: Conceptual and historical perspectives. *Philosophical Transactions of the Royal Society A: Mathematical, Physical and Engineering Sciences, 369*(1938), 842–867.

Steffen, W., Richardson, K., Rockström, J., et al. (2015a). Planetary boundaries: Guiding human development on a changing planet. *Science, 347*(6223), 1259855-1–1259855-10.

Steffen, W., Rockström, J., Richardson, K., Lenton, T. M., Folke, C., et al. (2018). Trajectories of the earth system in the Anthropocene. *PNAS, 115*(33), 8252–8259.

Turner, G. A. (2008). *Comparison of the limits to growth with thirty years of reality.* CSIRO.

Turner, G. (2014). *Is global collapse imminent?* (MSSI research paper no. 4) Melbourne, Australia: Melbourne Sustainable Society Institute, the University of Melbourne.

UN Department of Economic and Social Affairs. (2018). *2018 revision of World Urbanization Prospects.* Population Division, UNDESA. Retrieved from https://www.un.org/development/desa/en/news/population/2018-revision-of-world-urbanization-prospects.html.

US Congress. (1973). Energy reorganization act of 1973: Hearings. In *Ninety-third Congress, first session, on H.R. 11510.* p. 248.

Waters, C., Zalasiewicz, J., Summerhayes, C., et al. (2016). The Anthropocene is functionally and stratigraphically distinct from the Holocene. *Science, 351*(6269), aad2622-1–aad2622-10.

Watson, Sir Robert. (2019). *IPBES Chair - Quoted in UN Report: Nature's Dangerous Decline 'Unprecedented'; Species Extinction Rates 'Accelerating'.* Retrieved from https://www.un.org/sustainabledevelopment/blog/2019/05/nature-decline-unprecedented-report/.

Watts, N., Adger, N., Agnolucci, P., et al. (2015). Health and climate change: Policy responses to protect public health. *Lancet. Published Online June, 23,* 2015. https://doi.org/10.1016/S0140-6736(15)60854-6

WHO. (2005). *Ecosystems and Human Well-being: Synthesis* (Millennium Ecosystem Assessment) Washington, DC: Island Press. Retrieved July 9, 2014, from www.unep.org/maweb/documents/document.356.aspx.pdf.

WHO Commission on the Social Determinants of Health. (2008). *Closing the gap in a generation: Health equity through action on the social determinants of health* (Final Report–Executive Summary). Geneva: WHO. Retrieved from http://whqlibdoc.who.int/hq/2008/WHO_IER_CSDH_08.1_eng.pdf.

WHO. (2021). *The Geneva Charter for Well-being.* Geneva: WHO. Available at https://cdn.who.int/media/docs/default-source/health-promotion/geneva-charter---unedited---15.12.2021.pdf?sfvrsn=f55dec7_5&download=true Accessed 11 February, 2022

Williams, M., et al. (2016). The Anthropocene: A conspicuous stratigraphical signal of anthropogenic changes in production and consumption across the biosphere. *Earth's Future, 4,* 34–53. https://doi.org/10.1002/2015EF000339

WWF. (2014). In R. Mclellan, L. Iyengar, B. Jeffries, & N. Oerlemans (Eds.), *Living planet report—2014: People and places, species and spaces.* WWF International.

WWF International. (2018). In M. Grooten & R. E. A. Almond (Eds.), *Living planet report—2018: Aiming higher.* WWF International.

WWF. (2020). In R. E. A. Almond, M. Grooten, & T. Petersen (Eds.), *Living Planet Report 2020 - Bending the curve of biodiversity loss (Summary).* WWF.

Zalasiewicz, J. (2016). A history in layers. *Scientific American Special, 25*(5), 104–111.

Chapter 15
Health Promotion in the Anthropocene

Trevor Hancock

15.1 Health in the Anthropocene

Having considered in Chapter 14 the concept of Gaia as a setting—the ultimate setting—for health promotion, and the advent of the Anthropocene as a geological, ecological and socio-cultural phenomenon, it is time to consider what all this means for the health of the population, the work of health promotion and the emergence of a new field of work—planetary health.

15.1.1 The Health Implications of the Anthropocene

"Protect and preserve the source of human health: Nature".
Prescription 1, WHO Manifesto for a Healthy Recovery from Covid-19 (WHO, 2020a)

While the health impacts of climate change have received a lot of attention, it is only one part of the human-driven global ecological changes that constitute the Anthropocene. So it is the Anthropocene as a whole that is arguably the greatest threat—or at least second only to all-out nuclear war—to the health and indeed to the survival of both human and many non-human species in the twenty-first century.

Increasingly, the WHO recognises this, as the quote above from the WHO indicates, a sentiment that is repeated in the WHO's special report on climate change and health, (WHO, 2021a) and in the Geneva Charter for Well-being (WHO, 2021b). That recognition perhaps dates back to its participation in the UN's Millennium Ecosystem Assessment; writing in the health synthesis then the Director General noted "Nature's goods and services are the ultimate foundations of life and health"

T. Hancock (✉)
School of Public Health and Social Policy, University of Victoria, Victoria, BC, Canada
e-mail: Thancock@uvic.ca

© Springer Nature Switzerland AG 2022
S. Kokko, M. Baybutt (eds.), *Handbook of Settings-Based Health Promotion*,
https://doi.org/10.1007/978-3-030-95856-5_15

and called on the health sector "to ensure that the benefits that the natural environment provides to human health and wellbeing are preserved for future generations" (Millennium Ecosystem Assessment, 2005).

The health implications of climate change have been recognised for many years (IPCC, 1996) and WHO has been involved in addressing this issue since at least the early twenty-first century (WHO, 2003). In addition, WHO has a joint work program with the Convention on Biological Diversity on the health implications of the loss of biodiversity (see below for more on WHO's work on both these issues).

The health implications of the Anthropocene—especially climate change—are not hard to imagine. At their most extreme, as noted above, we may be facing an existential threat. While this does not mean that the human species will become extinct—although species routinely become extinct, and we should not imagine we are immune to the laws of nature—it means that we may be facing a threat to the stability and survival of many societies and civilisations around the world. Clearly, this would have profound adverse effects on the health of those populations.

Even if we can avoid this drastic outcome, we know there is a wide range of serious health impacts, which are well documented in the literature (see e.g. Hancock et al., 2015; Whitmee et al., 2015). There are five main categories of changes, each of which poses health threats in their own right:

- Global warming
- Ocean acidification
- Resource depletion
- Pollution and ecotoxicity
- Species extinction (Hancock et al., 2015)

However, since they often combine and interact in ways that multiply their effect, it is the combination of these changes—the Anthropocene—that poses the overall threat to health and wellbeing.

- These health threats are particularly well understood for climate change; the IPCC reported in 2014 with very high confidence that "if climate change continues as projected" there would be:

  - Greater risk of injury, disease and death due to more intense heat waves and fires
  - Increased risks of food- and water-borne diseases

  and with high confidence that there would be

  - Increased risk of under-nutrition resulting from diminished food production in poor regions
  - Consequences for health of lost work capacity and reduced labour productivity in vulnerable populations (Smith et al., 2014)

- WHO recognises that climate change is "the biggest global health threat of the 21st century" (WHO, 2015) and that it "threatens the essential ingredients of good health – clean air, safe drinking water, nutritious food supply and safe shelter – and has the potential to undermine decades of progress in global health". Thus WHO believes "the Paris Agreement on climate change is therefore potentially the strongest health agreement of this century" (WHO, n.d.). Its special report on climate change and health, prepared for COP26 in October 2021, provides a broad set of recommendations for what is, in essence, a dramatic transformation of our society, economy and communities that will yield not just health benefits but environmental, social and economic benefits (WHO, 2021a).

- Perhaps the greatest health concerns with respect to resource depletion are those associated with water and food supply: Depletion of fisheries, freshwater and soils, effects that are compounded by climate change, unsustainable farming and fishing practices, ocean acidification and other forms of pollution. Their impacts are already apparent, with the UN's Food and Agriculture Organisation warning in 2018 that hunger was increasing and that "climate change is among the leading causes of rising global hunger" because of "extreme weather events, land degradation and desertification, water scarcity and rising sea levels", among other factors (UNFCCC, 2018).
- The 2017 Lancet Commission on Pollution and Health (Landrigan et al., 2017) found that 16% of all deaths worldwide are attributable to pollution, but that this is "almost certainly" an underestimate, because the health impacts of large numbers of newer chemicals that have entered the market in the past 2–3 decades are not sufficiently well understood and cannot be estimated.
- It is harder to clearly estimate the health impacts of loss of biodiversity and species extinctions, although a report from the Secretariat of the Convention on Biological Diversity and WHO (2015)

"provides numerous examples of how biodiversity contributes to important ecological determinants of health, including water and air quality, food security, microbial diversity in the human microbiome, infectious disease control, pharmaceuticals and traditional medicines and mental, physical and cultural wellbeing" (Hancock et al., 2015)

while more recently WHO (2020b) has co-authored a report on integrating biodiversity in food-based interventions to support nutrition and health.

Commenting on a more recent report from the Intergovernmental Science-Policy Platform on Biodiversity and Ecosystem Services (IPBES), the Chair, Sir Robert Watson, noted:

"The health of ecosystems on which we and all other species depend is deteriorating more rapidly than ever. We are eroding the very foundations of our economies, livelihoods, food security, health and quality of life worldwide" (Watson, 2019).

15.1.2 Health Inequity in the Anthropocene

As noted in Chapter 14, the Anthropocene's ecological impacts are inequitably distributed both between and within countries, with the poor bearing the largest proportion of the burden. This means the health impacts will also be inequitably distributed, which is of course a significant concern for health promoters, and another example of the way in which the ecological and the social interact.

The Anthropocene, then, is an issue of health equity, and this will be seen at all levels from the local to the global. For example, the IPCC's 2014 *Synthesis Report Summary for Policymakers* notes:

> "Throughout the 21st century, climate change is expected to lead to increases in ill-health in many regions and especially in developing countries with low income" (Intergovernmental Panel on Climate Change, 2014, p. 15).

Similarly, the 2017 Lancet Commission on Pollution and Health noted:

> "Pollution disproportionately kills the poor and the vulnerable. Nearly 92% of pollution-related deaths occur in low-income and middle-income countries and, in countries at every income level, disease caused by pollution is most prevalent among minorities and the marginalized" (Landrigan et al., 2017).

15.1.3 Implications for Our Understanding of Health

"Health is a state of complete physical, mental and social wellbeing ..." (WHO, 1948)

As noted earlier, nature's goods and services constitute the ecological determinants of health, and are in many ways the most fundamental of all the determinants; without air, water, food, fuels and materials, life and health become difficult, if not impossible. So perhaps it is time to re-visit and revise WHO's 70-year-old definition of health to read "Health is a state of complete physical, mental, social *and ecological* wellbeing ...".

It is certainly time to recognise that the focus on the *social* determinants of health, while remaining blind to the ecological determinants, has been in part a mistake, a wrong path—or at least, only a partial path. In the background report for CPHA (Hancock et al., 2015), the authors note:

> "There is no mention of ecology, ecosystems or environment in the foundational work on population health in Canada, or in the various lists of Determinants of Health put forth by Health Canada, and later the Public Health Agency of Canada, which include 'the physical environment' as but one of a dozen or so determinants, but do not distinguish the built environment from the natural environment, nor recognize ecosystem goods and services as determinants of health."

This is not to suggest that we should turn away from the social determinants of health, but rather that we should recognise that the ecological and the social completely intersect, and this requires an eco-social approach to population health, which is what this report for CPHA calls for. Social and economic developments drive ecological changes, while ecological changes impact the wellbeing of societies, communities and individuals (see Fig. 15.1).

The CPHA report authors thus suggest that we need to expand our understanding of health to include the "health" of the ecosystems that support us, and the species that make up those ecosystems, as well as the wellbeing of future generations. They

Fig. 15.1 Eco-social model for public health action. (*Source*: Hancock et al., 2015, for the Canadian Public Health Association. Reproduced with permission)

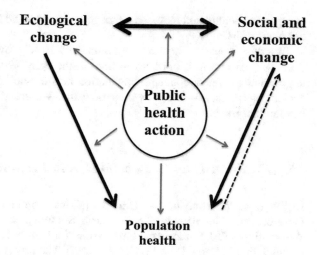

call for expanding our concept of public health ethics to include inter-species and inter-generational rights, the right of current and future generations of humans to a healthy environment and intergenerational equity and social justice, as well as the adoption and application of the precautionary principle (Hancock et al., 2015).

This expanded concept of health will need to be included in our population health models, in all health science/studies education, in research and in the development of indicators systems and the monitoring of population health. There are also clear implications for the framing of health impact assessments and the development of healthy public policy.

15.2   Health Promotion 2.0: From Social Determinants to Planetary Health

The Earth, I have argued, is the ultimate setting for health promotion. Earth System Science sees the Earth as an eco-social system, which means our interventions need to be eco-social interventions. So if we wish to improve the health and wellbeing of the Earth's population, health promotion must become an eco-social practice:

"the process of enabling the people of Earth to increase control over their own social, economic and technological systems, reduce the harm we do to ourselves and improve their health",

to reword the Ottawa Charter's definition.

In fact, this eco-social approach was embedded in the Ottawa Charter for Health Promotion (WHO, 1986), which included "stable ecosystems and sustainable resources" within the list of prerequisites for health, called for a socio-ecological approach to health, and included a pledge to "address the overall ecological issue of our ways of living".

But this aspect of health promotion was largely overlooked in the ensuing decades. The reason is not hard to find; in the early 1990s, health promotion was supplanted by a new concept—population health, with its heavy emphasis on the social determinants—and it is only now that we are slowly beginning to move beyond that fixation.

15.2.1 Towards an Eco-social Health Promotion

In 1992, at the time of the United Nations Conference on Environment and Development (the Rio de Janeiro Earth Summit), the Canadian Public Health Association's Task Force on the Implications for Human Health of Global Ecological Change reported on this issue (CPHA, 1992). The report noted in its introduction:

> "The harm that we are doing to this living planet – Gaia – and thus to ourselves . . . is the greatest challenge public health has ever faced".

The report went on to note that we now needed to apply public health concepts such as prevention, promotion and protection at the global level.

Then in 1993, the late Professor Tony McMichael, one of the world's leading environmental epidemiologists and Convening Lead Author of the Health Chapters for the Intergovernmental Panel on Climate Change for many years, published *Planetary Overload*, a ground-breaking review of the health implications of global ecological change (McMichael, 1993).

All of these issues were well understood as public health issues more than a quarter of a century ago, then, but they seemed to largely fall off public health's radar thereafter, as health promotion gave way to population health. While health promotion was rooted in political science and took an explicitly socio-political and action-oriented approach, population health was based in population epidemiology and evidence-based approaches, and was more interested in describing problems than in ways to address them; I used to describe population health as eloquent about causes, but silent on action.

Population health, however, found favour with governments across Canada and elsewhere, perhaps precisely because it was eloquent but silent, and was not advocating for significant social, environmental, economic and political change, as was health promotion. As a result, from 1993 to 2003, at least within Canada—home to both health promotion and population health—"health promotion went largely unnoticed. It was not positioned as a serious strategy within the health system" (Jackson & Riley, 2007).

Moreover, while claiming to be about "the determinants of the health of populations"—the subtitle of the leading book that launched the field (Evans et al., 1994)—population health's focus was on the *social* determinants of health. A search through the index reveals no mention of ecology or ecosystem; as Labonté (1995) observed, "population health arguments are largely silent on ecological issues". Thus, the discourse on the determinants of health quickly became a discourse on the social and economic determinants of health, culminating of course in the work and the report of the WHO Commission on the Social Determinants of Health (2008).

But while there is no question that the social determinants of health are vitally important and that the Commission did good work, we need to recognise that in focussing on the social and economic determinants, mainstream population and public health—including health promotion—became largely ecologically blind. It is only in the past few years that the ecological determinants of health have begun to again attract attention.

At the global level, this was in part spurred by the UN's Millennium Ecosystem Assessment, which was released in 2005. As noted earlier, not only did this report warn that "the ability of the planet's ecosystems to sustain future generations can no longer be taken for granted", but the Director General of the WHO noted "Nature's goods and services are the ultimate foundations of life and health". This point was reinforced by the reports on the health implications of climate change issued by the IPCC, and later by WHO's own reports on climate change and health and its participation with the Secretariat of the Convention on Biological Diversity in a report on the links between biodiversity and health (also noted earlier).

In response to the growing concern with the health implications of global ecological change, in 2012 the Canadian Public Health Association picked up where it had left off 20 years before, establishing a Working Group on the public health implications of global ecological change. The Working Group produced both a short position paper for the Association (CPHA, 2015) and a longer and more detailed background paper (Hancock et al., 2015).

Among the key points made in this report is that the ecological changes we see are driven by a combination of population growth, economic growth and technological development; that at the root of these socioeconomic and technological forces are a set of human values—emanating largely from the high income countries, but increasingly adopted by/imposed upon middle- and low-income countries around the world—that are not suited for the twenty-first century; and that we need to adopt an eco-social approach at all levels, across all sectors, that puts the wellbeing of people and the planet ahead of the economy.

The report presented a simple eco-social model for public health action (Fig. 15.1), which makes the point that both the natural ecosystems and the social and economic systems influence population health, and in turn they interact with each other. Moreover, while population health does not affect the natural systems (except that if the human population were drastically reduced it would benefit those natural systems), it does affect social and economic systems. A healthy population is good for society and the economy, while an unhealthy economy is bad for the health of the population. So ecological change that adversely affects health will likely adversely affect social and economic systems.

15.2.2 Public Health as (a Branch of) Human and Social Ecology

As noted above, when it comes to studying the relationship between humans and their environments, we have to deal with two interacting environments—the natural environment and the human-created social and built environment (note that the social environment includes the economy, which is simply a social construct). Together these create what we can think of as the human ecosystem; it is in fact an eco-social system.

The study of the human ecosystem is human ecology, which is "the study of the issues that lie at the interacting point of environment and culture" (Dansereau, 1966) or "the inter-disciplinary study of the relationship between human society and nature" (Commonwealth Human Ecology Council, 2017). In a much earlier pamphlet, the CHEC added that human ecology is

> "concerned with the philosophy and quality of life in relation to the development of biological and geological resources, of urban and rural settlements, of industry and technology, and of education and culture." (Commonwealth Human Ecology Council, n.d.).

According to Kartmann (1967), public health can be considered as that portion of human ecology concerned primarily with community problems of wellbeing. The idea that public health is part of or related to human ecology is hardly new; the distinguished Canadian public health scholar Dr. John Last wrote a textbook on *Public Health and Human Ecology* 35 years ago (Last, 1987).

An understanding of humans in these terms, and of public health as part of human ecology, has important implications for the way in which we approach population health issues and practise public health. In particular, it requires that we see the human ecosystem—and indeed, increasingly, the entire planet—as an eco-social system, where social and economic processes interact with natural processes.

Human ecology is closely related to the concept of social ecology, as developed by the late Murray Bookchin; social ecology argues that "nearly all of our present ecological problems originate in deep-seated social problems" and thus our ecological problems cannot be resolved without resolving the underlying social problems (Bookchin, 2007). He continues:

> "economic, ethnic, cultural, and gender conflicts, among many others, lie at the core of the most serious ecological dislocations we face today – apart, to be sure, from those that are produced by natural catastrophes." (p. 19)

Clearly, Bookchin's ideas are closely related to the concept of social determinants of health; substitute the words "health problems" for "ecological problems/dislocations" in the preceding paragraphs and they could have come straight from the report of the WHO Commission on the Social Determinants of Health (2008).

An eco-social approach to health, then, places health promotion within the realms of human and social ecology, with important implications for the practice of health promotion in the twenty-first century.

15.2.3   Planetary Health

At about the same time as the CPHA established its working group, Richard Horton, the Editor of *The Lancet*, gave a talk in Beijing at the centennial conference of the Rockefeller Foundation in which he called for a new approach that he called "planetary health"—"an investigation into the threats to human civilisations and to our survival from disturbances in planetary systems" (Horton, 2013). This was followed by a brief Manifesto for Planetary Health (Horton et al., 2014) and a joint Rockefeller-Lancet Commission on Planetary Health, which reported in 2015 (Whitmee et al., 2015).

The Rockefeller-Lancet Commission came to many of the same conclusions as the CPHA report, noting that while "Far-reaching changes to the structure and function of the Earth's natural systems represent a growing threat to human health . . . we have been mortgaging the health of future generations to realise economic and development gains in the present" (Whitmee et al., 2015).

The Lancet has since then established a new journal—*Lancet Planetary Health*— and with the Rockefeller Foundation has created the Planetary Health Alliance, "a consortium of over 200 universities, non-governmental organisations, research institutes, and government entities from around the world committed to understanding and addressing global environmental change and its health impacts" (https:// www.planetaryhealthalliance.org/mission).

15.3   Practising Health Promotion 2.0 in the Anthropocene

Planetary health can be thought of as the "new" health promotion—Health Promotion 2.0, if you like (Hancock, 2015a)—which takes an eco-social approach to public health in the Anthropocene at all levels from the setting of the home to the setting of our ultimate home, Gaia. In this final section, I will explore some of the key issues we will face in practising Health Promotion 2.0 in the Anthropocene.

In doing so, I will focus on what it means to *"enable the people of Earth to increase control over their own social, economic and technological systems, reduce the harm we do to ourselves and improve their health"*, as I re-framed the definition of health promotion for this purpose. In particular, I will focus on fundamental issues of governance that relate to the Ottawa Charter strategies of healthy public policy, including the economic system that has become the focus of governance, as well as supportive environments and community action, recognising that it will take new sets of personal skills to be engaged with and take action on these issues.

While I will not address the issue of re-orienting health services, I will just note that this means, on the one hand, that population and public health services must be fully engaged with monitoring and reporting on the ecological determinants of health and taking action to address these determinants at all levels, both through mitigation and adaptation measures (Hancock et al., 2015). On the other hand, the healthcare system needs to make environmental responsibility and carbon-neutral operation part of its code of practice (see Healthcare Without Harm and the Canadian Coalition for Green Health Care for examples), and also must prepare for dealing with the health consequences of the Anthropocene; WHO's initiative for low–carbon and net-zero health care systems, launched at COP26 in October 2021, has attracted a number of countries that have committed to these goals (WHO, 2021c).

But in line with health promotion's generally positive, hopeful and salutogenic orientation, I want to start with some thoughts about hope and opportunity.

15.3.1   Finding Hope and Seeing Opportunity in the Anthropocene

"Hope is finding positivity in the face of adversity" (Dutt & Brcic, 2014)

There is no question that we are facing serious, indeed severe ecological and social challenges, and that we need to move swiftly to make major changes in almost all aspects of our modern society and at all levels from the personal to the global. But while it is important to face reality—just as we believe people should if facing a terminal illness—simply telling people how bad things are and how much worse they are likely to get does not help. As we learned in the decades-long (and still ongoing) fight against tobacco, telling people they are going to get sick or die is not a very effective way to change behaviour.

So we need to find reason for hope, and to see the opportunities as well as the challenges that the Anthropocene poses. Indeed, so important is this that we devoted an entire chapter to the topic of "Signs of hope" in our report for CPHA (Hancock et al., 2015). In that chapter, we discussed five main sources of hope from a public health/health promotion perspective:

- There are important health co-benefits we can achieve by becoming a more ecologically sustainable society.
- We have helped to create major social and economic change in the past, most notably in the nineteenth and early twentieth century in response to the appalling health conditions of the industrialising countries.
- We have many partners—especially in the environmental movement, but in many other sectors, such as the emerging "green" economy—who welcome our engagement and support.
- We already have the much of the knowledge we need to make the changes we need to make, so we are not held back by a knowledge gap.
- We have made some progress in some areas in the past 50 years, and we can build on that.

In talking with young people in recent months about climate change, the climate strikes and the "Green New Deal" (New Economics Foundation, 2008; Wolf, 2019), I have found it helpful—and well-accepted—to both acknowledge the challenges their generation and their descendants will face, and the opportunities that will bring. Building on Naomi Klein's notion that climate change "changes everything"

(Klein, 2014), I point out that if we are to manage the transition to a healthy, just and sustainable future, we—and more specifically, young people today and the next couple of generations—are going to have to re-invent almost everything.

But while our notions of invention tend to turn to science and technology, the re-invention I am talking about is largely a social and indeed cultural transformation. Because our predicament is rooted in an unhealthy disconnect from nature and in a spiritual emptiness and a set of values that include greed, growth and acquisitiveness, and an equally unhealthy focus on individualism rather than a social awareness and conscience, we are going to develop new ethical and spiritual values to guide our actions. Philosophers, spiritual and political leaders are needed, as are artists of all kinds, who are much better placed to articulate and induce social and cultural change than scientists and technologists (Hancock, 2019).

In addition, we have to change our entire economic system, since it is not fit for purpose in the twenty-first century (as discussed below) and that means creating new businesses that are able to make money while protecting and improving the environment and at the same time increasing human and social development in an equitable manner. This new economy will provide all sorts of new opportunities for entrepreneurs and will demand new skills from the workforce (Hancock, 2020).

We are also going to have to re-invent our social system to provide a more positive and salutogenic environment for people throughout their lives, engaging them in meaningful activities and in decision-making. Ultimately, this means re-thinking the purpose and role of governance, as I discusss below. In all of this, there are countless opportunities.

15.3.2 A New Set of Values

The most important, but the most challenging task we face is to help to change the fundamental values that underpin the dominant world view or paradigm within which we operate—modernism. These values drive our economies and our societies, and thus lie at the heart of the Anthropocene; they are the root cause of our problems, and thus are not fit for purpose in the twenty-first century.

Modernism is rooted in two sixteenth century transformations in thought, according to Kumar (n.d.). The first was a religious transformation, the Protestant Reformation, with its attendant values relating to work (the Puritan work ethic), which led to modern capitalism. This was accompanied by a Scientific revolution that was based on rationalist thought and the scientific method, and resulted in "a sense of being superior to and/or apart from nature".

Kumar identifies a number of elements that comprise "modernism", but states "fundamentally, it is the economic changes that most dramatically affect industrial society." Those economic changes include "economic growth as the central defining feature of an industrial . . . economy". These transformations, and the growth in wealth, resources and power for the nations of the West that resulted led to a belief in the inevitability of progress.

But progress has been confused with economic growth, and two key values that relate to that; acquisitiveness and greed. We want more stuff, more wealth and power and we can never have enough. If you are a billionaire, you still are not a multi-billionaire. And if the acquisition of all that stuff, and wealth and the power that goes with it impoverishes others and harms the planet—well, that is just the cost of progress—a view that is strengthened because of our sense of being apart from nature. Moreover, as Leiss (1972) remarked:

> "If the idea of domination of nature has any meaning at all, it is that by such means, that is, through the possession of superior technological capabilities – some men [sic] attempt to dominate and control other men. The notion of a common domination of the human race over nature is nonsensical."

At the heart of our challenges, then, lie two sets of values that we have to change; acquisitiveness, greed and economic growth on the one hand, and our separation from nature on the other. With respect to the first, we need to replace growth with the concepts of adequacy or sufficiency—"enough" as a guiding principle (see below). Add to that a recognition that we are part of, not apart from, nature and must act accordingly, and we might have a fighting chance of getting to a society based on enough for all. It is thus gratifying to see that the Geneva Charter for Well-being, the product of the 10th Global Conference on Health Promotion, has as its first two areas of action "Value, respect and nurture planet Earth and its ecosystems" and "Design an equitable economy that serves human development within planetary and local ecological boundaries" (WHO, 2021b).

In developing new values, we should look to older sets of values, as the Indigenous Peoples' Statement from the 2019 IUHPE Conference notes:

> "Within Indigenous worldviews our relationship with the natural world is characterised by reverence and values that include sustainability, guardianship and love" (IUHPE, 2019).

These ideas are further explored by the IUHPE's Global Working Group on Waiora Planetary Health (Tuitahi et al., 2021).

Thus health promotion must work to change societal values and norms towards those values that are more compatible with achieving planetary health, learning from indigenous approaches (Ratima et al., 2019). While this may sound daunting, it is in fact something we do on a daily basis, and have always done, whether it be trying to change values and attitudes with respect to smoking, immunisation, substance use or poverty. We just need to raise our sights a bit!

15.3.3   Governance for Sustainable, Equitable Human Development

"Every system is perfectly designed to get the results it gets"[1]

---

[1] Variously attributed to quality-improvement guru W. Edwards Deming; Dr. Don Berwick, President and CEO of the Institute for Health Improvement, or Dr. Paul Batalden, one time Director

Governance, it must be understood, is more than government; it is "the process by which we collectively solve our problems and meet our society's needs. Government is the instrument we use" (Osborne & Gaebler, 1991), although I would say it is *an* instrument we use. There are other systems of governance in the private, institutional and community sectors, faith communities, etc. that are not government but that nonetheless are part of our overall societal or community systems of collective governance. At the urban level—but in fact at any level—governance is "the sum of the many ways individuals and institutions, public and private, plan and manage the common affairs of the city" (UN Habitat, 2002).

But this begs the question: Governance to what end, for what purpose? If we look at the world today, the answer would seem to be "to grow the economy and make us all rich"—meaning that we have lots of "stuff". But while a certain level of economic prosperity is needed to provide basic requirements for health (clean water, food, shelter, education, sanitation, basic health care, etc.), the evidence suggests that beyond about $20,000 GDP per capita ($10,000 in 1990 International dollars), further increases in GDP have little further impact on life expectancy[2]—but have a significant impact on expanding the ecological footprint.

So we do not need a high GDP to have a high life expectancy—countries such as Slovenia, Portugal, Malta, Cyprus and Greece do better than the USA while Chile, Lebanon and Cuba do about as well as the USA with much lower GDP per capita.[3]

What does seem to make a difference, certainly in high-income countries, is the degree of inequality; countries with lower levels of inequality have better results across a wide range of health and social outcomes (Wilkinson & Pickett, 2009).

Not only does life expectancy not increase as GDP increases beyond a certain point, but also in the USA—the country that puts the economy ahead of almost everything, and yet is also dedicated to "the pursuit of happiness"—another key measure of wellbeing—happiness—has actually declined in recent years in the USA as GDP has grown (Sachs, 2017).

This is important because "happiness is increasingly considered the proper measure of social progress and the goal of public policy" (Helliwell et al., 2017, p. 3). Indeed, the OECD committed itself in 2016 "to redefine the growth narrative to put people's well-being at the centre of governments' efforts" (OECD, 2016), while in 2019 New Zealand became the first country—at least among the high-income countries—to create a budget based on wellbeing.[4]

---

of The Center for Leadership and Improvement in The Dartmouth Institute for Health Policy and Clinical Practice (Susan Carr: "A Quotation with a Life of Its Own", http://www.psqh.com/julaug08/editor.html).

[2] See chart of LE and GDP pp in 1800, 1950, 1980 and 2012 at https://ourworldindata.org/life-expectancy.

[3] See chart of Life expectancy versus GDP per capita, 2015, at https://ourworldindata.org/grapher/life-expectancy-vs-gdp-per-capita?country=SDN.

[4] In her Budget message Prime Minister Jacinda Ardern commented "while economic growth is important – and something we will continue to pursue – it alone does not guarantee improvements

The USA is thus a case study of the failure of an economic growth-focussed agenda:

"The United States can and should raise happiness by addressing America's multi-faceted social crisis—rising inequality, corruption, isolation, and distrust—rather than focusing exclusively or even mainly on economic growth, especially since the concrete proposals along these lines would exacerbate rather than ameliorate the deepening social crisis." (Sachs, 2017, p. 179)

So to return to the opening quotation for this section, it seems that our governance and economic systems, and the values that underpin them, are perfectly designed to achieve high levels of environmental degradation and ecosystem harm, as well as high levels of poverty and inequality.

The question we must ask is: What would a system perfectly designed to achieve a healthy, socially just and ecologically sustainable society look like? What decisions would we make if the central purpose of governments at all levels, and of the societal and community processes of governance, was to maximise the health, wellbeing and level of human development of the entire population, in a manner that is indefinitely ecologically sustainable and socially just? Happily, these are the questions the WHO is now starting to ask, exemplified by the Geneva Charter for Wellbeing (WHO, 2021b).

The second key question for governance is "how do we do this"? Here we should recall that the first mechanism in the Ottawa Charter is to build healthy public policy, which is policy beyond the health sector that is intended to improve health (Hancock, 1985). So we need a process within government that places health, wellbeing and human development, along with ecological sustainability, at the heart of governance; the simple framework noted above (Fig. 15.1) would be a suitable way to frame this, as would the core concept of the Geneva Charter for Well-being: The creation of "sustainable well-being societies, committed to achieving equitable health now and for future generations without breaching ecological limits" (WHO, 2021b).

This constitutes a "whole of government" approach, in which all policies are assessed for their impacts on human development and ecological and social wellbeing. Such an approach has long been recommended by many organisations, but rarely put into practice; the case of South Australia (Baum et al., 2019) is a rare beacon of hope, although it lacked an ecological focus.

So at a national level, we should be asking what constitutes ecologically sustainable and health-promoting policies in key areas such as energy, transportation, housing and urban development, food, consumables and waste and in the industrial and resource sectors. (The final section touches on some of these at the local level.)

This understanding also needs to apply to the private sector, through what might be called "healthy private policy", and indeed across all sectors of society (public, private, non-profit, community, academic, faith); in other words, we also need a "whole of society" approach, in which the actions of corporations and citizens are assessed and managed so as to achieve these ends.

---

to our living standards". She went on to note "Nor does it measure the quality of economic activity or take into account who benefits and who is left out or left behind".

But this pre-supposes a societal agreement that such an approach is needed, so we also need a community-wide, society-wide and indeed, global process of engagement that presents the evidence of global ecological change and the social determinants of health, raises questions of fundamental values and goals and seeks some agreement on the way forward. A key part of that process will involve both dethroning the economy as the central focus of societies and their governments and at the same time replacing the existing economic system with a new system that is fit for the twenty-first century.

15.3.4   An Economics Fit for the Twenty-First Century

"Anyone who believes in indefinite growth in anything physical, on a physically finite planet, is either mad or an economist." (Boulding, US Congress, 1973, p. 248)

Our current economic system is simply not fit for purpose in the twenty-first century; as we can see very clearly in the USA, growth does not equate with happiness, neither necessarily with social justice, nor does it fit with the stability and sustainability of the ecological systems that are the ultimate determinants of our health. So what would a new economic system look like, one that was focussed on ecologically sustainable and socially just human development?

These ideas have been discussed for many years, not in mainstream economics, which has been largely taken over by the neo-liberal economics that lies at the root of our problems, but in the emerging field of ecological economics. Fritz Schumacher discussed them in his wonderful book *Small is Beautiful* almost 50 years ago (Schumacher, 1973) and Herman Daly has championed the concept of a steady state economy for decades (Daly, 1977).

In the foreword to a recent steady state economics book, *Enough is Enough*, Daly—the "elder statesman" of steady state economics—suggests that "enough", which means "sufficient for a good life", "should be the central concept in economics", while "the current answer of 'having ever more' is wrong" (Daly, 2013). Or as Gandhi said, "Earth provides enough to satisfy every [person's] need, but not every [person's] greed".

At its simplest, such an economy is one "where resource use is stabilized within environmental limits, and the goal of increasing GDP is replaced by the goal of improving human well-being. It's an economy where the goal is better lives, not more stuff." (Dietz & O'Neill, 2013). Note the very clear reference to "the goal of improving human well-being", which makes ecological economics of great interest to public health (Hancock, 2020).

A steady-state economy should not be thought of as a static economy, however. On the contrary, it is very dynamic; as more harmful activities are replaced by less harmful ones, there is plenty of scope for growth and innovation.

The concept of a steady state economy is finding new favour as the ecological crisis deepens. Kate Raworth (2017) has proposed an approach she calls "doughnut economics", in which we create an economy that is not too big and not too small; large enough to meet our societal needs, and yet small enough to meet those needs within the limits of the living planet. A number of changes are needed to achieve such an economy, including policies to conserve natural resources, stabilise population, reduce inequality, fix the financial system, create jobs, and change the way we measure progress (Dietz & O'Neill, 2013).

This latter point is a crucial one. As long as GDP remains the principal means of measuring societal progress—a purpose which its principal architect explicitly warned against (Kuznets, 1934) but which is how it is used at state/provincial, national and international levels—we are bound to follow the wrong path, because as we have seen above, growing GDP beyond a certain point does not add to life expectancy or otherwise improve health, nor does it lead to happiness. That is because it is fatally flawed in at least two important respects.

- First, GDP fails to distinguish between beneficial and harmful economic activity. Thus the entire economic activity of both the tobacco industry and the work of the healthcare system in treating tobacco-caused illness boosts GDP; so too do the clean-up costs of natural and human-created disasters such as hurricanes and oil spills, and also the economic activity of the fossil fuel industry, which is causing global warming.
- A second major problem is that it fails to include all the non-monetised activity such as raising kids, caring for a sick family member, volunteering and other actions that contribute to community wellbeing.

This is why there is a need to change our thinking about what constitutes "progress", and adopt new measures of progress (such as the Genuine Progress Indicator—GPI) that focus our attention on what matters (Hancock, 2015b). But at root, the economic system is only a social construct, built upon and driven by a set of social values. Changing those values is a more profound and more important task than changing the economic system.

15.3.5   WHO's Growing Interest in a Healthy, Green, Just Economy

Interestingly, the WHO was talking about the health co-benefits of a "green" economy in the areas of housing and transportation as long ago as 2011 (WHO, 2011a, 2011b). More recently, in response to the Covid pandemic and calls from many health organisations for a recovery that is not just green but also just and healthy—a sort of healthy Green New Deal—(Harvey, 2020) the WHO has begun to frame a societal post-COVID recovery in these terms. Its *Manifesto for a Healthy Recovery from COVID-19* (WHO, 2020a) offers six "prescriptions" for a healthy and green recovery, the first of which is "preserve the source of human health: Nature", while the others are:

- "Invest in essential services, from water and sanitation to clean energy in health-care facilities
- Ensure a quick and healthy energy transition
- Promote healthy, sustainable food systems
- Build healthy, liveable cities and
- Stop using taxpayers' money to fund pollution"

This last one is a blunt call for governments to stop subsidizing fossil fuels, which is quite a radical stance for an organistion such as WHO to take, and gives some sense of the seriousness with which WHO views the current situation (These ideas are taken even further in WHO's special report on climate change and health, prepared for COP26 in October 2021 - WHO, 2021a).

15.3.6   *Healthy Cities 2.0: One Planet Communities*

In closing, I want to bring all these issues down to a setting that has been a fruitful field for health promotion: Healthy cities and communities. The Healthy Cities approach was the first and arguably is the most successful of all the health promotion settings' approaches; in fact, its launch by WHO Europe predates the Ottawa Charter by almost a year, and it is now a large global movement (De Leeuw & Simos, 2017).

The Healthy Cities approach has always had an interest in ecological sustainability (see e.g. Hancock, 1996a, 1996b, 2000), but this has never been a central focus, perhaps in part because there are also sustainable city, green city and other environmentally focussed city movements. But an understanding that the Earth's living systems are in fact the most fundamental determinants of health make the "marriage" of health and sustainability both more possible and much more important.

As I argue in *Public Health Reports* (Hancock, 2000), a healthy community must also be a sustainable community. Given the rapid deterioration since then in the Earth systems upon which we depend, it is more apparent than ever that our communities, towns and cities must function within an ecological footprint equivalent to one planet's worth of biocapacity per person, their fair share of the Earth's biocapacity and resources. But at the same time, they still have to ensure everyone's basic needs are met and that all can enjoy a good quality of life and good health.

The concept of One Planet Living has been championed since 2002 by Bioregional (Desai & Riddlestone, 2002), a UK-based consultancy responsible, among other things, for developing BedZED, a socially and environmentally sustainable development in London. Since then, they have worked with communities around the world on how to become One Planet Communities (Desai, 2009). We have recently framed this idea as a One Planet Region (Hancock et al., 2017), linking it to the Healthy Cities approach: I think of this as Healthy Cities 2.0 (Hancock, 2018).

The challenge of becoming a One Planet City or Region is much greater for high-income cities, because they have large ecological footprints. Canada, for example, has a footprint of 4.75 planets (Global Footprint Network, 2019), although Victoria—where I live—may have a footprint closer to 3 planets (Moore & Hallsworth, 2018)—but even a 3-planet footprint would require a 67% reduction to get to a 1-planet footprint, while a 4-planet footprint requires a 75% reduction and a 5-planet footprint requires an 80% reduction.

Clearly these are all very large reductions and achieving them will be a major challenge, especially if at the same time we want to maintain, if not improve, health, wellbeing and social equity. But it is the high-income countries and cities that must lead the way, because: (a) historically they are responsible for most of the accumulated harm, (b) they continue to be the largest contributors and (c) if they cannot or will not shift their patterns of living, how can they plausibly urge others to do so?

Bioregional's One Planet approach is guided by a set of principles (Bioregional, 2016) that is notably different from many of the more standard "sustainable community" principles. That is because the first three principles are not about the environment at all but are about people, with health and happiness being the first principle, followed by equity and local economy and then community and culture (Fig. 15.2). For recent work on the application of the One Planet approach in the UK, Canada, Australia and elsewhere see Hancock et al. (2019).

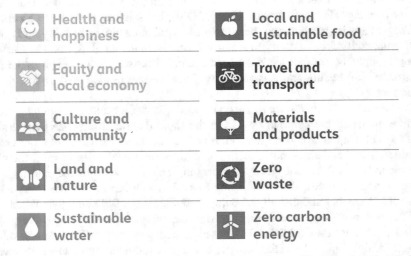

Fig. 15.2 Bioregional's ten principles of one planet living. (*Source*: Bioregional Annual Review, 2015–16. Available at http://storage.googleapis.com/www.bioregional.com/downloads/Bioregional-Annual-Review-2015-16.pdf © Bioregional)

15.4 Conclusion

Make no mistake, what I suggest above as the work of health promotion in the twenty-first century is a mammoth task—but then the challenges we face, as laid out in this chapter, are also mammoth. We will need to embrace an eco-social way of thinking and working at all levels and question such fundamental aspects of society as the underlying values that shape and drive it; our understanding of what constitutes progress and how we measure it; the economic system and the structure and process of governance and the collective good we seek to achieve.

We cannot do this alone, so we must find partners among those who are working to protect the Earth, achieve human development and social justice, re-imagine and re-design communities and economies and create a shift in values to respect and cherish each other and the Earth. We will find those partners not only in the environmental, social justice and peace movements but among economists, entrepreneurs, faith communities and many others.

One hundred and seventy years ago, Rudolf Virchow declared "medicine is a social science, and politics but medicine writ large" (Virchow, 1848). Today, we must recognise that health promotion requires a socio-ecological and socio-political approach and that societal organisation and functioning must be but health promotion writ large. Given both the scale and the urgency of the changes that are needed if we are to enable all the world's people to live lives of good quality, in good health, within the constraints of our living planet, health promoters everywhere, at every level, must start today to fashion a world in which our children and grandchildren can enjoy high quality lives in balance with each other and with the Earth.

Gaia truly is the ultimate setting for health promotion!

References

Baum, F., Delany-Crowe, T., MacDougall, C., van Eyk, H., Lawless, A., et al. (2019). To what extent can the activities of the South Australian Health in All Policies initiative be linked to population health outcomes using a program theory-based evaluation? *BMC Public Health, 19*, 88. https://doi.org/10.1186/s12889-019-6408-y

Bioregional. (2016). *Mapping Progress: Annual review 2015–16*. Retrieved from http://storage.googleapis.com/www.bioregional.com/downloads/Bioregional-Annual-Review-2015-16.pdf.

Bookchin, M. (2007). *Social ecology and communalism*. AK Press.

Commonwealth Human Ecology Council. (n.d.). *Human Ecology (brochure)*. London: The Commonwealth Secretariat. (This brochure was produced at around the time the CHEC was established in 1969, but is no longer available.)

Commonwealth Human Ecology Council. (2017). *Mission Statement*. Retrieved June 4, 2017, from http://www.checinternational.org/about-chec/who-we-are/.

CPHA. (1992). *Human & Ecosystem Health: Canadian Perspectives, Canadian Action*. Ottawa: The Association. Retrieved August 21, 2018, from https://www.cpha.ca/sites/default/files/assets/policy/ecosystem_health_e.pdf.

CPHA. (2015). The Ecological Determinants of Health Ottawa: CPHA Available at https://www.cpha.ca/sites/default/files/assets/policy/edh-discussion_e.pdf

Daly, H. (1977). *Steady-state economics: The economics of biophysical equilibrium and moral growth*. W. H. Freeman.

Daly, H. (2013). Foreword. In R. Dietz & D. O'Neill (Eds.), *Enough is enough: Building a sustainable economy in a world of finite resources*. Routledge.

Dansereau, P. (1966). *Proceedings, 1st Commonwealth Human Ecology Council Conference*. Royal Commonwealth Society.

De Leeuw, E., & Simos, J. (2017). *Healthy cities—The theory, policy, and practice of value-based urban health planning*. Springer.

Desai, P. (2009). *One planet communities: A real life guide to sustainable living*. John Wiley.

Desai, P., & Riddlestone, R. (2002). *Bioregional solutions: For living on one planet (Schumacher Briefings No 8)*. UIT Cambridge Ltd./Green Books.

Dietz, R., & O'Neill, D. (2013). *Enough is enough: Building a sustainable economy in a world of finite resources*. Berrett-Koehler.

Dutt, M., & Brcic, V. (2014). Medicare can still rise to meet its challenges. *Times Colonist* (Victoria BC), p. A11.

Evans, R., Barer, M., & Marmor, T. (Eds.). (1994). *Why are some people healthy and others not? The determinants of the health of populations*. Aldine de Gruyter.

Global Footprint Network. (2019). *National Footprint Accounts: Ecological Footprint and Biocapacity* (Data Year 2016). Retrieved January 29, 2020, from https://www.footprintnetwork.org/.

Hancock, T. (1985). Beyond health care: From public health policy to healthy public policy. *Canadian Journal of Public Health, 76*(Suppl 1), 9–11.

Hancock, T. (1996a). Planning and creating healthy and sustainable cities: The challenge for the 21st century. In C. Price & A. Tsouros (Eds.), *Our cities, our future: Policies and action for health and sustainable development*. WHO Healthy Cities Project Office.

Hancock, T. (1996b). Healthy, sustainable communities: Concept, fledgling practice and implications for governance. In M. Roseland (Ed.), *Eco-city dimensions: Healthy communities, healthy planet*. New Society Press.

Hancock, T. (2000). Healthy communities must be sustainable communities too. *Public Health Reports, 115*(2 and 3), 151–156.

Hancock, T. (2015a). Population health promotion 2.0: An eco-social approach to public health in the Anthropocene. *Canadian Journal of Public Health, 106*(4), e252–e255. https://doi.org/10.17269/CJPH.106.5161

Hancock, T. (2015b) Measuring what matters: Victoria's Vital Signs. In *Victoria's Vital Signs 2015*. Victoria BC: Victoria Community Foundation. Retrieved from https://victoriafoundation.bc.ca/wp-content/uploads/2015/10/2015_VitalSigns_LR_WEB.pdf.

Hancock, T. (2018). Healthy Cities 2.0: Transitioning towards 'One Planet' cities (Key challenges facing 21st century cities, Part 3). *Cities & Health, 1*(3). https://doi.org/10.1080/23748834.2018.1526659

Hancock, T. (2019). Beyond science and technology: Creating Planetary Health needs 'heart, gut and spirit' work. *Challenges, 10*, 31. https://doi.org/10.3390/challe10010031. https://www.mdpi.com/2078-1547/10/1/31/pdf.

Hancock, T. (2020) *Ecological economics and public health: An introduction*. Quebec: National Collaborating Centre for Healthy Public Policy (In press).

Hancock, T., Capon, A., Dooris, M., & Patrick, R. (2017). One planet regions: Planetary health at the local level. *The Lancet Planetary Health, 1*(3), e92–e93.

Hancock, T., Desai, P., & Patrick, R. (2019). Tools for creating a future of healthy One Planet cities in the Anthropocene. *Cities & Health*. https://doi.org/10.1080/23748834.2019.1668336

Hancock, T., Spady, D. W., & Soskolne, C. L. (Eds.). (2015). *Global change and Public Health: Addressing the Ecological Determinants of Health: The Report in Brief*. Canadian Public Health Association. Retrieved from www.cpha.ca/sites/default/files/assets/policy/edh-brief.pdf.

Harvey, F. (2020) World health leaders urge green recovery from coronavirus crisis The Guardian (26 May). The letter, from 350 organisations representing over 40 million health professionals and over 4,500 individual health professionals from 90 different countries. Retrieved from https://healthyrecovery.net/.

Helliwell, J., Layard, R., & Sachs, J. (2017). *World happiness report 2017.* Sustainable Development Solutions Network.

Horton, R. (2013). Offline: Planetary health—A new vision for the post-2015 era. *The Lancet, 382,* 1012.

Horton, R., Beaglehole, R., Bonita, R., Raeburn, J., McKee, M., & Wall, S. (2014). From public to planetary health: A manifesto. *The Lancet, 383,* 847.

Intergovernmental Panel on Climate Change (IPCC). (1996). Climate change 1995: Impacts, adaptations and mitigation of climate change. Contribution of Working Group II. In R. T. Watson et al. (Eds.), *Second assessment report of the intergovernmental panel on climate change.* Cambridge University Press.

Intergovernmental Panel on Climate Change. (2014). Summary for policymakers. In: Climate Change 2014: Impacts, Adaptation, and Vulnerability. In Field, C. B., Barros, V. R., Dokken, D. J., Mach, K. J., Mastrandrea, M. D., et al. (eds.), *Part A: Global and Sectoral Aspects. Contribution of Working Group II to the Fifth Assessment Report of the Intergovernmental Panel on Climate Change Change.* Cambridge University Press, Cambridge, United Kingdom and New York, NY. Retrieved April 12, 2021, from https://www.ipcc.ch/site/assets/uploads/2018/02/ar5_wgII_spm_en.pdf.

IUHPE. (2019). *Waiora–Indigenous Peoples' Statement for Planetary Health and Sustainable Development.* Retrieved from https://www.iuhpe2019.com/PicsHotel/iuhpe/Brochure/Indigenous%20Statement%20for%20Plenary%20Revised.pdf.

Jackson, S., & Riley, B. (2007). Health promotion in Canada: 1986 to 2006. *Promotion & Education, 14*(4), 214–218.

Kartmann, L. (1967). Human ecology and public health. *American Journal of Public Health, 57,* 737–749.

Klein, N. (2014). *This changes everything: Capitalism vs. the climate.* by Simon & Schuster.

Kumar, K. (n.d.). Modernization. In *Encyclopedia Britannica.* Retrieved March 10, 2014, from http://www.britannica.com/EBchecked/topic/387301/modernization.

Kuznets, S., (1934). *National Income, 1929–1932 73rd US Congress,* 2nd session, Senate document no. 124, p. 7. Retrieved from http://library.bea.gov/u?/SOD,888.

Labonté, R. (1995). Population health and health promotion: What do they have to say to each other? *Canadian Journal of Public Health, 86*(3), 165–168.

Landrigan, P., Fuller, R., Acosta, N. J. R., et al. (2017). The Lancet Commission on pollution and health. *The Lancet, 386*(10002). https://doi.org/10.1016/S0140-6736(17)32345-0

Last, J. (1987). *Public health and human ecology east Norwalk.* Appleton & Lange.

Leiss, W. (1972). *The domination of nature.* G. Braziller.

McMichael, A. (1993). *Planetary overload.* Cambridge University Press.

Millennium Ecosystem Assessment. (2005). *Ecosystems and human well-being: Synthesis.* Island Press. Retrieved from https://www.millenniumassessment.org/documents/document.356.aspx.pdf.

Moore, J., & Hallsworth, C. (2018). EcoCity footprint tool pilot summary report. *District of Saanich.* Retrieved August 27, 2019, from https://www.oneplanetsaanich.org/uploads/1/1/9/3/119346756/saanich_ecocity_summary_report_rev_june_2018.pdf.

New Economics Foundation. (2008). *A Green New Deal: Joined-up policies to solve the triple crunch of the credit crisis, climate change and high oil prices.* London: New Economics Foundation. Retrieved January 29, 2020, from https://neweconomics.org/campaigns/green-new-deal.

OECD. (2016). *Strategic orientations of the secretary-general: For 2016 and beyond Meeting of the OECD Council at Ministerial Level Paris, 1–2 June 2016.* Retrieved from https://www.oecd.org/mcm/documents/strategic-orientations-of-the-secretary-general-2016.pdf.

Osborne, R., & Gaebler, T. (1991). *Reinventing government.* Addison-Wesley.

Ratima, M., Martin, D., Castleden, H., & Delormier, T. (2019). Indigenous voices and knowledge systems—Promoting planetary health, health equity, and sustainable development now and for future generations. *Global Health Promotion, 26*(Supp. 3), 3–5.

Raworth, K. (2017). *Doughnut economics: Seven ways to think like a 21st century economist.* Chelsea Green Publishing.

Sachs, J. (2017). Restoring American Happiness (Chapter 7). In J. Helliwell, R. Layard, & J. Sachs (Eds.), *World Happiness Report 2017.* Sustainable Development Solutions Network.

Schumacher, E. F. (1973). *Small is beautiful: Economics as if people mattered.* Harper and Row.

Secretariat of the Convention on Biological Diversity and WHO. (2015). *Connecting global priorities: Biodiversity and human health, summary of the state of knowledge review.* Secretariat of the Convention on Biological Diversity.

Smith, K. R., Woodward, A., Campbell-Lendrum, D., Chadee, D. D., Honda, Y., et al. (2014). Human health: Impacts, adaptation, and co-benefits. In C. B. Field, V. R. Barros, D. J. Dokken, K. J. Mach, M. D. Mastrandrea, et al. (Eds.), *Climate Change 2014: Impacts, Adaptation, and Vulnerability. Part A: Global and Sectoral Aspects. Contribution of Working Group II to the Fifth Assessment Report of the Intergovernmental Panel on Climate Change* (pp. 709–754). Cambridge University Press.

Tuitahi, S., Watson, H., Egan, R., Parkes, M., & Hancock, T. (2021). Waiora: The importance of Indigenous worldviews and spirituality to inspire and inform Planetary Health Promotion in the Anthropocene. *Global Health Promotion 28*(4):73–82 (Special supplement for the IUHPE 2022 Conference, Montreal, on behalf of the IUHPE's Global Working Group on Waiora Planetary Health)

UN Habitat. (2002). *The global campaign on urban governance: Concept paper.* Nairobi: UN Habitat. Retrieved from http://mirror.unhabitat.org/content.asp?typeid=19&catid=25&cid=2097#What%20is%20governance.

UNFCCC. (2018) *UN Warns Climate Change Is Driving Global Hunger.* Retrieved from https://unfccc.int/news/un-warns-climate-change-is-driving-global-hunger.

US Congress. (1973). *Energy reorganization act of 1973: Hearings, Ninety-third Congress, first session, on H.R. 11510.* p. 248.

Virchow, R. (1848). Cited in Ackerknecht, E (1981) Rudolf Virchow New York; Arno Press.

Watson, Sir Robert (2019) IPBES Chair—Quoted in UN Report: Nature's Dangerous Decline 'Unprecedented'; Species Extinction Rates 'Accelerating'. Retrieved from https://www.un.org/sustainabledevelopment/blog/2019/05/nature-decline-unprecedented-report/.

Whitmee, S., Haines, A., Beyrer, C., Boltz, F., Capon, A. G., et al. (2015). Safeguarding human health in the Anthropocene epoch: Report of the Rockefeller Foundation—Lancet Commission on Planetary Health. *The Lancet, 386*(1007), 1973–2028. https://doi.org/10.1016/S0140-6736(15)60901-1

WHO. (1986). *Ottawa charter for health promotion.* WHO Europe.

WHO. (2003). In A. J. McMichael, D. H. Campbell-Lendrum, C. F. Corvalán, et al. (Eds.), *Climate change and human health: Risks and responses.* WHO.

WHO. (2011a). *Health in the green economy: Health co-benefits of climate change mitigation—Housing sector.* WHO.

WHO. (2011b). *Health in the green economy: Health co-benefits of climate change mitigation—Transport sector.* WHO.

WHO. (2015). *WHO calls for urgent action to protect health from climate change.* Retrieved January 21, 2021, from https://www.who.int/globalchange/global-campaign/cop21/en/.

WHO. (n.d.). *Climate change.* Retrieved January 21, 2021, from https://www.who.int/health-topics/climate-change#tab=tab_1.

WHO. (2020a). *Manifesto for a Healthy Recovery from COVID-19.* Geneva: WHO. Retrieved from https://www.who.int/docs/default-source/climate-change/who-manifesto-for-a-healthy-and-green-post-covid-recovery.pdf?sfvrsn=f32ecfa7_8.

WHO. (2020b). *Guidance on mainstreaming biodiversity for nutrition and health.* WHO.

WHO Commission on the Social Determinants of Health. (2008). *Closing the gap in a generation: Health equity through action on the social determinants of health (Final Report—Executive Summary)*. WHO. Retrieved from http://whqlibdoc.who.int/hq/2008/WHO_IER_CSDH_08.1_eng.pdf.

Wilkinson, R., & Pickett, K. (2009). *The spirit level: Why more equal societies almost always do better London*. Allen Lane.

Wolf, Z. (2019). *Here's what the Green New Deal actually says CNN* (Thu February 14, 2019. Retrieved January 29, 2020, from https://www.cnn.com/2019/02/14/politics/green-new-deal-proposal-breakdown/index.html.

WHO. (1948). Constitution of the World Health Organization Geneva: WHO

WHO. (2021a). COP26 special report on climate change and health: the health argument for climate action. Geneva: World Health Organization

WHO. (2021b). The Geneva Charter for Well-being. Geneva: WHO. Available at https://cdn.who.int/media/docs/default-source/health-promotion/geneva-charter---unedited---15.12.2021.pdf?sfvrsn=f55dec7_5&download=true Accessed 11 February, 2022

WHO. (2021c). COP26 health programme: country commitments. https://www.who.int/initiatives/cop26-health-programme/country-commitments Accessed 11 February, 2022

Index

A

Age-Friendly Cities, 98
Agentic- or actor-centred theories, 49
Aggregate health outcome indicators, 72
Airports
 authoritative declarations and
  statements, 230
 current situation, 228
 future, 229, 230
 healthy settings family, 230
 and public health, 228
AltspaceVR, 215
Annual international HPH
  conferences, 125
Annual reporting template (ART), 76
Anthropocene
 as an existential threat, 250–252
 definition, 245
 ecological phenomenon, 246
  ecological footprint, 247, 248
  Living Planet Index, 248
  planetary boundaries, 247
 geological phenomenon, 245, 246
 health implications of, 259–261
 health inequity in, 261
 implications for understanding of health,
  262, 263
 inequity in, 252–254
 sociocultural phenomenon, 249, 250
Anthropocene Working Group
  (AWG), 246
Anti-vaccination movement, 208
Aqueducts, 91
Assessment for healthy setting
 HIA, 70

Urban HEART (*see* Urban Health Equity
  Assessment and Response Tool
  (Urban HEART))
Assessment Program for Affective and Social
  Outcomes (APASO), 114
Australian Health Promoting Schools
  Association, 8

B

Balanced Scorecard (BSC), 77, 78
Beauty salons, 226
Bioregional's One Planet approach, 276
Black Death, 92
Blue Zone Project, 234
Bronfenbrenner's theory of human
  development, 27
Budapest Declaration, 9, 134

C

Centre for Health Equity Training, Research
  and Evaluation (CHETRE), 229
CHEP, 114
Child-Friendly Cities, 98
Cities Power Partnership, 101
Civic university, 161
Climate change, 246, 249, 251, 252
Complexity, 52
Consolidation approach, 6
Constitutive governance, 58
Core business' alignment, 36
COVID-19, 102, 218
 social media and, 212
Creative Cities, 98

D
DECiPHEr (Developing an evidence-based
           approach to city public health
           planning and investment in Europe)
           Program, 77
Declaration of Alma Ata, 4
Deep adaptation, 252
Dementia Friendly Gurdwara Project, 231
Digital divide, 207, 208
Digital health literacy, 205–209
Digital storytelling, 208, 209
Directive governance, 58
Doughnut economics, 273–274

E
Earth Summit, 6
Eastern Mediterranean
     HPS, 110
           Iran, school health in, 110, 111
           systems approach, need for, 111, 112
Ecological determinants, 244
Ecological footprint (EF), 247
Economic evaluation, 75
Economic globalization, 173
Economic growth, 50
Eco-social approach, 262, 263, 265–267, 277
EFQM Excellence Model and the Balanced
           Scorecard (HPH-EFQM-BSC), 134
Emerging settings
     airports (*see* Airports)
     healthy coastal communities (*see* Coastal
           communities)
     healthy workplace programme, 227
     traditional setting initiatives, 226
     weakness, 226
     worship place (*see* Places of worship)
Environmental Impact Assessment
           processes, 229
Equity, 96–98
Equity indicators, 72
Equity-oriented settings approach, 33, 39
Europe, HPS, 108–110
European Foundation for Quality Management
           (EFQM) model, 77, 79, 134
European Foundation for the Improvement of
           Living and Working Conditions
           (EFILWC), 9
European Healthy Stadia network, 190
European HPH Network, 139
European Network for Workplace Health
           Promotion, 9
European Network of Smoke-free Hospitals
           (ENSH), 127

European Pilot Health Promoting Hospitals
           Project, 9
European Sustainable Cities and Towns
           Campaign, 7
Evaluation for healthy setting
     BSC, 77, 78
     challenges, 84, 86
     EFQM model, 77
     elements, 73
     evaluation types and tools
           economic evaluation, 75
           impact evaluation, 75
           logic model, 75
           outcome evaluation, 75
           participatory evaluation, 74
           process evaluation, 75
     health-promoting hospital, 77
     health-promoting schools, 79, 81
     healthy university
           component activities and projects, 83
           levels of evaluation, 83
           overall "Whole System" approach, 83
           Self-Review Tool, 83
     MARI research framework, 76, 77
     participatory action research, 81
     realist evaluation, 84
     reasons for, 69
     steps and considerations, 73
     theory of change approach, 84
     Total Quality Management, 77
Evaluation in Health Promotion, 13
Evidence-based health care, 126
Expansion of healthy cities, 6, 7

F
Face-to-face (f2f) health interventions, 216
Festive Cities, 98
First Urban Planning Act, 92

G
GAA Healthy Club, 194
Gaia (Earth)
     determinants of health, 244
     earth system, 243
     history, 242
     living system, 243
     setting for health promotion, 244
General Evaluation Questionnaire (GEQ), 76
Genuine Progress Indicator (GPI), 274
Global ecological footprint, 248
*Global Evidence of Health Promotion
           Effectiveness*, 13

The Global School-based Student Health
Survey (GSHS), 80
Global School Health Promotion, 13
Google Ngram viewer, 47
GoSmart.net, 114
Governance
constitutive governance, 58
directive governance, 58
essence of, 57
in Google Ngram viewer, 47
multiple governance framework, 58
operational governance, 58
policy cube, 62
for settings-based health promotion,
58–60
values, 58
Governance for health, 271, 273
The Great Acceleration, 250
Greener on the Outside of Prisons
(GOOP), 182–185
Green New Deal, 268
Green Towns and Cities, 98

H
Happy Cities, 98
Healing rituals, 231
Health Behaviour among School-aged
Children (HBSC), 8
Healthcare Systems Core Strategies, 230
Health co-benefits, 268, 274
Health determinants, 167
Health impact assessment (HIA), 70
Health in all policy (HiAP), 53, 54, 56, 59,
60, 98, 151
Health inequalities, 185, 186
Health in Prisons Programme (HIPP),
180, 186
Health in Prisons Project (HIPP), 10
Healthism, 208
Health literacy, 108, 206, 208, 209, 216
Health professionals, 109
Health promoting hospitals, 8, 230
Health promoting schools, 8
Health promotion
in sports settings, 189, 190
application, 197
evaluation, 196, 197
framework and fundamental,
192–194
HPSC, 190, 191
history and development, 191, 192
international research, 194
strategies, 195, 196

Health Promotion 2.0
in Anthropocene
bioregional's One Planet approach, 276
economics fit for twenty-first century,
273, 274
governance for sustainable, equitable
human development, 271, 273
Healthy Cities approach, 275
hope and seeing opportunity in,
268, 269
modernism, 269
WHO's growing interest in healthy,
green, just economy, 274, 275
eco-social health promotion, 263–265
planetary health, 267
public health as human and social
ecology, 266
Health-promoting general practice, 226
Health-promoting higher education, 151, 152
challenges and opportunities, 160
context, concepts and theory, 154–157
history and development, 152, 153
sustainability and health promotion, 161
University of British Columbia, 157, 158
University of Central Lancashire,
158, 159
University of Puerto Rico, 159, 160
Health-promoting hospitals (HPH),
31, 77, 119
comprehensive framework, eighteen core
strategies as, 136
definition, 134
and EFQM, 134
European HPH Network, 139
five standards for, 138
future of, 141
globalizing, evaluation, and strategic
communication, 122
health care, 131
health care settings, health
promotion in, 142
health promoting, empowerment for, 135
historical background of, 120–128, 134,
137, 138
illness management, empowerment
for, 135
international HPH conferences, 131
international network, autonomy,
globalizing extending scope of, 122
international network structures,
development of concept and
initiation of, 121
national/regional HPH networks and
member hospitals, 141

Health-promoting hospitals (HPH) (*cont.*)
    phases and milestones of
            development, 121–123
    PRICES-HPH evaluation model, 140
    production, 132
    Putting HPH Policy, 135
    quality and evidence methodology,
            standardizing the concept and
            linking, 121
    regional/national networks, 130
    reorienting health services, 133
    setting approach, 120, 139, 142
    seven implementation strategies for, 138
    strategies, 130, 135
    success of, 129
    vision and mission, 133
Health-promoting school (HPS),
            79–81, 105–107
    Eastern Mediterranean, 110
        Iran, school health in, 110, 111
        systems approach, need for, 111, 112
    Europe, 108–110
    Hong Kong, 112–114
    initiatives of, 108
    settings approach, 115
Health-Promoting School Accreditation
            System (HPSAS), 114
Health-promoting settings, 48
Health-promoting sports club (HPSC), 190
Health-promoting universities, 10, 11, 31
Health-promoting workplaces, 9, 167, 168
    conceptualization and implementation of,
            170, 171
    international standards, 168, 169
    transformation of the world of
            work, 173–175
    WHP, elements and success factors
            of, 171–173
Healthy airports, 229
Healthy cities, 5
    approach, 275
    definition, 91
    development plan, 96
    foundation document, 98
    future, 100
    health promoting settings, 98
    history, 91, 94
    network, 124
    Ottawa Charter, 94, 97
    programme, 57
    theme cities, 98
    Twenty Steps, 230
Healthy coastal communities
    advantages, 233
    Blue Zone Project, 234

    coastal industries, 234
    contradiction, 234
    future, 235
Healthy islands, 7, 226
Healthy marketplaces, 226
Healthy prisons, 10
Healthy public policy (HPP), 53–55
Healthy Stadia, 202
Healthy stadium, 201
Healthy villages initiatives, 7
Healthy workplace programme, 227
High-income countries (HICs), 248, 252, 254
Hong Kong, HPS, 112–114
Hong Kong Health School Award Scheme
            (HKHSA), 81
Hong Kong Healthy School Award system
            (HKHSA), 113, 114
HPH Governance Board, 128
HPH network, 125
Human development model, 50
The Hygienists, 92

I
Immanuel Diakonie Group, 77
Impact evaluation, 75
Inclusive Cities, 98
Indigenous Peoples' Statement for Planetary
            Health and Sustainable
            Development, 242
Instant messaging (IM), 215
Institute of Leadership and Sustainability
            (IFLAS), 252
Institutions, 48, 49, 51
Instrumentalist, 49
Intergovernmental Science-Policy Platform on
            Biodiversity and Ecosystem
            Services (IPBES), 252, 261
International Civil Aviation Organisation
            (ICAO), 229
International Labour Organization (ILO), 168
International policy, 11
International Society for Quality in Health
            Care (ISQua), 138
International Standards
    health-promoting workplaces, 168, 169
International Union for Health Promotion and
            Education (IUHPE), 13, 31, 106
Internet for health promotion
    drawbacks to health promotion
            information on, 208
    health promotion, 207
Inter-sectoral steering committee (ISC), 57
Iran, school health in, 110, 111
Island of Rondraperina, 60

J
Jakarta Declaration, 11

K
Knowledge Cities, 98

L
2017 Lancet Commission on Pollution and
      Health, 261
Lancet Planetary Health, 267
Layers of settings, 30
Learning, 107, 112, 113
Lesbian, gay, bisexual, transgender, intersex,
      and questioning (LGBTIQ), 4
Lifestyle drift, 181
Liveability, 50
Living Planet Index (LPI), 248, 249, 254
Logic model, 75
Long-Range Planning unit, 93
Low-income countries (LICs), 254
Luxembourg Declaration, 9

M
Medizinische Polizey (medical
      police), 92
Mental health, 175
Metropolis.org, 102
Middle-income countries (MICs), 254
Ministry of Education, 108
Ministry of Health, 108
Monitoring, Accountability, Reporting, and
      Impact (MARI) research
      framework, 76
Mouvement hygiéniste, 92

N
Neoliberal welfare reforms, 232
Neolithic Demographic Transition, 93
Network, 52, 54, 57
New institutionalism, 48
Nutrition game, 217

O
Occupational health, 168, 170,
      171, 175
*Occupational Safety and Health
      Convention*, 168
Okanagan Charter, 155
One Planet Communities, 275
Operational governance, 58

Ottawa Charter, 169, 186
Ottawa Charter for Health Promotion, 4, 5,
      91, 94, 263
Ottawa Conference, 169
Outcome evaluation, 75
Overall "Whole System" approach, 83
Overcrowding, 177

P
Pacha Mama (Mother Earth), 242
Paris Declaration, 109
Participatory action research (PAR), 81
Participatory evaluation, 74
Physical world (PW), 214
Places of worship in UK
      current situation, 231, 232
      future of, 232
      historical developments, 231
      public health actors, 233
      timeline of settings-based health
            promotion, 231
Planetary boundaries, 247
Planetary health, 267
Planning, 91, 94, 100, 101
Policy
      definition, 46
      for health, 51, 52
      health in all policy, 53, 55, 56, 58
      healthy public policy, 53, 54, 56
      institutions, 48–51
      policy pancakes, 55
      politics and political science, 47, 48
      University of New South Wales, 46
      University of Sydney, 46
Policy cube, 61
Policy domain indicators, 72
Policy pancakes, 55
Policy transfer, 101
Political science, 46–48
Politics, 47, 49, 98, 99
Power, 49, 50, 54, 62
Praxis-based theory, 24
PRICES-HPH evaluation model, 140
Prisons
      as setting for health, 177
            challenges, 185
            GOOP, 182–185
            health-promoting prison, challenge, 182
            health-promoting prison concept,
                  178, 179
            health-promoting prison, strategic
                  policy implementation of, 182
            history and development, 180, 181
            lifestyle drift, 181

Prisons (*cont.*)
    majority of, 178
    overcrowding, 177
    principles for, 186
Prison Service Orders (PSOs), 180
Process evaluation, 75
Productivity, 50
Public health actors, 233
Public Health England, 231

R
Randomized controlled trials (RCTs), 211
Rarotonga Agreement, 8
Rational choice, 49
Realist and Theory of Change Evaluation, 84
Realist evaluation, 84
Regions for Health Network in Europe, 7
Reorient health services, 119, 131, 133
Resilient Cities, 98
Response component, 72
Reverse quarantine, 92
Rio Conference on Environment and
    Development, 6
Rockefeller-Lancet Commission, 267

S
Safe cities and communities, 98
Salutogenic orientation, 35
School Connectedness (SC), 106
Schools for Health in Europe (SHE)
    network, 109
Sea bathing, 233
Second United Nations Conference on Human
    Settlements, 7
Self-Review Tool, 83
Setting-based approach
    Bronfenbrenner's theory of human
       development, 26, 27
    conceptual framework for, 34
      checklist for, 38
      'core business' alignment, 36
      critical reflection, debate and
        research, 38–40
      ecological model, 36
      holistic change focus, 36
      salutogenic orientation, 35
      systemic perspective, 36
    conceptualization and theorization
      of, 28–33
    definition, 23
    healthy cities, 5, 6
      development and adaptation, 6, 7
      expansion of, 6

historical development, 3
liberation after Second World War, 4
new millennium
    application to new settings, 12
    documentation, evidence, guidance and
      cross-setting collaboration, 12, 14
    emerging themes for critical reflection,
      debate and research, 14, 15
Ottawa Charter for Health Promotion, 4, 5
praxis-based theory, 24, 26
from theoretical foundations to principles
    for practice, 37
typologies, 33, 34
wider application, 7
Setting-based health promotion approach,
    189, 190
    application, 197
    evaluation, 196, 197
    framework and fundamental, 192–194
    history and development, 191, 192
    HPSC, 190, 191
    international research, 194
    strategies, 195, 196
Shanghai Declaration, 12
Shanghai Statement on Healthy Cities, 230
Slow Cities, 98
Small island developing states (SIDS), 68
Smart Cities, 98
Social and Emotional Learning (SEL), 106
Social and Emotional Well-Being (SEWB),
    106, 115
Social determinants of health, 94
Social media for health promotion
    characteristics of, 210
    COVID-19 pandemic, 212, 213
    definition, 210
    health promotion setting, 209
    outlook, 213
    SNS, 211
    social support, 212
    theoretical considerations, 210, 211
Social networking sites (SNS), 211
Social Virtual Worlds (VWs), 214
Social wellbeing, 272
Space Cadets, 93
Stadia, 202
Stadiums, 190, 201–203
Staff well-being, 152
Student-focused guidance, 152
Sundsvall Statement on Supportive
    Environments, 6
Sustainability, 50
Sustainable Cities, 98
Sustainable community principles, 276
Sustainable development, 275

Sustainable Development Goals (SDGs), 102
Systemic perspective, 36

T
Theme Cities, 91, 98
Third Global Conference on Health
         Promotion, 11
3D multiuser virtual environments
         (MUVE), 214
Tinder Foundation, 208
Tipping elements, 251
Total Quality Management, 77
Transformation of the world of work,
         168, 173–175
Transition Towns and EcoDistricts, 98
Turn to faith, 232
Typology, 33, 34

U
UK Healthy Universities Network, 155
UK Healthy Universities Network Self-
         Review Tool, 83
UNESCO, 109
UNICEF, 109
United Cities and Local Governments
         (UCLG), 102
United Nations Advisory Committee of Local
         Authorities (UNACLA), 102
United Nations Framework Convention on
         Climate Change (UNFCCC), 101
University of British Columbia, 157, 158
University of Central Lancashire (UCLan),
         158, 159
University of Puerto Rico (UPR), 159, 160
UN's Millennium Ecosystem Assessment, 259
UN Sustainable Development Goals, 229
*The Urban Condition – People and Policy in
         the Metropolis*, 94
Urban health, 92, 94–96
Urban Health Equity Assessment and
         Response Tool (Urban HEART), 96
    assessment component, 72

    response component, 72
Urban planning, 91, 100
US Association of State and Territorial Health
         Officers (ASTHO), 56
US National Institute of Mental Health, 93

V
Values, 58
Vienna Recommendations, 9
Virbela, 215
Virtual immersive environment, 217
Virtual nature, 218
Virtual reality (VR), 215, 217
Virtual world (VW), 214, 216, 217
VITAL Lab, 216
VR chat, 215

W
Waste disposal management systems, 91
Wellbeing economics, 265, 272
Well-wrought governance, 58
Wessex Healthy Schools Award (WHSA)
         scheme, 114
Western Sydney Airport (WSA), 228
WHO Kobe Centre (WKC), 96
Whole system' approach, 29, 32, 36–38, 40
WHP, elements and success factors
         of, 171–173
Widening Digital Participation
         Programme, 208
Winter Cities, 98
Workplace health promotion (WHP), 167,
         170, 174
World Health Day, 96
World Health Organization (WHO), 80, 169
World Wide Fund for Nature (WWF), 248,
         249, 253, 254

Y
Yanuca Declaration on Healthy
         Islands, 230

Printed in the United States
by Baker & Taylor Publisher Services